The Comprehensive Guide to Inter
Veterinary Social Work

Sana Loue • Pamela Linden

Editors

The Comprehensive Guide to Interdisciplinary Veterinary Social Work

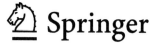 Springer

Editors
Sana Loue
Department of Bioethics
Case Western Reserve University
School of Medicine
Cleveland, OH, USA

Pamela Linden
Veterinary Social Work Program
University of Tennessee at Knoxville
Knoxville, TN, USA

ISBN 978-3-031-10332-2   ISBN 978-3-031-10330-8   (eBook)
https://doi.org/10.1007/978-3-031-10330-8

This Springer imprint is published by the registered company Springer Nature Switzerland AG
The registered company address is: Gewerbestrasse 11, 6330 Cham, Switzerland

Contents

About the Editors

Sana Loue, JD, PhD, MPH, MSSA, MA, LISW-S, CST-T, AVT, is a professor in the Department of Bioethics at Case Western Reserve University (CWRU) School of Medicine in Cleveland, Ohio. She holds secondary appointments in Psychiatry and Global Health at the School of Medicine and in Social Work at the Mandel School of Applied Social Sciences at CWRU. Dr. Loue served as the School of Medicine's inaugural Vice Dean for Faculty Development and Diversity from 2012 to 2020. Dr. Loue holds degrees in law (JD), epidemiology (PhD), medical anthropology (PhD), social work (MSSA), secondary education (MA), public health (MPH), and theology (MA). Her past research in both the domestic and international contexts has focused on HIV risk and prevention, severe mental illness, family violence, and research ethics. Her current research addresses the interplay between religion, society, and bioethics; the integration of cultural humility into clinical care and research settings; and past and current formulations of eugenics. She has authored or edited more than 30 books and more than 100 peer-reviewed journal articles. Dr. Loue served on the Board of the International Association of Veterinary Social Work and was the organization's inaugural Director of Education.

Pamela Linden, MSW, PhD, earned her MSW and PhD at Stony Brook University, New York. Dr. Linden holds a certificate in Veterinary Social Work from the University of Tennessee at Knoxville, where she is an instructor in the Veterinary Social Work and Veterinary Human Support Certificate programs. She is the founding President of the International Association of Veterinary Social Work. She administered programs for individuals with serious mental illness, conducted research on problem-solving courts for both juvenile delinquents and veteran's and, as a research scientist at the New York State Psychiatric Institute, studied mandated outpatient psychiatric treatment. Dr. Linden is the Director of Veterinary Social Work for the AlignCare Healthcare program, a part of the Program for Pet Health Equity at the University of Tennessee. Dr. Linden also administers a nationwide research project that explores experiences of veterinary medical students with diverse social identities and to improve mental health and well-being among veterinary students in the USA. Dr. Linden lives in Long Island, New York, with her husband, Steve, and dogs Dove and Lily.

Contributors

John Allgire, BA, is a detective with the Whatcom County Sheriff's Office, in Bellingham, Washington, where he has worked since 2001. Prior to being promoted to detective, he worked in uniform patrol and in Crime Scene Investigation (CSI). In the detectives' division, he works in the Sex Kidnap Offender Registration (SKOR) program and in major crimes. Detective Allgire is a polygraph examiner and also had been trained in computer and mobile forensics. He received his BA in Psychology from Western Washington University.

Sandra Brackenridge, LCSW, BCD, has been practicing Clinical Social Work since 1983 in various settings and in three states: Louisiana, Idaho, and Texas. She maintains a small private practice, and she supervises social workers for their clinical licensure. As Coordinator of Counseling Services at LSU School of Veterinary Medicine, 1990–1994, she developed a social work internship, a pet loss counseling program, an animal-assisted therapy program, and a counseling service for veterinary students. This was one of the first counseling programs in a school of veterinary medicine and the first program to offer all components. She left LSU to teach Social Work at Idaho State University from 1994 to 2008, and she continued as Associate Professor of Social Work at Texas Woman's University. She has published numerous articles, chapters, and two books, one about pet loss and the other about stress management for the veterinary practice team. She served as Pet Loss Consultant for the Idaho and for the Texas Veterinary Medical Foundations. She created and supervised the veterinary social work program and internship at the Center for Veterinary Specialty and Emergency Care from 2013 to 2020. Sandra provides consultation to other practices that wish to develop a veterinary social work program. She presents locally and nationally about issues in the veterinary profession, and she teaches for the University of Tennessee's certificate program in veterinary social work. In October 2018 Sandra received the Lifetime Achievement Award from the Texas state chapter of the National Association of Social Workers.

Athena Diesch-Chham, MSW, LICSW, earned her Master of Social Work degree from the University of Minnesota in 2011 and is currently licensed at the Clinical level in the state of Minnesota. As an Intern in the University's Veterinary Social Services program, Athena learned from the founder of the program Jeannine Moga, discovering her calling and passion for veterinary social work. Athena continues to attend to the "heart work" of veterinary medicine that was started at the Veterinary Medical Center many years ago.Athena has a wide range of professional interests, and is passionate about working with the veterinary community in learning how to manage stress, burnout, and moral injury and moral distress, as well as educating on the importance of sustainable practice and meaningful self-care. She delivers training on the topics of human-animal relationships to veterinary professionals, animal welfare organizations, and social service providers throughout Minnesota. Outside of her professional role, Athena spends time with her supportive husband, two young boys, and two pugs. Athena also enjoys traveling back to her parent's farm in southern Minnesota where her love of animals and the human experience began many years ago.

Joshua B. Friedman, MD, PhD, is a pediatrician at MetroHealth Medical Center and the Cleveland Clinic in Cleveland, Ohio, specializing in child abuse pediatrics. After completing university, he lived on the Masai Mara, Kenya, and researched hyena behavior. He completed his MD and PhD at Case Western Reserve University School of Medicine. Dr. Friedman completed his training in pediatrics at Case Western/MetroHealth. Since completing his training, he has worked at the Indian Health Service (in Montana) and worked in New Zealand. Dr. Friedman has researched topics including shaken baby syndrome, child abuse, and pediatric staff stress and has published various articles including about the economic and social benefits of shaken baby prevention programs and child murder by parents. He has presented nationally and internationally at conferences regarding child abuse.

Susan Hatters Friedman, MD, is a forensic and perinatal psychiatrist. She has practiced in forensic hospitals, general hospitals, court clinics, community mental health centers, and correctional facilities. Dr. Susan Hatters Friedman has served as Vice President of the American Academy of Psychiatry and the Law (AAPL) and as Chair of the Law and Psychiatry committee at the Group for Advancement of Psychiatry (GAP). She has received the AAPL Award for the Best Teacher in a Forensic Psychiatry Fellowship, the Red AAPL Award for outstanding service to organized forensic psychiatry, the Manfred Guttmacher Award for editing the book *Family Murder: Pathologies of Love and Hate*, and the Association of Women Psychiatrists' Marian Butterfield Early Career Psychiatrist Award for her contributions to women's mental health. She has published more than 100 articles (including in *World Psychiatry* and the *American Journal of Psychiatry*) as well as book chapters. Her research has primarily focused on the interface of maternal mental health and forensic psychiatry, including notably child murder by mothers. Dr. Susan Hatters Friedman currently serves as the inaugural Phillip J. Resnick Professor of Forensic Psychiatry at Case Western Reserve University, where she also has appointments in the departments of Pediatrics, Reproductive Biology (Obstetrics/ Gynecology), and Law. Dr. Susan Hatters Friedman also serves as honorary faculty at the University of Auckland in New Zealand.

Maya Gupta, PhD, MS, earned her MS and PhD in Clinical Psychology from the University of Georgia. Her primary area of expertise is animal cruelty, including its connections to domestic violence and other forms of violence. More broadly, she is also interested in the application of psychology and human service approaches to promoting animal welfare and the human-animal bond.Dr. Gupta is currently Senior Director of Research for the American Society for the Prevention of Cruelty to Animals, conducting applied research on veterinary forensics, animal behavior, law enforcement response to animal cruelty, community engagement, and policy issues. She previously served as Executive Director of both the Georgia-based Ahimsa House (a statewide animal safehouse program for victims of domestic violence) and the Animals & Society Institute. She is also an instructor for the University of Florida Veterinary Forensic Sciences Program and the Master's Program in Anthrozoology at Canisius College, and a guest lecturer/supervisor for the Veterinary Social Work Program at the University of Tennessee. She holds governance or advisory roles with the National Link Coalition, the Association of Prosecuting Attorneys' Animal Cruelty Advisory Council, the Section on Human-Animal Interaction in the American Psychological Association, Mojave Animal Protection, Pets for Vets, Ahimsa House, Paws Between Homes, and the Banfield Foundation's Safer Together Initiative for people and pets in domestic violence. She previously served on the Board of Directors of the Georgia Coalition Against Domestic Violence and was co-chair of the Cobb County Domestic Violence Task Force. Dr. Gupta has been a recipient of the Unity Award from the Association of Prosecuting Attorneys, the Angel Award from the ASPCA, and the Family Violence Task Force Member of the Year Award from the Georgia Commission on Family Violence. She lives north of Atlanta, Georgia, with six cats, two and a half horses, and an assortment of rescued/adopted pigeons and chickens.

Lisa Hacker is a licensed Advanced Practice Social Worker (APSW) in the state of Wisconsin. She earned her Master's degree in Social Work at the University of Wisconsin-Milwaukee in 2009. Lisa's postgraduate experience has been in pediatric, medical social work, as well as veterinary social work since 2018. She is the 2014 recipient of the Milwaukee BizTimes "Health Care Hero" Award for her work with the Make-a-Wish Foundation. Currently, Lisa is the Social Work Program Manager for a specialty and emergency veterinary hospital in the Milwaukee, Wisconsin area, which was featured in the June 2020 edition of the *Journal of the American Veterinary Medical Association* (*JAVMA*). She also established and manages a training program for MSW students for three area universities. Additionally, Lisa is working on her Grief Support Specialist Certification at the University of Wisconsin-Madison. At home, Lisa's pack includes her spouse, a 12-year-old black labrador retriever, a 4-year-old golden retriever, and a 7-month-old chocolate labrador.

Janet Hoy-Gerlach, PhD, is a licensed independent social worker with supervisory designation and is a social work professor at the University of Toledo in Ohio. She is lead author of *Human-Animal Interaction: A Social Work Guide*, published in 2017 by NASW Press. She developed and supervises graduate social work internships at the Toledo Humane Society, in collaboration with humane society staff. Her research focuses on mental health benefits of human-animal interaction using a One Health approach. Most recently she published a pilot study in which shelter animals were placed as emotional support animals for people with serious mental illness; the human participants experienced significant reductions in loneliness and mental health symptoms; and the animals gained permanent loving homes. She is the founder of OneHealth People-Animal Wellness Services (OHPAWS), which provides training and consultation on projects seeking to improve human and animal well-being.

Blair McKissock, PhD, CTRS, began as a Recreation Therapist 25 years ago, specializing in adventure therapy and animal-assisted therapy in mental health. Equine-assisted learning quickly became her preferred intervention. She earned certifications as a Certified Therapeutic Riding Instructor and Equine Specialist while training with many specialists in the field of equine-assisted services. She holds a Master degree in Education and a PhD in Applied EcoPsychology, studying the impact of equine-assisted work on those with trauma. She also holds certifications as a yoga teacher trainer, wellness coach, and a trauma specialist, all of which contribute to her practice and Breath Body Brain. Blair currently serves as the Director of Education at Strides to Success, where she partners with Debbie Anderson to provide consulting, professional education workshops, online courses, and resources in equine-assisted learning and therapeutic riding. Her research has been published in peer-reviewed publications and textbooks supporting the efficacy of equine-assisted work as a mainstream intervention option for learning and therapy. She is a passionate international speaker and advocate for the benefits of the human connection with nature, specifically equine interaction. She is very active with PATH International, supporting the development of professional competencies and educational opportunities in equine-assisted learning.

Jeannine Moga, MA, MSW, LCSW, is a licensed clinical social worker and Compassion Fatigue Specialist dedicated to the integration of human-animal relationships in social work practice. She has founded two veterinary social work programs (Veterinary Social Services at the University of Minnesota's Veterinary Medical Center, and Family & Community Services at NC State University's Veterinary Hospital) and works with animal care and social services professionals across the country to address the intersections of human and animal health and well-being. Her professional interests include occupational well-being; grief, loss, and life transitions; ethical decision-making; animal-assisted interventions; and moral distress in animal care professions. She currently serves as the Business Partner for Mental Health & Wellbeing for Banfield Pet Hospital, the Chief Happiness Officer for VETgirl, and teaching faculty at NC State University's School of Social Work.

Joelle Nielsen is the Program Coordinator for the Honoring the Bond program at the Ohio State University Veterinary Medical Center (VMC). (She started this role in September 2007.) In her role as a social worker, Joelle provides support to VMC clients as they encounter difficult situations regarding their beloved animals, especially during end-of-life stages. She also provides debriefing and consultation to the clinicians, staff, and students in the VMC. She has been responsible for developing and implementing the yearly Animal Remembrance Ceremony, which provides owners with a structured way to celebrate the lives of those animals they have lost. Joelle is very involved in collaborative relationships with other social workers and mental health professionals that work in (both academic and private/corporate) veterinary medical settings. Joelle received her BA in Psychology from Ohio University and her Master's in Social Work (MSW) from the Ohio State University College of Social Work and is a licensed social worker in the State of Ohio. When not at work, Joelle enjoys gardening, crocheting, and tending to her backyard pond. Joelle enjoys the company of her family, which always includes "at least one" cat.

Augusta O'Reilly, LCSW, received her bachelor's degree in Psychology from Appalachian State University in Boone, North Carolina, and a Master of Social Work and certificate for Veterinary Social Work from the University of Tennessee – Knoxville. She has professional experience with a wide breadth of animal settings, including veterinary clinics and research labs. Augusta's clinical experience predominately focuses on adolescents with behavioral diagnoses with whom she implements animal-assisted interventions when applicable. Augusta is a member of the International Association of Veterinary Social Workers, a Licensed Clinical Social Worker, and a Veterinary Social Worker. She currently resides in Southern Maine with her husband, daughter, two cats, Great Pyrenees, chickens, and two pigs. In her spare time, she enjoys camping, riding horses, and cooking.

Alyssa Pepe, LMSW, has been practicing Social Work since 2014 in New York State. She earned her Master's degree in Social Work at the University at Buffalo, the State University of New York, and has a Bachelor of Arts in Psychology and Sociology from Canisius College. She has worked in various settings including community mental health and substance use treatment and housing for individuals with severe, persistent mental illness. Alyssa began working at Orchard Park Veterinary Medical Center in 2019 as the Hospital's first Full Time Veterinary Social Worker. She developed a Field Placement with the University at Buffalo, School of Social Work, in the Fall of 2020 to provide graduate level students with the opportunity to learn about Hospital-Based Veterinary Social Work. Currently, Alyssa is enrolled in the Post-Graduate Veterinary Social Work Certificate Program at the University of Tennessee, Knoxville. Alyssa received the Exceptional Social Work Service Award from the New York State Chapter of the National Association of Social Workers. Alyssa lives with her fiancé and two rescue dogs in the Buffalo, New York area.

Bethanie A. Poe, PhD, LMSW, earned her doctorate from the University of Tennessee (UT) College of Social Work. She was a Fellow in UT's Veterinary Social Work program. During her fellowship, she helped to develop the Veterinary Social Work Certificate Program for concurrent and postgraduate students, and she has been an instructor in the program since its inception. Dr. Poe began her work in family violence almost 15 years ago, working first in a domestic violence shelter, then moving on to child protection, then working with batterers' intervention programs across the state of Tennessee. She also has experience in mental health and suicide prevention education. Dr. Poe is currently the Middle Tennessee Coordinator for UT's Human-Animal Bond in Tennessee (H.A.B.I.T) program and the Veterinary Social Work Certificate Programs Coordinator.

Addie Reinhard, DVM, is a graduate student in the Department of Community and Leadership Development at the University of Kentucky researching early-career veterinary well-being. She is a 2015 veterinary graduate from the University of Tennessee College of Veterinary Medicine and completed a certificate in Veterinary Human Support from the University of Tennessee in 2020. She is the Founder and Director of MentorVet, a mentorship and professional development program for new and recent veterinary graduates.

Jessica Ricker is a licensed social worker in the state of Ohio. She completed both her Bachelor of Social Work degree and Master of Social Work degree at Bowling Green State University in Bowling Green, Ohio. She has been practicing social work since 2017. Her work has primarily focused on assisting the older adult population. She currently practices full time at a senior center as their Social Services Specialist. Jessica thoroughly enjoyed her graduate social work internship at Community Pet Care Clinic. Jessica now has a passion for veterinary social work and is actively searching for opportunities to continue a path within a veterinary setting.

Renee M. Sorrentino, MD, is the Medical Director at the Institute for Sexual Wellness and Clinical Assistant Professor at Harvard Medical School in Boston, Massachusetts. Dr. Sorrentino is a board-certified forensic psychiatrist with expertise in the evaluation and treatment of individuals with paraphilias. Dr. Sorrentino received her medical degree from Boston University School of Medicine and completed her residency in adult psychiatry at Massachusetts General Hospital and McLean Hospital. Following her residency, Dr. Sorrentino completed a forensic psychiatry fellowship at Case Western Reserve University, School of Medicine, in Cleveland, Ohio. Dr. Sorrentino's practice is devoted to the treatment and evaluation of paraphilias and sexual offenders, as well as the hormonal treatment of paraphilias. Fifteen years ago she started one of the first multidisciplinary centers for the treatment of sexual offenders in the nation. Her vision was to incorporate the evidenced-based principles of sex offender recidivism by offering biological and psychological treatment modalities. In this capacity, Dr. Sorrentino has consulted with local and state agencies to provide treatment and evaluation to individuals who engage in problematic sexual behaviors. She is active in the local chapter of the Association for the Treatment of Sexual Abusers (ATSA) serving as a Board member for the past 10 years. She is also a councilor, editorial board member, and frequent presenter at the American Academy of Psychiatry and the Law.Dr. Sorrentino has authored book chapters and journal articles in the areas of general forensic psychiatry as well as paraphilic disorders. Her research is focused on establishing a technology to better understand an individual's sexual interest using thermo cameras. She has spoken both nationally and internationally on the topic of paraphilias. Dr. Sorrentino is one of few psychiatrists in the United States who provides biological treatment to individuals with problematic sexual behaviors. Recognizing the impact that treatment has on reducing sexual violence, training and mentorship has been a central focus of her career. To this end she has been instrumental at introducing the paraphilic disorders in six of the psychiatry residency training programs in Massachusetts. In addition, she mentors trainees and general psychiatrists in the treatment of paraphilias with the goal of decreasing sexual violence with the help of psychiatrists.

Aimee St. Arnaud is a business partner in two full-service veterinary clinics (Community Pet Care Clinic in Ohio and Open Door Veterinary Care in North Carolina) that focus on removing barriers to care and increasing access to veterinary services while still maintaining a net positive revenue. She has created a nonprofit mentorship training called Open Door Veterinary Collective for clinics that want to replicate their business model, which includes giving back through their revenue, providing incremental care and creating strong community partnerships with human social service and animal nonprofits. She has experience in mentoring from her time at the ASPCA Spay/Neuter Alliance where she helped develop six training programs that mentored over 170+ clinics to open that perform 1.5 million spay/neuter surgeries annually and trained over 1000 veterinary professionals annually in efficient spay/neuter techniques to help more dogs and cats.

Debbie L. Stoewen, DVM, MSW, RSW, PhD, hails from the rural town of Ayr, Ontario, Canada, where she raised her daughter with "all things feathered, finned, and furred," and with her daughter now a zookeeper, she's privy to the most intriguing behind-the-scenes tours – and feeding carrots to rhinos! Life never ceases to be wondrous with the deep and profound connection that we have with animals.It was that connection that influenced her life's work. Upon graduating from the University of Guelph, Debbie spent the first years of her career as a veterinarian in general and emergency practice, upon which she founded the Pioneer Pet Clinic, a family-centered companion animal hospital in Kitchener, Ontario. With room in her heart for helping children as well as animals, she began fostering with Family and Children's Services. Introduced to, and inspired by, an alternate helping profession, she returned to school to take undergraduate coursework in social development studies, completing a Master of Social Work at Wilfrid Laurier University. As the first person in North America to be a veterinarian and social worker, she merged her unique expertise with a PhD in Epidemiology (University of Guelph), specializing in communication.Since then, Debbie has held various positions within industry, wherein she developed a fully accredited, evidence-based veterinary continuing education program called *The Social Side of Practice*. This program specializes in the areas of wellness, communication, teamwork, organizational culture, and leadership. She has given over 400 presentations internationally and published close to 30 articles in veterinary and social work journals and news magazines, including numerous articles (and a book chapter) on compassion fatigue. Debbie has a special interest in the topic, and supporting the animal care community, not just from her expertise as a social worker but also from her experience of it as a veterinary practitioner at a time when it was not yet recognized, when there was no name for it. She is a caregiver, healer, and teacher by nature, with a passion for supporting the health and welfare of people and animals at the intersection of the human-animal bond. She volunteers with various organizations, from local charities and nonprofits to international professional associations, and all in all, in all that she does, seeks to make the world a better place.

Elizabeth B. Strand, PhD, is the Founding Director of Veterinary Social Work (VSW) at the University of Tennessee College of Veterinary Medicine. She is a licensed clinical social worker, experienced family therapist, Grief Recovery Specialist, and a Mindfulness-Based Stress Reduction Teacher. She has been working in the field of social work for 25 years. Dr. Strand is also trained as a Rule 31 Mediator, Child, and Adult Anicare Animal Abuse Treatment counselor, a Compassion Fatigue Specialist and holds a Doctor of Philosophy in Social Work.Dr. Strand's areas of interest include the link between human and animal violence, animals in family systems, the development of veterinary social work, communication skills, conflict resolution, and stress management techniques in animal-related environments. Her professional mission is to encourage the humane treatment of both people and animals and to care for those professionals who care for animals.

Aviva Vincent, PhD, is a doctoral graduate of Case Western Reserve University, Mandel School of Social Welfare, in veterinary social work. Her research focuses on the biological impact that animals have on children, specifically in the reduction of fear and anxiety in stressful situations. Additionally, her research includes integration of physiological measures in social science research (e.g., saliva collection for measures of oxytocin, alpha-amylase, and cortisol). She is co-owner and founder of Healing Paws LLC, the only Veterinary Social Work practice in Northeast Ohio. Her background in veterinary social work informs her practice as the Director of Program Quality at Fieldstone Farm Therapeutic Riding Center in Chagrin Falls, Ohio. In this capacity, she is responsible for ensuring high-quality programs in adaptive riding, hippotherapy, carriage driving, and ground lessons offered to over 1000 participants annually. She is an instructor of Animal-Assisted Interventions at the University of Tennessee in the Veterinary Social Work Certificate Program. Aviva served as cofounder of the human-animal interactions workgroup with the National Association of Social Workers – Ohio chapter, and is on the board of the International Association of Veterinary Social Work. She authored a chapter in the text *Career Paths in*

Human-Animal Interaction for Social and Behavioral Scientists. Aviva enjoys time with her wife and dog, Shaina, horseback riding, running, and cycling.

John Volk, BS, is senior consultant with Brakke Consulting, serving the global animal health, veterinary, and pet care markets. John is principal author of five landmark studies of the veterinary profession: Brakke Study of Financial and Economic Behaviors of Veterinarians (1998), AVMA-Pfizer Business Practices Study (2005), Bayer Veterinary Care Usage Study (2011–2013), VPI-Veterinary Economics Financial Health Study (2014), and Merck Animal Health Veterinary Wellbeing Study (2018, 2020). He has authored several articles for veterinary journals and is highly sought after as a speaker at veterinary conferences. In 2019 VetPartners, the association of veterinary practice management consultants, presented John with its Pioneer Professional Award his "vision and contributions to the business of veterinary medicine."Prior to joining Brakke in 1994, John was president of The John Volk Company, one of the leading advertising and public relations firms in agriculture and animal health; he sold that firm in 1992. John is a graduate of the University of Illinois where he earned a BS in agricultural communications and did graduate work in marketing. He also served on the faculty of the University of Illinois College of Veterinary Medicine as communications director. John currently serves on advisory councils for the University of Illinois College of Agricultural, Consumer and Environmental Sciences and for the Chicago High School for Agricultural Sciences, a unique public school for inner city students.

Ellen Kinney Winston, MA, LPC, NCC, CAAP, received her Bachelor's degree in Psychology from Washington University in St. Louis, Missouri, and her Master's degree in Counseling Psychology from the University of Denver in Colorado. She holds a Certificate in Animals and Human Health from the University of Denver and a Certification in Animal Assisted Psychotherapy (CAAP) and is a Licensed Professional Counselor (LPC) in Colorado and a National Certified Counselor (NCC). Ms. Winston has counseling experience in a variety of settings, including residential treatment for adolescents, substance abuse treatment for adults, school counseling, Head Start centers, early childhood education centers and daycares, home-based family therapy, and private practice settings. In 2010, Ms. Winston cofounded Animal Assisted Therapy Programs of Colorado (AATPC), helping to create the unique programs, recruit and train staff and interns, conduct individual and family therapy for clients, and train professionals. Currently, Ms. Winston is the Training Director for AATPC, managing the online Certificate in Animal Assisted Psychotherapy. For more information about AATPC, please visit www.animalassistedtherapyprograms.org

Part I
Foundations of Veterinary Social Work

Chapter 1
Introduction to Veterinary Social Work

Sana Loue

Introduction

Historically, concern for animals during disasters has focused on issues related to their importance as secure food sources, such as in the case of poultry and cattle, and their potential to lead to outbreaks of infectious diseases, such as cholera and anthrax, as the consequence of the illness and death of roaming animals (Federal Emergency Management Agency, n.d.). It was not until Hurricane Katrina in 2005 that the nation became attuned to the lack of protection for animals during major natural disasters and the importance of the human-animal bond (Wan, 2006). Indeed, not only are pets often considered to be members of the family, but for some individuals, pets can represent extensions of the self (Hill et al., 2007; Serpell, 2003). Forty-four percent of individuals who refused to evacuate during the storm remained in place because they did not want to abandon their pets, which were initially denied entrance into New Orleans' emergency shelters (Bruillard, 2017). Even so, it has been estimated that more than 100,000 pets were left behind, and perhaps as many as 70,000 died. The trauma suffered by those forced to leave their animals behind was made all the more evident by the scene captured by the Associated Press of a young boy whose small, white dog Snowball was confiscated by a police officer as the boy boarded an evacuation bus; the child was so traumatized by and cried so hard at the loss of his beloved animal that he vomited (Associated Press, 2005, 2010). Cindy Meyers, then-board president of the Humane Society of Southeast Texas in Beaumont, castigated those responsible for the evacuation effort for their failure to recognize that pets are family members and need to be evacuated with their families (Associated Press, 2005). Importantly, the lack of attention to the

S. Loue (✉)
Department of Bioethics, Case Western Reserve University School of Medicine,
Cleveland, OH, USA
e-mail: Sana.Loue@case.edu

© The Author(s), under exclusive license to Springer Nature Switzerland AG 2022   3
S. Loue, P. Linden (eds.), *The Comprehensive Guide to Interdisciplinary Veterinary Social Work*, https://doi.org/10.1007/978-3-031-10330-8_1

needs of animal family members during the Hurricane Katrina evacuation efforts and the consequent trauma to individuals and communities highlighted how the accommodation of pets in emergencies can actually enhance human safety and well-being (Leonard and Scammon, 2007).

The traumatic scenes of families being separated from their pets and the pain caused by their inability to later find them prompted the bipartisan promulgation of the federal Pets Evacuation and Transportation Standards Act (PETS) in 2006, amending the Robert T. Stafford Disaster Relief and Emergency Assistance Act (1988). PETS provides for the availability of federal disaster relief contingent on states' planning for the needs of people with service animals and/or pets and specifically authorizes the Federal Emergency Management Agency (FEMA) to provide rescue, care, shelter, and essential needs for individuals with household pets and service animals, and to the household pets and animals themselves following a major disaster or emergency.

Veterinary Social Work as a Profession

Veterinary social work had come into being just a few short years prior to Hurricane Katrina and was not widely recognized at that time. The plight of individuals, families, and their animal family members during and following Katrina evacuation and shelter efforts underscored the importance of two of veterinary social work's four pillars: grief and pet loss and human-animal interaction. Less visible during Katrina, but no less important, were reflections of the other two pillars: the link between animal and human violence and compassion fatigue and conflict affecting veterinary personnel.

What Veterinary Social Workers Do

Veterinary social workers (VSW) work in a variety of settings and in diverse roles. They may be employed in hospitals that tend to the needs of people, animal hospitals, animal clinics, veterinary practices, universities, schools of social work, veterinary colleges, research enterprises, private social work practices, group mental health practices, camps, nonprofit organizations, foundations, and policy think tanks. In each of these settings, veterinary social workers must interface and effectively engage and collaborate with members of other professions including, depending upon the specific setting, veterinarians, veterinary technicians, physicians, nurses, scientists, social workers, psychologists, policymakers, funders, faculty members, administrators, and support teams.

Accordingly, veterinary social work is interprofessional by its very nature. Interprofessional practice focuses on improving healthcare quality, accessibility, and outcomes while reducing associated costs by leveraging the coordination, collaboration, and cooperation of professionals from multiple backgrounds (Interprofessional Education Collaborative, 2016). Four competencies underlie interprofessional practice:

- The ability to work with other professionals to maintain mutual respect and values
- The ability to use one's knowledge of one's own role and those of other professions to appropriately assess and address the healthcare needs of patients and to promote and enhance the health of populations
- The ability to communicate with patients, families, communities, and professionals in health and other fields in a responsive and responsible manner that supports a team approach to the promotion and maintenance of health and the prevention and treatment of disease
- The ability to utilize relationship-building values and the principles of team dynamics to perform effectively in different team roles to plan, deliver, and evaluate patient/population-centered care and population health programs and policies that are safe, timely, efficient, effective, and equitable (Interprofessional Education Collaborative, 2016, p. 10)

Depending upon the particular setting and the role of the veterinary social worker, the VSW must be prepared to address any number of situations that range widely in terms of their immediacy and severity. They may be asked to consult with a veterinary practice with respect to the office organization and staffing, to plan with a family for their pet's demise, or to intervene with a suicidal student or veterinary team member. They may present professionally at national and international conferences, conduct research, prepare manuscripts for publication, or collaborate with state legislators to draft relevant legislation. Each of these situations presents exciting opportunities and challenges.

Standards of the Profession

Not surprisingly in view of the wide range of settings in which VSWs work and the diversity of situations that may be called upon to address, there have been some calls for the development of standards for the profession. Currently, there are no enunciated standards for veterinary social work or for the credentialing of veterinary social workers. Although the use of the professional labels "social work" and "social worker" is often regulated under state law (see, e.g., Ohio Revised Statute section 4757.02, 2014), there are no existing guidelines or rules for who may call themselves a veterinary social worker. Indeed, social workers may utilize animal-assisted interventions in their practices without a firm understanding of the nature of human-animal interaction and without a full understanding of the ethical obligations that arise in such situations, with respect both to the human client and to the animal. Other mental health professionals who are not social workers may also work in animal-related settings, underscoring the need to delineate what veterinary social workers can do and the need for subspecialty training in social work.

Whether the credentialing of veterinary social workers would or should require passage of a standardized examination remains controversial. Some VSWs may focus on only one of the four pillars of veterinary social work, raising questions as to whether they should be required to demonstrate competency in all four domains. Additionally, a focus on only the four pillars does not necessarily encompass the wide range of skills that may be needed by VSWs working in areas that are less frequent within social work, such as the development and promulgation of legislation and appearance as an expert witness to a legislative or judicial body. Although a certain level of competence in such areas may be required as elements of one's training, the level of training may not adequately prepare a social worker with the skills necessary for practice in a defined subspecialty.

Veterinary Social Worker Training

Students must graduate from an accredited social work program in order to obtain licensure and practice social work in the United States. Although licensure varies by state, graduation from an accredited program is a requirement in most states (Council on Social Work Education, 2022). The social work education degree program must meet the standards enunciated by the Council on Social Work Education (CSWE), which is the national accreditation organization for social work degree programs in the United States and its territories.

Social work students in accredited social work graduate and undergraduate programs are required to complete field placements, which are essentially internships. These placements provide an opportunity for social work students to apply their classroom learning and to develop skills and mastery of specified social work competency areas. The CSWE has identified nine foundational social work competencies that students must master by the conclusion of their social work degree program. Some graduate social work programs also develop advanced competencies that they then submit to CSWE for approval. Each competency has related practice behaviors which further delineate dimensions that need to be developed and mastered. Below provides a listing of the foundational competencies required to successfully complete an accredited social work degree program (Council on Social Work Education, 2015, pp. 8–9).

Competency 1. Demonstrate Ethical and Professional Behavior

- Make ethical decisions by applying the standards of the NASW Code of Ethics, relevant laws and regulations, models for ethical decision-making, ethical conduct of research, and additional codes of ethics as appropriate to context.
- Use reflection and self-regulation to manage personal values and maintain professionalism in practice situations.

- Demonstrate professional demeanor in behavior, appearance, and oral, written, and electronic communication.
- Use technology ethically and appropriately to facilitate practice outcomes.
- Use supervision and consultation to guide professional judgment and behavior.

Competency 2. Engage Diversity and Difference in Practice

- Apply and communicate understanding of the importance of diversity and difference in shaping life experiences in practice at the micro-, mezzo-, and macro-levels.
- Present themselves as learners and engage clients and constituencies as experts of their own experiences.
- Apply self-awareness and self-regulation to manage the influence of personal biases and values in working with diverse clients and constituencies.

Competency 3. Advance Human Rights and Social, Economic, and Environmental Justice

- Apply their understanding of social, economic, and environmental justice to advocate for human rights at the individual and system levels.
- Engage in practices that advance social, economic, and environmental justice.

Competency 4. Engage in Practice-Informed Research and Research-Informed Practice

- Use practice experience and theory to inform scientific inquiry and research.
- Apply critical thinking to engage in analysis of quantitative and qualitative research methods and research findings.
- Use and translate research evidence to inform and improve practice, policy, and service delivery.

Competency 5. Engage in Policy Practice

- Identify social policy at the local, state, and federal level that impacts well-being, service delivery, and access to social services.
- Assess how social welfare and economic policies impact the delivery of and access to social services.
- Apply critical thinking to analyze, formulate, and advocate for policies that advance human rights and social, economic, and environmental justice.

Competency 6. Engage with Individuals, Families, Groups, Organizations, and Communities

- Apply knowledge of human behavior and the social environment, person-in-environment, and other multidisciplinary theoretical frameworks to engage with clients and constituencies.
- Use empathy, reflection, and interpersonal skills to effectively engage diverse clients and constituencies.

Competency 7. Assess Individuals, Families, Groups, Organizations, and Communities

- Collect and organize data, and apply critical thinking to interpret information from clients and constituencies.
- Apply knowledge of human behavior and the social environment, person-in-environment, and other multidisciplinary theoretical frameworks in the analysis of assessment data from clients and constituencies.
- Develop mutually agreed-on intervention goals and objectives based on the critical assessment of strengths, needs, and challenges within clients and constituencies.
- Select appropriate intervention strategies based on the assessment, research knowledge, and values and preferences of clients and constituencies.

Competency 8. Intervene with Individuals, Families, Groups, Organizations, and Communities

- Critically choose and implement interventions to achieve practice goals and enhance capacities of clients and constituencies.
- Apply knowledge of human behavior and the social environment, person-in-environment, and other multidisciplinary theoretical frameworks in interventions with clients and constituencies.
- Use inter-professional collaboration as appropriate to achieve beneficial practice outcomes.
- Negotiate, mediate, and advocate with and on behalf of diverse clients and constituencies.
- Facilitate effective transitions and endings that advance mutually agreed-on goals.

Competency 9. Evaluate Practice with Individuals, Families, Groups, Organizations, and Communities

- Select and use appropriate methods for evaluation of outcomes.
- Apply knowledge of human behavior and the social environment, person-in-environment, and other multidisciplinary theoretical frameworks in the evaluation of outcomes.
- Critically analyze, monitor, and evaluate intervention and program processes and outcomes.
- Apply evaluation findings to improve practice effectiveness at the micro-, mezzo-, and macro-levels.

Although students who attain these competencies are able to practice and conduct research in the field of social work, they may not have developed the specific skills necessary to be effective and succeed within the subspecialty of veterinary social work. Although some social work programs may offer courses that address one or more of the four domains of veterinary social work, at the present time, to the best of this author's knowledge, there is only one program in the United States that currently offers a comprehensive, integrated training program in veterinary social work.

- The University of Tennessee, Knoxville, offers the Veterinary Social Work Certificate Program, a joint program between the Veterinary College and the College of Social Work. The program focuses on the four modules of animal-assisted interventions, animal-related grief and loss, the link between human and animal violence and animal abuse and compassion fatigue and conflict management. The University of Tennessee launched a second certificate program, the Veterinary Human Support Certificate Program.
- The University of Denver offers several specialized educational certifications through the Institute for Human and Animal Connection: Animal-Assisted Social Work, Animal and Human Health Certificate, Canine-Assisted Intervention certificate, Equine-Assisted Mental Health Practitioner, and Humane Education Practitioner.

As with all social workers, veterinary social workers are encouraged to further expand their knowledge and skills through continuing professional education opportunities. These are often available through programs sponsored by state chapters of the National Association of Social Workers and by professional organizations.

There is a growing need for training programs in veterinary social work beyond those that currently exist. The increasing frequency of natural disasters with their impact on families and their animal members, the concerning rate of suicide among veterinarians, the high levels of burnout and compassion fatigue experienced by veterinary students and personnel, and the need to de-escalate conflicts between human clients and veterinary providers and within veterinary practices, all call for increased numbers of trained veterinary social workers who are able to effectively intervene. This training includes, as well, the need to develop additional field placement opportunities and identify associated competencies.

Future Directions

Veterinary social work is a relatively nascent professional area, recognized only 20 or so years ago. Numerous challenges and opportunities present themselves.

Although social workers are to understand and welcome diversity, the subspecialty of veterinary social work itself is characterized by the absence of diversity. Additional outreach is needed within the social work profession and to students contemplating social work as a career to make them aware of this subspecialty and encourage and support their development and participation in this field.

We have relatively little knowledge about various issues that are directly relevant to veterinary social work. Research is urgently needed to address issues such as:

- The impact of veterinary social work interventions on the retention of veterinary technicians and nurses
- The effectiveness of veterinary social workers in addressing burnout, compassion fatigue, and depression among veterinarians and other veterinary personnel
- Strategies to better integrate VSWs into the healthcare team, both for humans and animals
- Potential roles for veterinary social workers in less traditional settings, such as zoos and municipal animal control agencies
- Strategies to expand access to VSW services, which entail expanding access to veterinary care for lower-income pet owners
- Variations and similarities across populations with respect to their understanding and acceptance of veterinary social work services
- Pet owner experiences with veterinary social work

This volume is intended to serve as a resource for veterinary social workers, veterinary practice managers, veterinarians, veterinary technicians, veterinary practice staff, policymakers, faculty, and students by exploring the contributions to knowledge, practices, policies, published research, and scholarship for the areas of veterinary social work. In its 16 chapters, we not only provide a detailed review and discussion of the many dimensions of practice and research within the field but also highlight those areas that require additional consideration and research.

Chapter 2, authored by Poe and Strand, provides an in-depth discussion of how the field of veterinary social work came into being and gained professional recognition and acceptance. They bring the field's short history alive through their interviews with the founders of the field.

Stoewen explores in Chap. 3 the growing issue of compassion fatigue and burnout in the animal care community. She offers strategies not only for the recognition of compassion fatigue but for interventions at the levels of the individual and the organization. Her exploration of these issues underscores the need for trained veterinary social workers who can help address these issues.

Susan Hatters Friedman and colleagues integrate the perspectives of psychiatry, pediatrics, and law enforcement in their comprehensive discussion in Chap. 4 of the link between animal and human neglect and violence. The chapter focuses not only on research relating to this connection but also on available interventions and on relevant law enforcement procedures.

Several subsequent chapters focus our attention on veterinary social work in a variety of different settings. Vincent and colleagues (Chap. 5) look at the use of animal-assisted interventions across a wide range of settings, including airports, hospitals, and dental offices. They examine the theoretical basis for these interventions and point us to training programs for both the human and the animals involved in their delivery. Their interviews with currently practicing VSWs provide concrete examples of how and why an understanding of the theoretical basis of animal-assisted interventions is important. Winston's examination in Chap. 6 of the use of animal-assisted interventions in the psychotherapeutic setting not only speaks to the methods and its associated benefits but also raises important ethical and legal issues associated with animal-assisted interventions in this setting, astutely noting the complete absence of guidance to social workers from their professional organizations with respect to the ethical obligations to the animals relied upon in practice. Moga's chapter on the ethics of interprofessional practice (Chap. 7) expands on these issues.

Brackenridge, Hacker, and Pepe explain in Chap. 8 how VSWs can effectively be integrated into the veterinary hospital setting. They provide a vivid picture of what a day in such a setting might look like. Strand and colleagues identify in Chap. 9 the numerous settings in which conflict may arise and the role that can be played by the VSW in de-escalating and mitigating these conflicts. Their discussion is augmented by their strategic selection of various case examples that serve to highlight the important role of the VSW and the many situations in which their assistance may be critical.

Volk (Chap. 10) focuses on yet another aspect of veterinary social work: the provision of interventions and support to veterinarians' well-being and mental health. The chapter provides suggestions not only for VSWs who may wish to develop an intervention but also to veterinary-aligned professionals who may be searching for strategies to enhance their well-being.

Linden's chapter (Chap. 11) takes us to animal-related practice management. She explores service delivery models, the roles and responsibilities of VSWs in such settings, and barriers to reliance on VSWs.

Chapters 12 and 13 address veterinary social work in educational settings. Diesch-Chham focuses on the roles of VSWs in the veterinary college, with specific attention to the need for VSWs to address student mental health and well-being and to assist students to develop proactive strategies to avoid compassion fatigue, burnout, and depression. Hoy-Gerlach and colleagues explore the development and implementation of veterinary social work internships in veterinary settings, specifically noting the need for interprofessional collaboration and the resulting benefits not only for the student in training but also for the staff of the veterinary setting.

Loue engages us in Chap. 14 with an exploration of the ethical and legal issues that may arise in the context of conducting research that involves both humans and animals. Gupta expands on the discussion of research by examining in Chap. 15 the current state of research in veterinary social work, noting the ongoing need for additional research to bring us answers to unresolved questions. In the final chapter, Chap. 16, Loue presents the findings of cross-cultural studies while underscoring the relative dearth of knowledge regarding the understanding, acceptance, and use of veterinary social work across cultures and societies.

References

Associated Press. (2005, September 9). *Has snowball finally been found?* NBC.com. https://www.nbcnews.com/health/health-news/has-snowball-finally-been-found-flna1c9440911. Accessed 21 Aug 2021.

Associated Press. (2010, August 24). *Horror stories about pets in the aftermath of Hurricane Katrina prompted new evaluation rules.* https://www.foxnews.com/us/horror-stories-about-pets-in-the-aftermath-of-hurricane-katrina-prompted-new-evacuation-rules. Accessed 21 Aug 2021.

Bruillard, K. (2017). How the chaos of Hurricane Katrina helped save pets from flooding in Texas. *Washington Post*, August 31.

Council on Social Work Education. (2015, June 11). *Education policy and accreditation standards.* https://www.cswe.org/getattachment/Accreditation/Accreditation-Process/2015-EPAS/2015EPAS_Web_FINAL.pdf.aspx. Accessed 21 Aug 2021.

Council on Social Work Education. (2022). 2022 Educational policy and accreditation standards. https://www.cswe.org/accreditation/standards/2022-epas/. Accessed 30 July 2022.

Federal Emergency Management Agency. (n.d.). *IS-0010.a Animals in disasters: Awareness and preparedness: Lesson 1: Introduction.* https://emilms.fema.gov/is_0010a/curriculum/1.html. Accessed 22 Aug 2021.

Hill, R. P., Gaines, J., & Wilson, R. M. (2007). Consumer behavior, extended self and scared consumption: An alternative perspective from our animal companions. *Journal of Business Research, 61*(5), 553–562.

Interprofessional Education Collaborative. (2016). *Core competencies for interprofessional collaborative practice: 2016 update.* Interprofessional Education Collaborative.

Leonard, H. A., & Scammon, D. L. (2007). No pet left behind: Accommodating pets in emergency planning. *Journal of Public Policy & Marketing, 26*(1), 49–53.

Ohio Revised Statute § 4757.02. (2014).

Pets Evacuation and Transportation Standards Act, Pub. L. No. 109–308. (2006).

Robert T. Stafford Disaster Relief and Emergency Assistance Act, Pub. L. 100–707. (1988).

Serpell, J. A. (2003). Anthropomorphism and anthropomorphic selection: Beyond the "cute response". *Society & Animals, 11*(1), 83–100.

Wan, W. (2006). A lesson from Katrina: Pets matter: Disaster plans include first aid, evacuation options for four-legged victims. *Washington Post*, January 2.

Chapter 2
History of Veterinary Social Work

Bethanie A. Poe and Elizabeth B. Strand

The Development of the University of Tennessee Veterinary Social Work Program

Elizabeth Strand, PhD, LCSW, coined the term "veterinary social work" in 2002 and is the founder and director of the University of Tennessee, Knoxville (UT), Veterinary Social Work program.

The development of veterinary social work as a field of practice and the UT Veterinary Social Work program are inextricably linked. For Strand, the journey toward developing the UT Veterinary Social Work program began when she was working on her PhD at the UT College of Social Work.

> I was going to study family systems because I love family therapy. That is what I did between my masters and Ph.D. I was going to study the relationship between daughters and their fathers, but there was this kind of fascinating woman named Dr. Catherine Faver. She had bunnies and she was interested in the Link between human and animal violence and was turning her...academic attention to animals. I had never considered it before, but she was such a unique person, and her passion was so clear and true that I got involved in studying the Link between human and animal violence. My dissertation research was on domestic violence victims and their concern for pets before leaving their abusive situations (Strand, 2021).

In 2000, the UT College of Veterinary Medicine obtained a new dean, Dr. Michael Blackwell. Blackwell would bring a unique perspective to the position:

> ...before I came to the university of Tennessee, I was both running a private practice and I was, at this point in time, Chief of Staff of the Office of the Surgeon General of the United States, and we were working on issuing the first Surgeon General's report on mental health.

B. A. Poe (✉) · E. B. Strand
University of Tennessee, Knoxville Colleges of Veterinary Medicine and Social Work,
Knoxville, TN, USA
e-mail: bpoe2@utk.edu

© The Author(s), under exclusive license to Springer Nature Switzerland AG 2022
S. Loue, P. Linden (eds.), *The Comprehensive Guide to Interdisciplinary Veterinary Social Work*, https://doi.org/10.1007/978-3-031-10330-8_2

So, during my tour through that office, I became more sensitized about mental/emotional health issues in America.

As I would go to my practice in the evening, increasingly, I was recognizing as I looked across the table into the eyes of my clients, I was sometimes seeing what appeared to be depression or certainly anxiety about what's going on, and I felt so inadequate.... I felt inadequate because it's painful when people are struggling in a moment, whether it's an end-of-life decision or a treatable problem... and they're just worried sick. Or the financial concerns... I wanted to do something about that.... I had a mission reason for coming [to UT], but one part of that mission was to do something about this gap in our ability to serve our clients. (Blackwell, 2021).

Upon coming to UT, Blackwell would be introduced to and would go on to become friends with the then dean of the UT College of Social Work, Dr. Karen Sowers. The idea for having social workers in the UT College of Veterinary Medicine would arise one evening over a casual conversation.

...It's amazing to me what great creativity can come out of relationships and sitting around having a glass of wine, unwinding, and just talking about stuff. And we were doing that, and he said, 'you know, we really need social workers in college of vet med' and I was intrigued.

We started the conversation. It really started [by] talking about the high level of suicide among veterinarians, and the level of depression among veterinarians, and I became very concerned when he started talking about that. I had had the kind of traditional view of 'wouldn't it be great to be a veterinarian? You get to play with the little animals all the time!' No, they're experiencing death at such a high rate among their clients and...being an animal lover myself, I was able to put myself in those shoes and recognize what he was talking about.

Serendipitously, as wonderful things happen by chance sometimes, Elizabeth Strand was a doctoral student....and she was doing her dissertation in this area.... Quite frankly, in the beginning, our faculty was not readily accepting. [They were] wondering, you know, is this really social work? Is this a legitimate area for research, etc.? But, with Elizabeth's wonderful, exuberant personality, she, of course, slowly started winning people over. So, it was things coming together at the right time, and [Strand] adding her vision to Michael [Blackwell's] and my vision. So, we started talking actually housing a social worker at the College of Vet Med (Sowers, 2021).

By the end of the year, Dean Sowers would introduce Dean Blackwell to Elizabeth Strand, who was still a PhD student at the time.

And so, people at the College of Social Work knew I was studying animals, and I was the first person-I think that maybe there was one other Ph.D. student that was kind of co-occurring with me, maybe came a little after me, that was studying animals, so it was a little tough....to study something so outside of the box. But, Catherine Faver was there, and she was my support, so I could do it.

There were two masters [of social work] students [who] wanted to do a field placement regarding animals; no doubt they were influenced by Dr. Catherine Faver. At the time, there were some really important people: Michael Blackwell was the Dean of the [UT] College of Veterinary Medicine and he came in with a vision of having mental health present in veterinary settings. Catherine Faver, of course, who was studying animals...Karen Sowers [Dean of the UT College of Social Work] who was receptive to Dr. Blackwell's vision. And then there was John New who founded the HABIT [Human Animal Bond in Tennessee] program, so he was receptive and had written about mental health professionals [in veterinary medicine] as well. So, kind of all that came together and I was able to take this student desire and negotiate that my Ph.D. stipend would go towards me supervising these two [social work] students at the College of Veterinary Medicine. I was paid ten hours a week, but I clearly worked forty hours, no doubt, a week in building the program and building the partnership between the [UT Colleges of Veterinary Medicine and Social Work] (Strand, 2021).

Strand's first day on the UTCVM Hospital floor was May 2, 2002; and so, what would become veterinary social work was born.

The transition from Strand being a doctoral student supervising two MSSW interns in the College of Veterinary Medicine to becoming the director of the Veterinary Social Work program was an intricate one. While being the result of a collaboration between the Colleges of Social Work and Veterinary Medicine meant that there were more resources and expertise to engage, it also meant that there were two sets of administrators, regulations, and budgets to navigate. Dean Blackwell had a clear vision of what he wanted veterinary social work to be:

> The vision that I had was that... I want to be able to stand on the east coast of the United States and look across this country to west coast, and most veterinary practices either have a veterinary social worker on staff or they have a formal relationship with a social worker to service their clients.... The other charge was the program needed to address a diverse population, that being students, staff, faculty, and clients. (Blackwell, 2021).

To accomplish this mission, Strand had to enlist the help of others that were doing similar work. She contacted Dr. Susan Cohen at The Animal Medical Center (AMC) in New York City to see if she could observe how Cohen practiced in the veterinary hospital.

> I wrote to Susan Cohen and asked, 'can I follow you around?' and she said yes...I went back two days in a row...you know, I felt like a field student. She is such a good teacher... I remember her taking me to the room with all the blood donor dogs...and I remember [Cohen's] energy was very clinical... it wasn't dispassionate or cold, it was just par for the course, if you will. And I remember vividly that feeling inside of 'wow, this is different social work' because I went in with my hat of...dog love and she was showing me what it is to be a professional social worker in [the veterinary] environment. Not that you don't have positive feelings but...you have a different kind of clinical engagement with the animals (Strand, 2021).

> We were building the concept of Veterinary Social Work, which involved a lot of logic models, and strategic planning meetings with this Dean, and that Dean and this student, and this person from human medicine about how they run things in human medicine...there were a lot of strategy meetings, and who was at the table was key....
>
> In those meetings, we would review these logic models, so I would be up all night writing .... You know, it was all in my head, but I had to get it on paper and present it to everyone... (Strand, 2021).

Naming Veterinary Social Work

It was important to everyone involved in the program's development that the field have a name. "...once you define it and you nail it down and you say 'these are the ethics of the practice, there are our principles', then you gain legitimacy" (Sowers,

2021). But why call it "veterinary social work"? The name "veterinary social work" was consciously selected to embody the interdisciplinary, mutually dependent partnership between two fields that, while having obvious differences, have similarities in their scope of practice and core values.

Practice

The word *veterinary* is an adjective, and it means "of, relating to, practicing, or being the science and art of prevention, cure, or alleviation of disease and injury in animals and especially domestic animals" (Merriam-Webster, n.d.). This is an important point because while many associate the term *veterinary* only with the clinic to which they take their pets, that is not an accurate view of the profession. Not only are veterinary professionals in hospitals and clinics working to improve the lives of individual animals but also on the ground during disaster relief efforts, developing and maintaining standards in the food production industry, and creating policy in our local, state, and national legislative bodies; veterinary professionals are present and working hands-on at all levels of our society for the health, safety, and betterment of humans and animals. To collaborate effectively with such an active, applied profession like veterinary medicine, one must be equally as proactive.

> I became a social worker on purpose. I chose social work on purpose because of its nitty-gritty, boots-on-the-ground, systems perspective, strengths perspective, micro/macro, really nice model of how to influence the world…Looking at the careers of social workers throughout the ages, I'm proud of my heritage as a social worker. I really believed that paradigm, that framework [of social work] was one that was very well suited to serving the goals and needs of veterinary medicine (Strand, 2021).

Dean Blackwell also had strong feelings about the appropriateness of social work as a partner for veterinary medicine. "…[before coming to UT] I met a mental health social worker and that relationship really grounded me in the belief that [social work] was really the best suited for veterinary medicine because of the breadth of your scope, of your focus, and the methods that you use to address [challenges]. In other words…the fire that is burning right now on my desk; how do I address the reality of where the person is right now? So it just made immense sense that we needed to partner with social work" (Blackwell, 2021).

Core Values

Upon graduation, veterinarians take the following oath:

> Being admitted to the profession of veterinary medicine, I solemnly swear to use my scientific knowledge and skills for *the benefit of society* through the protection of animal health and *welfare*, the *relief of* animal *suffering*, the conservation of livestock resources, the *promotion of public health*, and the advancement of medical knowledge. I will practice my

profession conscientiously, with *dignity*, and in keeping with the principles of veterinary medical *ethics*. I accept as a lifelong obligation the *continual improvement* of my *professional knowledge and competence*. (American Veterinary Medical Association, *emphasis added*).

Meanwhile, the set of standards that guide the professional conduct of social workers are below:

- Service.
- Social Justice.
- Dignity and worth of the person.
- Importance of human relationships.
- Integrity.
- Competence.
  (National Association of Social Workers, Code of Ethics)

When looking at the comparison between the Veterinarian's Oath and the ethical principles enunciated in the Code of Ethics of the National Association of Social Workers (NASW) above, the parallels between the two are easily discernible. Each demonstrates a dedication to improving conditions for the public good, and treating others with dignity, while also practicing ethically and competently. Given social work's ethical mandate to practice only within one's area of competence, partnering with the profession with the most expertise regarding non-human animals becomes apparent if we are to truly address the challenges that arise from human and animal relationships. Therefore, the name "veterinary social work" establishes the connections between the two fields of expertise, setting the expectations of collaboration while maintaining appropriate boundaries of practice between the two professions.

Contention Around the Term "Veterinary Social Work"

The term *veterinary social work* has not been without its detractors and has caused great debate on both the human and animal sides. Even Dean Blackwell wasn't sure about the term in the beginning:

> I was concerned about the biases that exist in the name 'social worker'. We live in a society where people are ignorant about the profession and when you push them to tell you 'what is a social worker?', [they say] 'well, they take your children away, right? Isn't that what they do?' or some of these more negative, provocative roles that social workers fulfill. And yet, there's this big ol' universe of what the profession fulfills that's just off the radar.... We had to overcome a bias about having social work in veterinary medicine. Veterinary was okay, but it's a claimed term... I was concerned that it might be a limiting factor.... (Blackwell, 2021).

For some people, the problem is the word "veterinary"; they feel it is too limiting as not all veterinary social work practice occurs within a veterinary hospital or clinic. As described in the Practice section, this can be addressed with education about the wide array of roles veterinary professionals fulfill.

Others take issue with "social work," citing the fact that there are many types of licensed mental health professionals including licensed professional counselors, marriage and family therapists, psychologists, and psychiatrists that are involved in addressing the needs that arise in human-animal relationships. While these other mental health professionals cannot claim to be veterinary social workers as social work is a title-protected profession, they can and do make great contributions to the field on both the micro- and macro-levels. UT Veterinary Social Work acknowledges this difference in the Veterinary Social Work Certificate Programs by training other mental health professionals in the program but makes note of the distinction by writing the title on their certificate as "Veterinary Mental Health." The use of "social work" in "veterinary social work" is not to malign other mental health professions, but rather to embrace the complementary ethics and methods of practice between veterinary medicine and social work.

> The intention of veterinary social work, in my heart at least, was that it would be a marriage between veterinary medicine and social work such that each profession is better. I know that I am certainly a more humane social worker because of my exposure to veterinary medicine (Strand, 2021).

The Four Areas of Veterinary Social Work Practice

As veterinary social work is currently defined, there are four general areas of a practice which the needs from human-animal relationships typically arise: animal-related grief and bereavement, the Link between human and animal violence, compassion fatigue management, and animal-assisted interventions.

- *Animal-related grief and bereavement*, also commonly referred to as "pet loss," refers to the reactions one may experience due to the loss of an animal. The loss may be due to the death of the animal or for any other reason that the animal is no longer with the person.
- *The Link between human and animal violence* is the name given to the idea that animal abuse is correlated with other types of violence. Topics typically discussed in this area include intimate partner violence, child abuse, elder abuse, animal fighting, and animal hoarding.
- *Compassion fatigue management* refers to the knowledge and skills needed to address compassion fatigue, or secondary traumatic stress, which is a form of burnout that manifests itself as physical, emotional, and spiritual exhaustion (Strand et al., 2012). UT Veterinary Social Work also includes conflict management in this category as conflict is often a source of compassion fatigue.
- *Animal-assisted interventions* refer to the deliberate inclusion of an animal as part of the therapeutic process. Interventions must be goal oriented and structured (Kruger & Serpell, 2006).

Work in the field of human-animal relationships had been occurring since the 1960s. Leo K. Bustad, veterinarian and founder of the Delta Society (now Pet

Partners©) in the 1970s, is credited with introducing the term "human-animal bond" into the nomenclature. However, Dr. Boris Levinson, often referred to as the "father of animal assisted therapy," had articulated the concept, if not the exact phrase, earlier in his books[1]*Pet-Oriented Child Psychotherapy* (1969) and *Pets and Human Development* (1972).

In the 1970s and 1980s, early studies about the Link (Tapia, 1971; Tingle et al., 1986; Wax & Haddox, 1974a, b) and the therapeutic benefits of animals (Netting et al., 1987) were published. Articles about pet loss and mental health in veterinary settings also began appearing in journals in the 1980s (Cohen, 1985; Quackenbush & Glickman, 1983; Lagoni et al., 1988; Lagoni & Hetts, 1989; Butler & Lagoni, 1995). The concept of compassion fatigue would appear in 1992 (Joinson, 1992), and Figley's work on compassion fatigue would soon after be applied to animal-related professionals, leading him to write *Compassion Fatigue in the Animal-Care Community* (Figley, 2006).

Strand discerned these themes that would become the four areas of veterinary social work practice as she reviewed the available literature on human-animal relationships for her dissertation research. She also found that what she was reading in the literature was reflected in her experiences in the UT College of Veterinary Medicine:

> I was doing my dissertation work on the link between human and animal violence and because of that I was reading all the literature that social work had given to the human-animal bond, and I was also looking in other disciplines as well. [The four areas of veterinary social work practice] were the themes that I noticed in the literature, but I found that they correlated with boots-on-ground in the clinic because at that same time... I was reading and I was watching at the front desk of the small animal clinic. I was listening to the kinds of cases that disturbed the veterinary team. I was on the phone with clients. I was talking to clients. We were having pet loss support groups.... I was interacting with the Knoxville community around domestic violence and pets. (Strand, 2021)

While it was obvious in the literature and from experience that veterinary teams were experiencing stress and burnout, it was a fellow PhD student at the UT College of Social Work at the time, Tracy Zaparanick, who identified compassion fatigue management as a crucial part of veterinary social work practice.

> [Tracy] knew Michael [Blackwell] and she came up with the idea of building out the compassion fatigue component of veterinary social work. She and I worked on a couple of things together, and so that's really how compassion fatigue became a large part [of veterinary social work]. I added the conflict [management] piece on because, of course, that's a big part of what causes teams so much distress (Strand, 2021).

What makes veterinary social work unique is not that it considered human-animal relationships. Instead, it was that, for the first time, all of these areas of practicing in the space where humans and animals connect were brought under one encompassing term. Even more unusual in comparison to human-animal studies at the time, veterinary social workers are expected to be competent in all of the areas of

---

[1] For a detailed history of the development of the human-animal bond as a field, these authors suggest Hines' 2003 article, *Historical Perspectives on the Human-Animal Bond.*

veterinary social work practice. Many students are attracted to the predominantly positive field of animal-assisted interventions. While animal-related bereavement and compassion fatigue have sad implications, one can ultimately connect those experiences with positive experiences of caring about animals. On the other hand, studying the dark side of human-animal relationships, the Link, can make students profoundly uncomfortable.

> …there are many students that got angry that I was asking them to pay attention to the Link between human and animal violence….If you're a social worker, you don't get to cream from the top about what clients you serve. You're there to take care of the whole bit, and the whole bit of the human-animal relationships is not all pretty. And so, if ethically, to me, if we are going to integrate and attend to animals, then we need to attend to all of it, not just the part of it that makes us feel cozy (Strand, 2021).

Early Days at the UTCVM

While a few other veterinary colleges had social workers or psychologists on staff— University of Pennsylvania, Louisiana State University—it wasn't a common practice. Strand describes her early days in the UT College of Veterinary Medicine:

> …It was just this feeling of 'what are you doing here?'. I had no desk. And in the beginning, … I would get permission from the senior clinician to go and observe, so I would just stand in the treatment rooms and observe everything going on in the treatment rooms. I learned a lot… I didn't get involved very much. Over a few months… if I saw that there was something that was needed, like you know, people need this trash taken out or something like that, you know, I would do that! …I would try to look at what was needed, within my scope of practice, was there something I could contribute that would help, and I would help in those little ways.
>
> I also…sat at the front desk of the small animal clinic and I learned from the front desk staff about the kinds of clients that came in and heard them talk to clients and got a sense of what were the sort of stressors that came in. Mostly, it was a lot of shadowing; a lot of standing around; a lot of being quiet; a lot of observing… and then [I] slowly started a pet loss support group. So, it was all pet loss back then, right? I mean, everybody in the vet hospital knew they had…psychological distress, and they knew it was everywhere, but the only name they had for it was 'pet loss'… but I could see it was way bigger than that.
>
> They didn't actually call me Dr. Death, but you know it was kind of like 'we don't want the social worker to come in the room because then that means something is dying…People made fun of the concept of veterinary social work, and that was hard. (Strand, 2021).

Like their counterparts in the College of Social Work, faculty in the College of Veterinary Medicine were unsure about this partnership between the two professions:

> I think the biggest word on a word cloud would be 'confusion'… but then, through time I came to appreciate that some were really bothered because I was introducing—I literally heard this—'voodoo science' into veterinary medicine…. It [was] ignorance… I was understanding of all that, because veterinary medicine has operated in a silo, and when you go into a veterinary college, it's an ivory tower in a silo, very disconnected from reality in many respects. So, I was okay with that. And when I say Dr. Strand was the right person, it starts with the fact that we needed someone with the skill set and the personality, and just

the spirit to weather that kind of environment and yet still nudge it in the direction we need to go. It took only a bit of time before the messaging started to come back to my office indicating that she was being effective…. By the time I left [in 2008, Veterinary Social Work] was the one program that the faculty were in agreement that they would never want to lose. (Blackwell, 2021).

Strand made it a point to conduct yearly program evaluations, gathering information from not only faculty and staff in the college but also from the clients served. These reports would reflect how many people were accessing veterinary social work, which lent support to the hiring of a part-time Assistant Director, Dr. Geneva Brown, in 2006. Brown provided clinical support in the veterinary hospital, ran the pet loss support group, and supervised clinical MSSW students, which left Strand free to do more work with the College of Veterinary Medicine faculty and expand the veterinary social work program. After about a year, Brown retired and was replaced by Danielle Groeling, LCSW. Groeling left in 2008, and due to a global financial crisis happening at that time, the position was not filled, leaving Strand as the only veterinary social worker on staff once again.

The Impact of Students

Staying true to its origins, the UT Veterinary Social Work program's services have always been student driven. While trying to get the program off the ground, it presented some challenges:

It was hard to build a program while having interns there at the same time. [The interns] were also shadowing… I would be in one treatment room, and [the interns] would be in another treatment room, and then we would all kind of come back together and talk about what we [had] learned…. I didn't feel like I could completely let them turned loose because I didn't know the environment…. [As the sole social worker on staff] that meant that everything was just about [which] students wanted to participate and [if] could we put a team together. So every year there was a new team…it was very hard to build…a sustainable structure because each year there were new students, but you know, we were still able to be of service to the College in meaningful ways. (Strand, 2021).

While the program remained adaptable for students' particular interests related to veterinary social work, standard activities for the MSSW interns began to solidify. Students would begin their internship with a "scavenger hunt" to familiarize themselves with the layout of the hospital and meet the people they would need to know throughout the College. They received training on communication skills and stress management; self-care practices would be required in their learning plan. They visited the local animal shelter and did a ride-along with an animal control officer.

Clinical MSSW students spend most of their time in the veterinary hospital, providing client support during patient treatment and euthanasia, co-facilitating the pet loss support group, and engaging with veterinary students, interns, and house officers regarding not only their cases but also academic and personal issues. Macro-practice interns focus much of their time on program development, evaluation, and event coordination, such as the Spring Learning Series, which was a lunch-and-learn-type educational series provided to the faculty, staff, and students on veterinary social work-related topics that could be useful in their day-to-day work, as well as earn them continuing education credit.

Expanding Veterinary Social Work's Reach

UT Veterinary Social Work expanded its reach by hosting a day-long workshop for the Tennessee Chapter of the National Association of Social Workers on February 16, 2007. Dean Blackwell gave a welcoming address, and then participants were educated about the four areas of veterinary social work practice by Drs. Strand and Brown; Dr. John C. New, who was a Professor and the Head of Comparative Medicine and the founder of Human Animal Bond in Tennessee (HABIT); two doctoral fellows with veterinary social work, Dr. Janelle Nimer, LCSW, who is now the director of 4 Healing Center in Utah, and Dr. Jan Yorke, who was a professor Laurentian University; and three MSSW interns, Erin Allen, MSSW, now working at the Argus Institute; Teresa Nolan Pratt, LCSW, who has a private practice; and this chapter's co-author, Dr. Bethanie Poe, LMSW.

The NASW workshop served as a launch point for the International Veterinary Social Work Summit (IVSWS), a biennial interdisciplinary conference for professionals who are interested in veterinary social work. The first Summit was held in April 17–20, 2008, at the University of Tennessee, Knoxville. Speakers included Susan Cohen, Catherine Faver, Stephanie, Johnson, Christina Risley-Curtiss, Ken Shapiro, Bert Traughton, and Tracy Zaparanick; presentations addressed animal-related bereavement, the Link, animal-assisted interventions, and compassion fatigue, as well as diversity, spirituality, and teaching communication skills. The first Summit had a total of 43 attendees, including speakers and UT Veterinary Social Work staff and students. "The first Summit was just an opportunity to bring people together to meeting in a different way that integrated that aspect of what we love so much about animals, which is play, into the way that we engage each other on the topic of veterinary social work" (Strand, 2021). Subsequent Summits were held in 2010, 2013, 2015, 2018, and 2020.

The 2010 Summit was very similar to the 2008 Summit, as it was also held on the UT campus, covered the same range of topics, and had a similar number of participants. In 2013, the Summit grew exponentially in several ways. First, the 2013 Summit had a specific theme: "Is there a role for social work in the care and welfare of animals?" Second, it was the first time that abstracts were submitted for the Summit, and there were multiple tracks to choose from during the conference. Third, this Summit had a variety of sponsors in addition to departments of the University of Tennessee and local sponsors, such as Young-Williams Animal Center, the Knoxville Animal Clinic, and the Knoxville Zoo. The Summit also received support from PetSafe, the American Society for the Prevention of Cruelty to Animals

(ASPCA), Zoetis, Merial FVS, Purina, Banfield Pet Hospital, Hills, and the Society of Animal Welfare Administrators (SAWA). These sponsorships allowed the Summit to engage two high-profile keynote speakers, Temple Grandin and Hal Herzog. These keynotes additionally distinguished the 2013 Summit from earlier Summits. The presence of these keynote speakers led to an increase in the attendance of the third Summit—almost triple what it had been in 2006 and 2008. In addition to speaking at the Summit itself, Grandin and Herzog also presented an evening lecture that was open to the public, followed by a book signing that attracted attention both to the event and to the field of veterinary social work.

The fourth IVSWS evolved once again. In 2015, UT Veterinary Social Work collaborated with the Association of American Veterinary Medical Colleges (AAVMC) to present the Veterinary Wellness & Social Work Summit. It was a combination of two meetings: the Health & Wellness Summit that had been hosted at The Ohio State College of Veterinary Medicine and the IVSWS. The goals of this inter-professional meeting were to:

- Develop a common understanding of the health and wellness issues faced by veterinary medical students and recent veterinary graduates.
- Engage in inter-professional dialogue about health and wellness factors in the veterinary profession.
- Share and formulate interventions for enhancing and protecting health and wellness within the veterinary profession (AAVMC & VSW, 2015).

Like the previous Summits, the conference consisted of keynote presentations, workshops, podium and poster presentations, table topic discussions, and play and wellness activities. More than 200 people attended.

In 2018, the Summit reverted to UT Veterinary Social Work, this time focusing on the topic of "Animals & Poverty." While the Summit has always been interdisciplinary, the 2018 Summit went beyond animal-related professionals and mental health professionals to include a keynote by Dr. Don Bruce, the Douglas and Brenda Horne Professor of Business in the Haslam College of Business at the University of Tennessee with a joint appointment in the Department of Economics and the Boyd Center for Business and Economic Research, to provide a different lens on poverty for Summit participants.

The theme of the 2020 Summit was also "Animals & Poverty." Due to the COVID-19 pandemic, the 2020 Summit was held virtually. Despite the change in delivery method, the content and atmosphere of the Summit remained intact and had the silver lining that more than 200 people were able to attend, versus the slightly more than 100 people that were able to travel to Knoxville in 2018.

Since its inception, the purpose of IVSWS has been to provide an opportunity for professionals with an interest in veterinary social work to come together to learn from one another and continue to grow the field. "[The Summits] have continued to be fairly small…but people leave bright-eyed…and inspired, so I think we have a good thing going in terms of how we run the Summits" (Strand, 2021).

Pioneers in the Field

Veterinary social work is an inherently interdisciplinary field, bringing together professionals from both animal-related professions and mental health practitioners to address the challenges that arise in and from human-animal relationships. Although it is not possible to mention all who have influenced the field of veterinary social work from its inception to the present, this section presents prominent mental health professionals whose contributions have formed the foundation of what has become veterinary social work.

The authors of this chapter gathered perspectives from mental health professionals who have made major contributions to the field. These pioneers describe how they became a mental health professional in a veterinary setting, their experiences with burnout and self-care, their most memorable and most difficult experiences, and what advice they would give to anyone entering the field of veterinary social work.

James "Jamie" Quackenbush, M.S.W. (1948–2005), is recognized as the first social worker in a veterinary hospital. Starting in the late 1970s, Quackenbush was the social worker in the Veterinary Hospital at the University of Pennsylvania. Dr. Susan Cohen (2021) recalls that the idea originally came from Dr. Louise P. Shoemaker, the Dean of the School of Social Work from 1971 to 1985 (Lloyd, 2008). Upon walking through the Veterinary Hospital, she noticed that the clients often looked worried. After sitting down to speak with them, she decided that this was a population with an unmet need. Quackenbush is quoted as saying he came into his position "kind of by mistake" while looking for financial aid to complete his doctorate (Rovner, 1986). The project he was going to work on fell through, and he found himself in a conversation with Dean Shoemaker who said, "maybe they should have a social worker at the vet hospital" (Cohen, 2021). Described by *The Washington Post* as "the nation's first full-time pet bereavement counselor," Quackenbush estimated that he counseled about 1000 people coping with the death of their pets during the last year alone in his position at the University of Pennsylvania Veterinary School's Center for the Interaction of Animals and Society (Rovner, 1986). Quackenbush's book, *When Your Pet Dies: How to Cope with Your Feelings,* (Quackenbush & Graveline, 1985) received media attention from The Today Show, the BBC, *People Magazine*, and Oprah Winfrey (*Ann Arbor News,* 2006). Quackenbush was awarded the Delta Society Beyond Limits Award in 1986 for "contributions to the study and promotion of the human-animal bond" (*Ann Arbor News,* 2006).

Susan P. Cohen, DSW, was the first social worker in the Animal Medical Center (AMC) in New York City. Hired in 1982, AMC was, at the time, one of the busiest animal hospitals in the world and one of the few that was open 24 hours a day. In 1983, she started the first Pet Loss Support Group. During her over 28 years as the Director of Counseling, she helped develop the field of pet loss counseling and veterinary training in communication skills and stress management (Cohen, n.d.-a).

Cohen has mentored numerous social workers who would later go on to be innovators in the field. She has taught social work courses at Columbia University and Long Island University and was a consultant for Pfizer Animal Health (now called Zoetis) and Purina (Cohen, n.d.-a). She has authored numerous articles and book chapters on social work in a veterinary setting, pet loss, and compassion fatigue. Cohen has also made television appearances related to her work on "The Today Show," "The Oprah Winfrey Show," and "20/20" and had her work featured in *The New York Times*, *The Wall Street Journal*, *The New Yorker*, and *Smithsonian Magazine* (Cohen, n.d.-b).

Cohen retired from AMC in 2011. She went on to develop her consulting practice, Pet Decisions, where she provides education, media, and practice help regarding communication, compassion fatigue, human-animal interactions, as well as transitions and loss. She currently facilitates six different veterinary social work-related support groups and continues to share her work through writing and speaking engagements. She also created Social Workers Advancing the Human Animal Bond (SWAHAB), a special interest group of NASW-NYC, the New York City chapter of the NASW. The group's mission is to "…recognize and promote the health relationships individuals have with animals and the powerful bond that can exist between them" (SWAHAB, n.d.) .

Cohen remembers that ever since childhood, she has had an intense attachment to her animals and grieved each loss deeply. In her early 20s, she had an experience that began to pique her interest in the human-animal bond:

> … I was in my early 20s, and I had a cat that I was very attached to that was getting a little older… I took her to the vet for a checkup which, again, people didn't do so much [at this time], and I realized how anxious I was. The veterinarian was new to me, and she spent a lot of time looking into my cat's eyes, at which point, I decided that my cat had gone blind and that I didn't know it. So, I'm quietly crying, 'oh, my poor blind cat! Oh, how I've neglected her!'
>
> And I asked the vet about it and she said, 'she's not blind!'. And I said, 'her eyes look funny!', and she said 'If she were a person, she'd be getting reading glasses. This is just what happens to cats.'
>
> And I thought as I left 'Wow, I'm really super attached!' …I tried to lecture myself: 'You've got a husband and a child and a job—what's the matter with you?!' and it was having no effect. I said, I can't be the only one that feels this way. There must be a lot of other people who don't have any of these kinds of social supports. You know, somebody ought to really do something about this….

Several years later, in her first social work position working with college students with disabilities, Cohen found herself once again faced with the intensity of the human-animal bond. During her team's weekly meeting, she noticed that she was "…always the one that knew if [the students] were grieving a pet or service dog…. And after a number of those kind of episodes, you say [to yourself], 'everybody here is wonderful. They are all well trained. How come I'm the one that knows that it's been six months and they're still grieving that pet? What's going on here? …. And again, I started thinking 'wow, you know, somebody really ought to do something about that!' And again, I said [to myself] 'that's a crazy idea… nobody's going to pay you to do that!'

The final moment of truth was I picked up a book that I was going to use to work with students called *Guerilla Tactics of the Job Market* [Jackson, 1978].... I'm sitting on the subway and I'm reading this chapter, and [the author] says 'A question you should ask yourself [is] what are two or three job duties that you would enjoy so much you would practically pay somebody to let you do them?' And this voice in my head, as though I thought you'd never ask, says: talking to people, and animals."

A few months later, Cohen found a brochure about a conference on the relationship between people and animals happening at the University of Pennsylvania. On this brochure, there was a name of one veterinarian from New York City: Dr. William J. Kay. Unknown to Cohen at the time, Dr. Kay was the Chief Executive Officer at the Animal Medical Center (AMC) (1975–1996). He was aware of the program that had been started at the University of Pennsylvania, and he himself had had a similar experience as Dr. Shoemaker. While obtaining specialized training in the neurology department at Bellevue, Dr. Kay noticed that he was seeing the same reactions in the waiting rooms there as he was at the AMC, and he was able to make the connection that Bellevue had social workers. After originally bringing Cohen in to help plan another conference, Dr. Kay decided that what might be needed was a social worker in the AMC, and as Cohen was a social worker, he asked her to write the job description.

> I always laugh, but I had nothing to lose, so I wrote it the way I really thought it should be! I invented a pet loss group which had never been done. I'm not saying no one would have ever thought of it, but in those days, there was [Alcoholics Anonymous] and that was it.... I wrote in various community outreach things. I wrote in teaching young veterinarians because they were getting zero training in this. In some of the schools... [students] were discouraged if they said anything about...the client. It was 'forget the client! Your job is the animals.' And they didn't know what to do! If somebody cried, that was like a failure... and it was an absolute belief in the profession [at the time] that if you allow people to be present for euthanasia, they would faint and hit their head and sue you, and then they would hate you forever. So, of course, you can't let [clients] back there.... I wrote in everything I could think of as a social worker about how to reach people, and I tripled spaced it because they would be crossing stuff out and laughing....

It was several months later after turning in the proposal that the job offer came. It turned out that other mental health professionals had been brought in, but they had not been a good fit in the veterinary setting. She left the security of her university job and started in September 1982 to build the program at the AMC. She knew that she had been truly accepted that December at the traditional holiday party.

> At some point I get called up, and Santa says to the crowd, 'You know, we're a teaching hospital. Everybody here has fancy equipment; they've got stethoscopes and they've got microscopes... but the newest member of our team doesn't have any equipment at all, and they gave me... a jewel encrusted, gold sprayed box of Kleenex with a cord around it so I can hang it around my neck and just hand out tissues, because they didn't even have tissues in exam rooms. Everybody's crying, but, of course, you want to pretend that nobody was going to cry.... After this, they started putting tissues in the room. That's when I knew, 'oh, this is going to work out'.

Cohen says that she has not experienced burnout in her work. "There's so much work to be done and there [are] so many places to do it! It's one of the things that made me pick social work over all the other mental health disciplines, which are all wonderful and have great people in them, but it seemed to me that social work really dealt with the whole person in their whole situation.... So, for me, this has not been a burnout situation because there is always a way to help; there is always a place to intervene."

However, she is concerned about compassion fatigue and burnout in the veterinary profession, particularly the effects of the internet reviews, social media, and the pressure to be available 24/7.

> ...there are new challenges in veterinary practice...in the past 10 years that have really contributed to burnout and compassion fatigue.... I absolutely believe in the importance of teaching self-care and providing mental health services.... I think there is still a great need for mental health support, for continuing to be creative in the way we prepare people to be in [the veterinary] profession...and we have to prepare people for...transitions.

For those wishing to enter the field, she has this advice: "Get yourself a degree where you can get a job, and then become the human-animal interaction expert wherever you are—whether it's physical therapy or a public school—and bring that in and create your own situation."

> I just want to say how really grateful I am for having been able to be in this field and to contribute, to be a part of making things new and watching other people do new things and create new things.... All the people who have come at it, whether from the veterinary side or the mental health side... to watch it grow and become useful....
>
> To be who I actually am all the time at work; to live out my values with people who share those values; to have room to create without a lot of rules and constraints and people competing and looking over your shoulder and trying to stab you in the back; to spend my life working that way is one of the greatest gifts I will ever have (Cohen, 2021).

Bonnie S. Mader, M.S., started the first phone hotline for pet loss support at the University of California, Davis School of Veterinary Medicine, with Kelly Palm, DVM, in 1988. Inspired to start the hotline by the success of local pet loss support groups, the Hotline was staffed by veterinary students as part of an elective class. Over the Pet Loss Support Hotline's 20-year history, more than 15,000 calls were received (Features Editor, 2009). Mader continues to work to promote mental health for people in the veterinary field.

Stephanie LaFarge, PhD, was hired as a psychologist for the American Society for the Prevention of Cruelty to Animals (ASPCA) in New York City in 1997, and she held that position until her retirement in 2020.

As a child, LaFarge loved animals and wanted to be a veterinarian but found herself discouraged by high school math. Instead, she changed her focus to psychology, although her interest in and attachment to animals never faded.

Her first PhD project was a 1973 experiment which became the subject of documentary entitled *Project Nim (2011)*. A baby chimpanzee, referred to as NimChimpsky, was separated from his mother and raised in LaFarge's home to see if he could be taught sign language and, then, like a human child, communicate first using words and then sentences.

After the Nim experiment, her focus changed to child psychology. LaFarge would go on to work with terminally ill adolescents for 10 years, and then another 30 years, working in end-of-life thinking and planning for people dying of HIV/ AIDS, substance abuse, and other causes.

> And then I was walking in New York City where I live and I realized, the only thing I was interested in were the dogs on the street. So, I thought, you know, I just really have to get back to animals somehow in my career. At that time, the ASPCA was just beginning to expand into a number of areas of New York City. I had volunteered there as a teen-ager, and I went there and got hired and was there for 20 years. (LaFarge, 2021)

In addition to providing support to everyone in the veterinary community at the ASPCA, she also ran a toll-free, 24/7 pet loss hotline that received over 2000 calls a year and the number to which was once a Jeopardy! clue: "…it just put the phone number up on the screen. I had no idea about this, I never watched Jeopardy! but somebody called me and said so…. I didn't put that in my resume', but that was exciting." (LaFarge, 2021)

Shortly after being hired there, the ASPCA began to focus on animal cruelty and hoarding. LaFarge developed an alternative sentencing option for people convicted of animal cruelty; this was the only such program in the United States at the time. She also deployed with ASPCA first responder program, both for man-made disasters such as dog fighting rings and animal hoarding situations and natural disasters. "That was a very important part that I hadn't anticipated, but it became a very important part of my job there….like everyone else in mental health, I was trying to figure out a way to build in compassion fatigue support and all those things."

> …this is not true in all cultures, but in our culture [people] have a kind of a split brain between 'I'm an animal person' or 'I'm a people person'. Even many veterinarians would say 'You know, I don't like people. That's why I went into veterinary medicine'. And donors have that same thing 'I'm committed to animals.' However, that's not a practical thing when you think about it. How are you going to fund and support animals? You have to integrate, ultimately, the well-being of the animal with the well-being of the person. The tension between the animal welfare and the people welfare, that's a barrier. …small examples of where the needs or the animal and the needs of the people diverge, and you have to decide how you're going to handle that. … [You need to]be prepared for that case, or several cases, that break your heart. (LaFarge, 2021)

Laurel Lagoni, M.S., is a co-founder, with Carolyn Butler and Suzanne Hetts, and director of the pet loss support program, Changes: Support for People and Pets at Colorado State University (CSU). Established in 1984, Changes would grow into what is now the Argus Institute at the James L. Voss Veterinary Teaching Hospital.

After what she describes as a "very sterile and medical" euthanasia experience with her golden retriever along with the lack of body care for pets at the time, Lagoni found herself wondering if she could put her masters in family therapy with an emphasis in grief counseling to use at the CSU College of Veterinary Medicine.

Dr. Stephen Withrow, who would go on to become the Founding Director of the Flint Animal Cancer Center, had come to CSU in 1978 with the intention of building a clinical oncology service, which was new in the field of veterinary medicine.

> About a month later, Steve Withrow called Dr. Cook [her advisor] and said, 'you know, I'm a veterinary oncologist. I'm just starting out in my career building a program here. We have people bringing their animals here from all over the country for cancer treatment and they're crying and they're upset. I don't know what to do. (Lagoni, 2021)

Lagoni and two other volunteers started visiting the waiting room at the Veterinary Teaching Hospital two mornings a week. Occasionally, Dr. Withrow would refer a client if something came up or ask Lagoni to follow up with a client on the phone.

> …it was very informal. We didn't know what we were doing. We didn't know if anyone would be interested…it was really just kind of 'okay, let's just stick our toe in.' [Withrow] told us about Susan Cohen at AMC in New York who definitely had a program going, and Jamie Quackenbush at Penn, who was a Post Doc [postdoctoral fellow], I think. At that point he was doing research in the field and I think had a small clinical program going on. So, we called and talked with them and got some ideas on maybe how to set up a program. And, you know…from that sort of very bumbling, amateurish beginning…we just little by little, started to establish ourselves. (Lagoni, 2021)

Eventually Lagoni resigned her faculty position in the Human Development and Family Studies Department to begin working part-time at the vet school. "From there, it started to take off because I could be there on a more permanent basis and people knew where to find me, and started calling me into cases….Eventually, we built our own office right in the middle of the waiting room. We became a part of the fabric of every day clinical visits, so we were called into cases all the time, and we were just part of the interdisciplinary team." (Lagoni, 2021)

Lagoni also put her degree in journalism to use. "I was eager to document everything, so I wrote everything down, and we published a lot…because we did that, we got very well established and very well known. It just unfolded, really kind of step-by-step, and of course, other programs began to arise around the country. A lot of the pet loss hotlines came about at the at time at different universities." (Lagoni, 2021)

Not only did Lagoni face challenges when it came to funding, but also when it came to early attitudes about addressing pet loss and grief.

> …there was sort of the 'old guard' of veterinary medicine when we began who thought even talking about [pet loss] was not only silly, but wrong…that it would cause more upset for the clients, for their staff, that it would take more of their time if they started to address these topics.
>
> One of the first things we were asked to do is, we were invited to be keynote speakers at one of the regional conferences, for, I believe it was AAHA…we didn't know until we got there, but the conference was boycotted that year because we were going to be giving a talk on [pet loss support]…We had a much smaller audience than they were used to having at that conference. To their credit, they kept us on the program…. We got a letter after our first article was published… we honestly got hate mail, and one of them…started his letter by saying "Dear High Priestesses of Grief". He said we are bringing a death culture into the field and that…it doesn't belong there and should never be talked about and on and on. I still have the letter. (Lagoni, 2021)

After 20 years at CSU, in 2004, Lagoni left her position as the Director of Argus. "[By] the time those 20 years kind of rolled around, I just was exhausted. I had just gotten to the point where I just couldn't do it anymore.... Quite honestly, I came home and, as I remember it, I sat on my couch for about 2 months and stared out the window, you know, and just watched the birds kind of fly by the window because I was just exhausted...I think that self-care is so vitally important.... It was a different time, and it just wasn't...as acknowledged and validated and talked about [as it is now]." (Lagoni, 2021)

She went on to co-found World by the Tail, Inc., which distributes Veterinary Wisdom© brand products to animal care professionals and animal owners, including ClayPaws©, the original paw print kit, from which she retired in 2020.

> We started talking about a phrase that we coined, which was called 'bond centered care' and developing a 'bond centered practice', what we were really trying to help people understand is that dealing with the emotions and dealing with the clients and their needs is every bit as vital to the success of their practice as dealing with the medicine.... I think it's so well grounded now, it's such a part of veterinary medicine that people think it's always been this way, and it's really just the last three, four decades...You know, it wasn't always this way at all!...anybody coming into the field needs to...make sure [they] keep speaking up about that, because it's easy to forget, and easy to...take for granted. (Lagoni, 2021)

Gail Bishop was the clinical coordinator for the Argus Institute and co-founder of Colorado State University's (CSU) Pet Hospice Program. While she retired in December of 2020, she is still active in development for the Argus Institute.

After working for 15 years doing grief work in a variety of settings including hospice, a funeral home, and a suicide resource center, Bishop felt the need to take a sabbatical after the death of her father. When she felt ready to return to work, she wanted to use her skills, but in a different way.

> ...it really was not just my interest and passion for helping individuals who are grieving. It was also my skill level of program development and fundraising, and my desire to work students, teaching, and work around animals. So, it's kind of like I put all the pieces of...what would feed my soul.... I reached out to Laurel [Lagoni] to say 'hey...do you need anybody?" And so next thing you know, I got hired on a part time basis to try me out, and 19 years later I retired! (Bishop, 2021)

Early on in her position, Bishop found that while accepted, Argus was often pigeonholed as only being needed if a patient was dying. She spent time educating the veterinary teams about what other resources and support Argus could offer not only to clients but to them; "and then, once that happened, it was just a well-oiled machine!"(Bishop, 2021)

Bishop encourages those who are interested in working in a veterinary hospital to be sure they know what they are getting into.

> Can I handle this emotionally and honestly, physically, too? ...We've had...two counselors and an intern, [who] ended up leaving us fairly quickly, even though we did two days of a working interview so they could get an idea of how intense it can be, that left us because they had difficulty with the smells of death, the sights of blood, the intensity, and the lack of structure...see what [you're] actually getting into. (Bishop, 2021)

While she acknowledges that this pet loss is not the field for everyone, Bishop loved her work.

> …I know not everybody has this luxury, but what I loved about my work and my career at CSU is that I got to juggle a lot of balls. You know, you work on the clinic floor; you get to facilitate rounds; you get to teach students. I started the first university based veterinary hospice program, so I started a program that never existed! (Bishop, 2021)

Planning for CSU's Pet Hospice Program began in 2002, when veterinarians Charles Johnson and Jack Lebel formed a task force of interested parties, including Bishop. After the first year of planning, the task force was reduced to Bishop and Julia Brannan, with Johnson and Lebel retained as consultants. The program launched with 18 veterinary student volunteers in 2004. CSU' Pet Hospice Program was the first of its kind to be established in a veterinary teaching hospital (Gore et al., 2019).

Sandra Brackenridge, LCSW, BCD, has been a clinical social worker since 1983. She was the Coordinator of Counseling Services at Louisiana State University (LSU) School of Veterinary Medicine from 1990 to 1994, which was one of the first counseling programs in a school of veterinary medicine. She left LSU to teach social work at Idaho State University from 1994 to 2008, when she took a position as an Associate Professor of Social Work at Texas Woman's University. She retired from teaching in 2017. Brackenridge has published two books—one about pet loss and one about veterinary team stress management—as well as numerous other articles and chapters. She was awarded the Lifetime Achievement Award from the Texas state chapter of the National Association of Social Workers in 2018.

Brackenridge's journey started while she was getting her master's in social work. She wanted to do a study for her thesis in which she would interview members of the community with or without her dog and compare the amount of disclosure. She found a professor willing to let her do the project and set out to find an agency to do it in.

"…Nobody would let me in! In 1980, nobody would allow animals in a school, or a hospital, or a nursing home, or anything! People called me crazy." Eventually she was able to conduct the study in a Catholic Girl's Home where the children were wards of the state. "If I had had a bigger sample, [the results] would have been significant."

It would not be until almost a decade later that Brackenridge's focus would return to human-animal interactions. She attended a conference hosted by The Delta Society, the North American Riding for the Handicapped Association, and Canine Companions, which inspired her to start using her dog in her private practice, as well as for therapy visits.

Shortly after moving to New Orleans, her dogs were tragically killed on the highway. The loss inspired her to write a children's book, *Because of Flowers and Dancers* (Brackenridge, 1994), to help caregivers explain humane euthanasia and the emotions of grief to children. It also made her realize the lack of support for people experiencing pet loss.

"…I started reaching out to vets in the New Orleans area, and they just ate it up!" (Brackenridge, 2021) She would go into veterinary clinics and talk to the staff, and she started a pet loss support group.

This work inspired her to contact Dr. William Jenkins, the Dean of the LSU School of Veterinary Medicine, to explore other possibilities.

> I got his secretary, and [she] said, 'well, actually we're hiring a counselor, but I think the applications have closed.' She put me on hold and went to check, and said 'if you get your resume' here by tomorrow morning, then we'll consider it.'…. There was no internet; it was early 1990…. LSU was actually 73 miles exactly from my house. So, I took my resume in the next day.
>
> …I ended up getting hired by Dr. Jenkins. We had a joke, because when I interviewed with him, his bathtub was overflowing and his son was locked out of his house, and I had just delivered puppies the night before and I had puppy poop on my clothes, and so, you know, we hit it off! (Brackenridge, 2021)

The Dean's original vision was to have a counseling service for everyone in the building, which encompassed around 800 staff, faculty, and students. He also wanted a pet loss service for the clinic and for alumni. Brackenridge envisioned having a pet therapy program. However, her position was originally only 20 hours a week, so they started off with seeing students and crisis counseling for other people. She left LSU to go to Idaho State University in 1994, and the program was taken over by her former intern, Stephanie Johnson, who is also featured in this section.

While Dr. Jenkins may have been all in, that was not the case for every veterinarian Brackenridge encountered.

> I'll never forget at LSU when I gave my first presentation…. I don't remember what it was [for], but there was this guy in the audience, a crotchety, old vet. And I was talking about pet loss and grief due to pet loss and he stood up and said 'why can't we just tell them to get a grip?'
>
> Getting buy-in was the most difficult [part] and it's not as hard today. Part of it is because of everything I've done and my reputation,,…but people are used to social workers now…. they're in the schools, they're in human hospitals, they're in nursing homes, they're in hospice… also because a majority of veterinary schools have some sort of mental health service, I think among veterinarians, it's not as hard to get buy-in anymore. (Brackenridge, 2021)

While there have been times she has been physically exhausted because of the amount of work she had, Brackenridge says she's never experienced burnout.

> I found it very rewarding. I've heard other people say 'I couldn't do pet loss counseling all the time' but I find it to be an honor to there in people's personal moments like that…. One of the biggest reasons I kept going at LSU was back when was because these veterinary professionals are so important in people's lives, and nobody cares for them, or back then certainly, nobody was caring for them. They still are…one of my favorite populations of people. (Brackenridge, 2021)

Today, Brackenridge mains a small private practice and provides clinical supervision for social work licensure. She also provides veterinary hospitals and practices with veterinary social work consultation services that include trainings and debriefings, as well as veterinary social work program development. Her consultation practice grew out of interest from students who wanted to complete the UT Veterinary Social Work program and needed placements for their field hours. After this happened a few times, she set up a website, and she started to get inquiries from all over the country.

> It's been a long road…. But I think I'm just really happy that veterinary social work is taking off; it's a real thing…. The whole veterinary field is learning about it…and I'm just really happy with where it is. (Brackenridge, 2021)

Stephanie Johnson, LCSW, is an assistant professor in Veterinary Clinical Sciences at the Louisiana State University (LSU) School of Veterinary Medicine. She began her journey in veterinary social work in 1990 while getting her Master of Social Work.

> …long story short, there were two [social work students] left trying to find internships because our first placements didn't work out, and it was either the LSU Vet School or the rape crisis center…. Both of us were thinking the opposite. She was thinking 'Oh, gosh, nobody's [going to] want to go to the vet school. She's going to want to do rape crisis, too' and I was thinking 'How cool is that! She's going to want to be with the animals as well, so I'm going to have to go to rape crisis.' So, it worked out absolutely perfectly! (Johnson, 2021)

As her first year's internship was coming to a close and it was time to find a new placement, Johnson found that she didn't want to leave, nor did her supervisor, Sandra Brackenridge, want her to leave.

> … I talked to our…field supervisor. Her name was Dr. Betty Stewart; she has since passed away…. She was a huge human-animal bond proponent at the time, and she said 'if you can create a different experience, then you can stay.' So, I started our pet therapy program, or that's what I told her I was going to do and spelled it all out…she rubber stamped me and let me stay for a second year. (Johnson, 2021)

After her second-year internship was complete, Johnson continued to work at LSU part-time from 1992 to 1994 and took over full time after Brackenridge left in 1994. "I've never left, and they haven't asked me to, so I'm assuming it's still a good fit!" (Johnson, 2021)

Johnson's role has evolved over time as circumstances and the needs at the LSU School of Veterinary Medicine have changed. Today, her focus is working with the veterinary students. She provides crisis-oriented support and coaching as well as some ongoing counseling in some cases. She teaches throughout the vet school curriculum on topics such as communication skills, the human-animal bond, animal-related bereavement, ethics, and problem-based learning. She also provides limited grief counseling for clients of the vet school and manages the pet therapy program with the assistance of a volunteer coordinator.

While her advice to people going into veterinary social work is not to try to do it all, doing it all seems to have worked out well for Johnson. "I haven't experienced [burnout]…and I think some of it is—as much as I would tell anyone not to do everything… not to do teaching, not to do counseling, not to do grief counseling all together--I do think [the variety] was helpful for me…. No day was ever the same, and I got a break from doing one thing or the other. And then, once teaching came in, I think that…added another facet to it which made it not the same old, same old sort of thing." (Johnson, 2021)

For Johnson, the most rewarding experiences have also been the most challenging. When working with pet loss clients, "being there and holding that story in your hands.... I'm listening to those stories, hearing those stories, knowing the impact that that animal has had, knowing that impact that that grief, that loss has had is hard to sit with as well, even though sitting with it is also very rewarding." (Johnson, 2021)

While having the support of the veterinarians and staff at LSU, the inherently different role a social worker plays and not having someone with whom to share and process on a day-to-day basis can be challenging at times, as is balancing the dual roles she has as she puts on her different hats at the vet school. Johnson says she found support in the early years from people doing similar work in the field such as her supervisor, Sandra Brackenridge, even after she left, as well as Elizabeth Strand, Jennifer Brandt, and Kathleen Ruby, and today "...there's a whole group now, which I never thought we would have had before!" (Johnson, 2021)

Maureen MacNamara, MSW, PhD, is best known for creating the Pet Partners© program, the first comprehensive, standardized training in animal-assisted activities and therapy for volunteers and healthcare professionals.

Growing up in a family of veterinarians, animals and animal behavior have always been a love of MacNamara's.

> I went to an introductory meeting of Delta Society, which at the time was called Delta Group, and it was one of two meetings. They did one in Irvine, California, and one in the University of Minnesota, and so I went out to the Irvine, California one.... I talked to Leo Bustad...and he said 'you have a lot of skill in animal behavior and understanding animals...but you need to learn about human behavior.... So, I headed off to social work to do that. (MacNamara, 2021)

She also met Susan Cohen at that meeting and learned about her work at the Animal Medical Center in New York City. Since she was in New York for graduate school, MacNamara opted to go to AMC to work with Cohen during her second-year internship.

> It was very interesting because [Cohen] was at Animal Medical Center in essentially a clinical social work, or veterinary social work position, and I was macro practice concentration. So, what I did...instead, I worked with one of the specialties... I was a part of the cardiology team, much to their dismay at the time! Because, you know, why would you have social worker? And they really didn't know what I was going to do and didn't know why I was there. (MacNamara, 2021)

However, MacNamara found that due to her life experience, she was comfortable with veterinary medicine and was able to "speak veterinarian." This enabled her to help the cardiology team learn to better communicate with clients.

Another task during MacNamara's internship was to provide an in-house training about suicide and suicide prevention in response to two suicides by veterinary technicians, one of whom was also a veterinary hospital client who killed herself after having her pet euthanized.

> ...the veterinarians and line staff were pretty freaked out by this. So, I gave this presentation on suicide and suicide prevention, and I'll never forget... The director, after I finished, said 'well, that's not going to happen here!' And a couple of veterinarians said 'well, it already has!'. Apparently, it had never bubbled up to the director that there were these two suicides. About 3 weeks later, one of the veterinarians took home euthanasia solution in a drip and was found after she had passed. So that then increased my credibility, unfortunately.

> And the different veterinarians then would come to my office, and it was so interesting to watch. They would stand with their toes kind of on the threshold of the doorway, and they would keep looking up and down the hall as they talked to me about stuff. I would say 'well, you could come in'. [They would say] 'no', because they knew once they came in, it was a problem, and everyone would know they had a problem, but as long as they stood in the doorway, they perceived that as being interpreted as 'just chatting'. (MacNamara, 2021)

MacNamara remembers crafting the Pet Partners© program (Pet Partners, 2021) as one of her most enjoyable experiences:

> It's so delightful to see people go, 'Oh! We could do that!' Like, 'yeah, we could!'. Crafting the Pet Partners program for Delta was just a hoot because my consulting team was about 200 people, 250 people nationwide. It was just amazing. And what was really fascinating was nobody knew anything; none of us knew anything, because it was so new! We kind of wrote it as we went along…then a year later we'd go 'wow, that didn't really work' and we'd go erase it and start over…. A failure was not seen as a bad thing. Failure was 'note to self: don't do that again!'… To now, all these years later to go, 'we did it.' Because the goal was to help people understand the potential health capacity of animals, and we're there now. (MacNamara, 2021)

She encourages people who want to be in veterinary social work to "be a good social worker first…understand what social work does before you start including an animal in social work." For those who want to engage in animal-assisted interactions, she says "You need to have an understanding of animals other than your pets…. I have made a practice of working with 'animal colleagues'…we had… a lot of different animals on these farms, and different dogs and so they were my colleagues, not my pets. And in that way I can look at them with a critical eye, and I can say 'you're doing a great job' or 'you're not doing your job so well' then…we could strategize about 'does this animal need to be retired?'" (MacNamara, 2021)

Today, MacNamara is an Associate Professor at Appalachian State University in North Carolina focusing on macro-practice.

Michele Gaspar, DVM, DABVP (Feline), MA, LCPC, is a member of Vets4Vets where she works one on one with veterinarians on personal and professional challenges.

> I am somewhat unique in that I am a veterinarian and I am a mental health professional. So, I'm a 1994 graduate of the University of Wisconsin School of Veterinary Medicine…in our training in a very progressive school, I really don't think that much was given to considering the stresses and the self-care and the work that needs to be done in order for us to be healers. (Gaspar, 2021)

In the early 2000s, Gaspar joined the Veterinary Information Network and found herself faced with veterinary professionals experiencing mental health crises.

> [I] would read posts from colleagues and would also talk to some colleagues on the phone, and it was very clear that there was significant anxiety, significant depression, lots of burnout, even suicidality. And I thought that my interest in psychology and my career path in veterinary medicine could be melded into something that would be useful for my colleagues. (Gaspar, 2021)

Gaspar returned to school in 2009 at Loyola University in Chicago, IL, and graduated in 2012 with a degree in pastoral counseling.

I think there are few professions that can really match [veterinarians'] ability to heal not only the patient in front of us, but the individuals who come into our consultation rooms. And it takes quite of bit of good boundary building. It takes a very large dollop of understanding who we are in order to make that happen. (Gaspar, 2021)

For the past 10 years, Gaspar has facilitated a yearly mindfulness meditation retreat for veterinary professionals; however, she wants to be sure to avoid, as one of her colleagues put it, being "awash in meditation, yoga, and bagels" as the only method of addressing burnout and self-care. "I think veterinarians and health providers in general take much of the burden on themselves, but I think the fact of the matter is that burnout is specifically a institutional problem… [meditation, yoga, and bagels are] a very classic way that most institutions try to make people feel affirmed…that's not what our veterinarians and our staffers need." (Gaspar, 2021)

Today, she is a psychotherapist with a private practice in Chicago. She continues to be involved with the Veterinary Information Network as a consultant in the feline internal medicine folder and a member of Vets4Vets, where she offers one-on-one consultations for veterinary professionals.

Jeannine Moga, LCSW, has developed and led two veterinary social work programs: one at the University of Minnesota's Veterinary Medical Center and the other at Family & Community Services at the North Caroline State University's Veterinary Hospital.

As a second year master of social work student in 2003 at the University of Minnesota, Moga was looking for a field placement that would allow her to specialize in human-animal relationships with the goal of becoming a canine and equine assisted therapist. One of the social work faculty members had done some volunteer work at the College of Veterinary Medicine and suggested that the Moga talk to the hospital administrator.

The hospital administrator was an RN who had spent a lot of time managing in human hospitals and said, 'I know what social workers do. I can find a place for you for your field.' And so they gave me a cell phone and locking file cabinet, and put me on the floor and I figured it out! (Moga, 2021)

After graduation, she was hired on a 1-year limited pilot contract to see if she could develop programming for the veterinary teaching hospital. She stayed at the University of Minnesota for 8 years as their program director during which time she provided case management, crisis intervention, and short-term grief counseling; facilitated a pet loss support group; provided community and professional education on topics related to human-animal relationships; and was a field instructor for social work students. She went on to do similar work at North Carolina State University Veterinary hospital for another 6 years.

For Moga, the most meaningful experiences have not always been pleasant or easy. "[The most meaningful experiences] come out of a lot of challenge and a lot of self-evaluation, critical thinking, and trying to solve problems in unique ways. And then getting to a point where you maybe come up with an idea that resonates for people in a way that nothing else has…." (Moga, 2021)

A lack of understanding about what social workers do and their skill set in the veterinary community presented Moga with challenges in her work:

> I think the big challenge, and also the opportunity, is that we have to go where the resistance is, and there's lots of resistance. In my first few years within the veterinary hospital, I had a mental health colleague who had done some work in the veterinary space a long time prior and we were having a conversation about the challenges of the work. She started to laugh and said, 'it's not compassion fatigue; it's Sisyphus fatigue. It's trying to roll the boulder up the hill every day, and being the one, and oftentimes THE one person to do it, because you might be the only social worker in the college or building or the practice. And then, at the end of the day, you've worked so hard, and you watch the boulder roll back down. And you're just doing it, day after day after day. And that can be really exhausting, but you know, this is where the opportunities are if we can learn to engage that resistance and really lean into being change agents. (Moga, 2021)

Moga encourages new social workers to develop their general practice toolkit and to expose themselves to as much of the field of social work as they can before trying to specialize. She also encourages social workers in veterinary settings to model learning into challenging feelings.

> I think one of our most important tasks in this entire professional work is encouraging people who work with animals as their calling to lean into their own humanity. …What we can do to model and to encourage people to lean into those human responses can actually enhance the work and actually can lead to resilience. And so I would love to see us really try to do more teaching in that area of leaning into what your human response to pain is and that is not going to break you down, but that actually strengthens your skills and it strengthens your connection to your work and your sense of meaning in your work, and your ability to connect to other people in pain. (Moga, 2021)

Moga left the veterinary hospital setting in 2018 and recently accepted a position with Banfield Pet Hospital where she will continue to focus on mental health and well-being in the veterinary setting.

Sandra B. Barker, PhD, is a Professor Emeritus in the Department of Psychiatry at Virginia Commonwealth University (VCU). During her career, she was the Bill Balaban Chair in Human-Animal Interaction on the Medical Campus of VCU, the Associate Director of Inpatient Psychiatry Programs, an Affiliate Scientist with the VCU School of Nursing Center for Excellence in Biobehavioral Approaches to Symptom Management, and the founding director for the Center for Human-Animal Interaction.

Barker's journey into the field began in the 1980s while she was working as a counseling program director and faculty member at a university in West Virginia.

> My vet's office happened to be right down the street [from where she worked], and I was in his office one day waiting to be seen… This young man came out that was so distraught. Soon after the veterinarian came out and said the gentleman had just signed a permit to euthanize his pet. He said [to me], 'Can't you help with this?!' And this light bulb went off in my head. (Barker, 2021)

After getting the appropriate approvals, pet loss counseling was then added to the list of services provided. The ensuing publicity attracted the attention of the Virginia Veterinary Medical Association's and the Virginia-Maryland College of Veterinary

Medicine at Virginia Tech. She collaborated with them to do some local presentations and seminars.

About a year after joining the Department of Psychiatry at Virginia Commonwealth University (VCU), she brought up the idea of adding pet loss counseling to their services. She then worked with local veterinarians to set up a community pet loss support group.

As many others have expressed, securing resources was a barrier Barker had to face. "When our Center for Human-Animal Interaction was established in the School of Medicine in 2001, it was established with no funding, no time allotted, no resources, no space, and so it was really starting from scratch... Even today, fundraising to support the Center, to support efforts that...aren't in the mainstream is always a huge challenge."

In contrast, that same year, Barker received a prestigious invitation.

> As I think back, one experience that stands out that was just so amazing for me was being invited to present some of my human-animal interaction research to the U.S. Surgeon General David Satcher up in his office in Washington, D.C. It was just a remarkable time! It was 2001, so the field was still in its infancy and to be among a handful to be recognized in that way was just humbling, and also such a boost to think that this gave such credibility to the field....(Barker, 2021)

And so, Barker advises, "Be patient if you're starting a new program and you're in an area that it's not already well-known and accepted. Start small and include all the major stakeholders, the people that can help get you the approvals and support you need. And as you slowly grow (and I emphasize 'slowly'), don't ever forget your core."

As of this writing, Barker is still in clinical practice part-time as a trauma therapist and providing EAP counseling. She is also an adjunct professor of small animal sciences at Virginia Tech where she teaches about grief counseling and the human-animal bond. Barker was also an early member of The Delta Society (now Pet Partners). She joined in 1985 and served on many of their boards including the Human-Animal Bond Advisory Board, of which she is still a member.

> I'm still so passionate and excited about being involved in this field! But I think that's partly because of the priority I've always placed on balance....as hard as you work, make sure you play as hard, and take care of yourself. (Barker, 2021)

Jennifer Brandt, MSW, PhD, was hired in 2017 by the American Veterinary Medical Association (AVMA) in the newly created position of Director of Member Wellness and Diversity Initiatives to continue her work to improve mental health and well-being among veterinary professionals. She is responsible for "identifying, developing, implementing and coordinating activities and programs that enhance the wellbeing of its members, and advancing the association's commitment to diversity and inclusion in all aspects of the profession" (American Veterinary Medical Association, 2019). Since 2003, Brandt has served as a master trainer and facilitator for the Institute for Healthcare Communication and has presented national and internationally at veterinary schools and conferences (American Veterinary Medical Association, 2017). Before entering her role at the AVMA, Brandt served in multiple roles at The Ohio State University College of Veterinary Medicine. She was the Director of Individual and Organizational Development, Director of Health and Wellness, Director of Student Services, and the founding coordinator of the Honoring the Bond Program, which is a support service for animal owners (American Veterinary Medical Association, 2019).

Veterinary Social Work Today

The field of veterinary social work continues to grow, not only in terms of the number of practitioners but also in terms of the breadth and depth as health-related professions move toward a One Health model of understanding and practicing in the world, and the significance of the role of non-human animals play in the experience of being human is acknowledged.

As a collaboration between the UT College of Veterinary Medicine (UTCVM) and the UT College of Social Work (UTCSW), the University of Tennessee, Knoxville's Veterinary Social Work program continues to thrive and is a linchpin in the field. UT's Veterinary Social Work program serves the clients, faculty, and staff of the UTCVM as well as the wider community by providing counseling and coaching services, a dedicated helpline, and routine support groups for animal-related issues, including pet loss while also serving as an educational hub for the profession.

Veterinary Social Work Education

The demand for education in veterinary social work grew as the field became more well-known. UT Veterinary Social Work's first step in this direction was in 2008 with the development of two, 2-hour elective graduate seminar courses within the College of Social Work. Guided by human-animal bond course outlines from Dr. Risley-Curtiss, a professor at Arizona State University, and Dr. Cheryl Resnick-Cortes, a professor at Georgian Court University (Lakewood), these chapter co-authors as well as Danielle Groeling, who was the Assistant Director of VSW at the time, and Janelle Nimer put together syllabi for the two courses. The first was, as one might expect, was entitled "Introductory Seminar to Veterinary Social Work" and familiarized students with the four areas of veterinary social work. Those wishing to delve deeper could continue their studies in the "Advanced Seminar in Veterinary Social Work," in which students would have experiential exercises such as interviewing animal-related professionals, attending order-of-protection court hearings, and volunteering in an animal-related setting. These two classes would serve as the foundation for the Veterinary Social Work Certificate Program.

As of this writing, UT Veterinary Social Work offers three certificate programs for those interested in the field: the concurrent Veterinary Social Work Certificate

Program, the post-graduate Veterinary Social Work Certificate Program, and the Veterinary Human Support Certificate Program.

The Veterinary Social Work Certificate Program (VSWCP) was launched in 2013. The concurrent VSWCP is for students currently working on their master's degree in social work. To earn the certificate during their course of study, students use their elective courses to follow a track of courses designed to educate them about the field of veterinary social work and develop necessary skills for practice, which are then applied in their field practicum. For some students, their field placement may be an explicitly animal-related host setting such as a veterinary clinic or animal shelter. For others, the field placement may be what is thought of as a traditional social work setting such as a school, hospital, or other human service agency. In those cases, the student must incorporate some element of veterinary social work into their placement to earn the certificate.

The post-graduate VSWCP is a continuing education certificate that provides education for licensed mental health professionals. Like the concurrent VSWCP, it is designed to provide the student with education about the four areas of veterinary social work practice and the skills to put that education into use. Students in the post-graduate certificate complete self-paced online modules, participate in live workshops, and complete a 250-hour service-learning Keystone Project. Similar to the concurrent student's field practicum, the Keystone Project requires the student to create a service-learning project highlighting at least one of the four areas of veterinary social work and, with the help of a consulting veterinarian, develop and implement measurable objectives. The results of the Keystone Project are then presented at the International Veterinary Social Work Summit, a biennial inter-professional conference.

The Veterinary Human Support Certificate Program (VHSCP) was launched at UT in 2018. This certificate is designed for animal-related professionals who wish to help others as they navigate the challenges that arise around animals, but do not wish to become mental health professionals. Instead, this certificate is geared toward providing animal-related professionals with knowledge and skills that can be used daily to promote well-being for both clients and staff in animal-related settings. As in the post-graduate VSWCP, these students complete self-paced online modules, live workshops, and a service-learning Keystone Project that is presented at the International Veterinary Social Work Summit. However, instead of a consulting veterinarian on their project like the VSWCP students, VHSCP students must have the input of a consulting licensed mental health professional.

As of this writing, there are 48 graduates of the VSWCP and 99 students currently enrolled and 13 graduates of the VHSCP and 33 students currently enrolled. Applications are evaluated on a rolling basis.

International Association of Veterinary Social Work

In 2017, Colleen Crockford, MSW, LICSW, developed a proposal to create an association for "individuals and organizations practicing social work in the areas of human-animal bond and veterinary communities." Crockford presented this proposal to Elizabeth Strand, who then held a working group meeting at the 2018 International Veterinary Social Work Summit for those interested in potentially forming an association. That working group helped identify what the goals of a veterinary social work association should be, as well as potential members of a formation committee to begin the work of developing the mission, vision, and structure of the potential organization.

Members of the formation committee included, in alphabetical order by last name, Sandra Brackenridge, Katherine Goldberg, Maya Gupta, Pamela Linden, Sarina Manifold, Joelle Nielson, Bethanie Poe, Rebecca Poplawski, and Aviva Vincent.

The International Association of Veterinary Social Work (IAVSW) made its debut at the sixth International Veterinary Social Work Summit in 2020. The IAVSW is an interdisciplinary membership organization that supports and promotes professionals who tend to the human needs that arise in the relationship between humans and animals by creating and maintaining professional standards, encouraging research, and advocating for a better world for all species. Its stated vision is "A world where professionals work together to honor and understand the impact of the human-animal relationship" (IAVSW, 2020).

The inaugural Board of the IAVSW was:

- President: Pamela Linden.
- Vice-President: Aviva Vincent.
- Treasurer: Maureen McNamara.
- Secretary: Angie Arora.
- Board Director of Communications &Social Media: Isabel Ballard.
- Board Director of Ethics & Standards of Practice: Jeannine Moga.
- Board Director of Education: Sana Loue.
- Board Director of Fundraising & Development: Robin Peth-Pierce.
- Board Director of Membership and Member Services: Hanna Mamzer.

Conclusion

Since Jamie Quackenbush and Susan Cohen first began working in veterinary hospitals in the late 1970s and early 1980s, until this field of practice was named "veterinary social work" in 2002, until today, almost 20 years later, veterinary social workers have been making things better for people who care for animals. Pet loss groups are a resource found in many communities. Domestic violence shelters that allow pets are slowly becoming more common. Talking about mental health is expected in veterinary schools around the country. As veterinary social work continues to grow, one can only imagine the strides the field will make in the next 20 years. This chapter ends with this thought from Michele Gaspar:

> There are incredibly creative people doing some really wonderful things in this field. And you know, I'm certainly at the tail-end of my career, not at the beginning, and there's a certain amount of envy that I have for people coming up through the ranks. And it's a well-placed envy because I think the future is bright.

References

American Association of Veterinary Medical Colleges and Veterinary Social Work (2015, Nov 2–3). Veterinary Wellness & Social Work Summit program. University of Tennessee, Knoxville.

American Veterinary Medical Association. (2017, September 13). *Social worker joins AVMA staff.* Retrieved from: https://www.avma.org/javma-news/2017-10-01/social-worker-joins-avma-staff. Accessed 24 Apr 2021.

American Veterinary Medical Association (2019). *Mission possible: Creating a culture of well-being.* Retrieved from: https://axon.avma.org/local/catalog/view/product.php?productid=11. Accessed 24 Apr 2021.

American Veterinary Medical Association (nd): Veterinarian's oath. Retrieved from: https://www.avma.org/resources-tools/avma-policies/veterinarians-oath. Accessed 21 Mar 2021.

Ann Arbor News. (2006, January 5). *James E. "Jamie" Quackenbush.* Retrieved from https://obits.mlive.com/obituaries/annarbor/obituary.aspx?n=james-e-quackenbush-jamie&pid=16223258. Accessed 20 June 2021.

Barker, S. (2021, April 27). Video interview.

Bishop, G. (2021, Feb 22). Video interview.

Bishop, G., Long, C., Carlsten, K., Kennedy, K., & Shaw, J. (2008). The Colorado State University pet hospice program: End-of-life care for pets and their families. *Journal of Veterinary Medical Education, 35*(4), 525–531. https://doi.org/10.3138/jvme.35.4.525

Blackwell, M. (2021, May 12). Video interview.

Brackenridge, S. (1994). *Because of flowers and dancers.* Veterinary Practice Publishing.

Brackenridge, S. (2021, March 5). Video interview.

Butler, C., & Lagoni, L. (1995). Facilitating owner-present euthanasia. In J. D. Bonagura (Ed.), *Kirk's current veterinary therapy XII.* W.B. Saunders.

Cohen, S. P. (1985). The role of social work in a veterinary hospital setting. *The Veterinary Clinics of North America. Small Animal Practice, 15*(2), 355–363. https://doi.org/10.1016/s0195-5616(85)50307-1

Cohen, S. (2021, February 26). Video interview.

Cohen, S. P. (n.d.-a). Susan Cohen DSW, SWAHAB Chair (n.d). http://swahab.org/uploads/6/5/1/0/65109377/susancohenprofile.pdf. Accessed 10 June 2021.

Cohen, S. P. (n.d.-b). *About Dr. Susan. Pet decisions.* https://www.petdecisions.com/about/. Accessed 20 June 2021.

Crockford, C. (2017). *Creating an association for individuals and organizations practicing social work in the areas of human-animal bond & veterinary communities: Association formation proposal.* Submitted to University of Tennessee Veterinary Social Work.

Features Editor. (2009, November 12). Pet loss support hotline closes after 20 years of service. *The California Aggie.* Retrieved from: https://theaggie.org/2009/11/12/pet-loss-support-hotline-closes-after-20-years-of-service/. Accessed 27 Apr 2021.

Figley, C. (2006). *Compassion fatigue in the animal-care community.* Humane Society Press.

Gaspar, M (2021, April 21). Video interview.

Gore, M., Lana, S. E., & Bishop, G. A. (2019). Colorado State University, pet hospice program. *Veterinary Clinics of North America Small Animal Practice, 49*(3), 339–349. https://doi.org/10.1016/j.cvsm.2019.01.002. Epub 2019 Mar 4. PMID: 30846381.

Hines, L. M. (2003). Historical perspectives on the human-animal bond. *American Behavioral Scientist, 47*(1), 7–15. https://doi.org/10.1177/0002764203255206

International Association of Veterinary Social Work. (2020). *About Veterinary Social Work.* Retrieved from: https://veterinarysocialwork.org/about-iavsw

Johnson, S. (2021, April 27). Video interview.

Joinson, C. (1992). Coping with compassion fatigue. *Nursing (Jenkintown, Pa.), 22*(4), 116–121. https://doi.org/10.1097/00152193-199204000-00035

Kruger, K. A., & Serpell, J. A. (2006). Animal-assisted interventions in mental health: Definitions and theoretical foundations. In A. H. Fine (Ed.), *Handbook on animal assisted therapy: Theoretical foundations and guidelines for practice* (2nd ed., pp. 21–28). Elsevier.

LaFarge, S. (2021, February 24). Video interview.

Lagoni, L. (2021, February 25). Video interview.

Lagoni, L. & Hetts, S. (1989) Pet loss counseling in veterinary medicine. *Trends,* October/November, 33–36.

Lagoni, L., Arguello, S., Withrow, S., & Pike, C. (1988). Patient death and dying. In D. McCurnin (Ed.), *Veterinary practice management* (pp. 308–319). J.B. Lippincott Company.

Levinson, B. M. (1969). *Pet-oriented child psychotherapy.* Thomas.

Levinson, B. M. (1972). *Pets and human development.* Thomas.

Lloyd, M. F. (2008). *100 years: A centennial history of the school of social policy & practice.* University of Pennsylvania School of Social Policy & Practice. https://repository.upenn.edu/centennial/?utm_source=repository.upenn.edu%2Fcentennial%2F1&utm_medium=PDF&utm_campaign=PDFCoverPages. Accessed 30 Mar 2021.

MacNamara, M. (2021, April 19). Video interview.

Merriam-Webster. (n.d.). Veterinary. In *Merriam-Webster.com dictionary.* Retrieved May 23, 2021, from https://www.merriam-webster.com/dictionary/veterinary

Moga, J. (2021, April 22). Video interview.

Netting, F. E., Wilson, C. C., & New, J. C. (1987). The human-animal bond: Implications for practice. *Social Work, 32*(1), 60–64.

Pet Partners. (2021). *The Pet Partners Story.* https://petpartners.org/about-us/petpartners-story/. Accessed 11 June 2021.

Quackenbush, J., & Glickman, L. (1983). Social work services for bereaved pet owners: A retrospective case study in a veterinary teaching hospital. In A. H. Katcher & A. M. Beck (Eds.), *New perspectives on our lives with companion animals* (pp. 377–389). University of Pennsylvania Press.

Quackenbush, J., & Graveline, D. (1985). *When your pet dies: How to cope with your feelings.* Simon & Schuster.

Rovner, J. (1986, March 10). Coping. *The Washington Post.* Retrieved from: https://www.washingtonpost.com/archive/lifestyle/1986/03/10/coping/bee59a55-312f-4a77-b254-3e8ad686c2c8/

Social Workers Advancing the Human-Animal Bond. (n.d.). Retrieved from: http://swahab.org/httpswwwfacebookcomanimalbond.html

Sowers, K. (2021, May 8). Video interview.

Strand, E. B. (2021, May 6). Video interview.

Strand, E. B., Poe, B., Lyall, S., Allen, E., Nimer, J., Yorke, J., Brown, G., & Nolan-Pratt, T. (2012). Veterinary social work: A specialized social work practice. In C. N. Dulmus & K. M. Sowers (Eds.), *Fields of social work practice: Historical trends, professional issues, and future opportunities* (pp. 245–271). John Wiley & Sons, Inc.

Tapia, F. (1971). Children who are cruel to animals. *Child Psychiatry and Human Development, 2*(2), 70–77.

Tingle, D., Barnard, G. W., Robbins, L., Newman, G., & Hutchinson, D. (1986). Childhood and adolescent characteristics of pedophiles and rapists. *International Journal of Law and Psychiatry, 9,* 103–116.

Wax, D. E., & Haddox, V. G. (1974a). Sexual aberrance in male adolescents manifesting a behavioral triad considered predictive of extreme violence: Some clinical observations. *Journal of Forensic Science, 19*(1), 102–108.

Wax, D. E., & Haddox, V. G. (1974b). Enuresis, fire setting, and animal cruelty: A useful danger signal in predicting vulnerability of adolescent males to assaultive behavior. *Child Psychiatry and Human Development, 4*(3), 151–156.

Part II
The Practice of Veterinary Social Work

Chapter 3
Compassion Fatigue in the Animal Care Community

Debbie L. Stoewen

Introduction

Over the last two decades, compassion fatigue has increasingly come to be recognized as a significant stress-related occupational hazard for those in the animal care community (Figley & Roop, 2006; Scotney et al., 2015; Lloyd & Campion, 2017; Hill et al., 2020; Rohlf, 2018). This includes those who work in veterinary practices, humane societies, animal shelters, animal control services, animal rescues and rehabilitation services, and biomedical research laboratories. Anecdotal and early research evidence suggests that those who work on farms and in zoos could also be susceptible, although less so (Scotney et al., 2015; Hill et al., 2020; Shearer, 2018).

Many people choose to work in animal care because they love and feel a kinship with animals. Those who work in *animal health* examine, diagnose, and provide treatment to animals, preserving quantity and quality of life and the human-animal bond (HAB). Those who work in *animal welfare* rehome or reunite lost and abandoned animals, conduct cruelty investigations, rescue/rehabilitate domestic or native wild animals, engage in feral cat trap-neuter-return, and/or provide health services. And those who work in *biomedical research* care for, and oversee the welfare of, animals in research, significantly contributing to advances in science and medicine to protect human and animal health and the environment. Despite the diversity in roles, all of these animal care providers share the duality of providing care to animals and being exposed to trauma as a part of their work (Rohlf, 2018), and it is this precise combination from which compassion fatigue may arise. First coined by Joinson (1992), compassion fatigue arises from the various stressors

D. L. Stoewen (✉)
University of Guelph, Guelph, ON, Canada
e-mail: stoewend@uoguelph.ca

© The Author(s), under exclusive license to Springer Nature Switzerland AG 2022
S. Loue, P. Linden (eds.), *The Comprehensive Guide to Interdisciplinary Veterinary Social Work*, https://doi.org/10.1007/978-3-031-10330-8_3

experienced by those in the caregiving professions who help, or want to help, others in need (Joinson, 1992).

Helping naturally starts from a place of compassion. Compassion is a term derived from the Latin roots *com*, which means "together with," and *pati*, which means "to bear or suffer" (Singer & Klimecki, 2014; Fernando et al., 2016). Thus, it is understood as "suffering with," and more specifically, "a deep awareness of the suffering of another coupled with the wish to relieve it" (Hoad, 1996; Nunberg & Newman, 2000). Compassion is a core value and ethical imperative within any helping profession (Monk, 2021) and the essential quality in caring for others (Geppert & Pies, 2019).

Caring for others can be tremendously satisfying, offering immense joys and a sense of meaning, purpose, and difference-making in the world (Stoewen, 2019; Radey & Figley, 2007), what is known as compassion satisfaction. This is the sense of joy, pleasure, or fulfillment that can be experienced from helping others which can lead to feeling satisfied, gratified, or invigorated by one's work (Figley & Roop, 2006; Radey & Figley, 2007; Stamm, 2005, 2010). At the same time, caring for others can incur a cost, "the cost of caring," known as compassion fatigue (Figley, 1982). Compassion fatigue is understood as a deep physical, emotional, and spiritual exhaustion that diminishes the ability to empathize or feel compassion for others (Figley, 2002; Showalter, 2010). Defined by necessary variables, it requires a caregiving relationship within which there is an exchange of empathy, emotions, and information, along with the desire on the part of the caregiver to alleviate the pain and suffering of the other (Figley & Roop, 2006). Although compassion satisfaction and compassion fatigue are conceptually distinct – not opposite ends of the same continuum – they are both influenced by emotional engagement with others (Polachek & Wallace, 2018; Stamm, 2002, 2005, 2010). Compassionate work can be both greatly rewarding and costly. Almost everyone who cares for "others in distress" will eventually experience some degree of compassion fatigue (Mathieu, 2011). As Remen (1996) so appositely stated, "The expectation that we can be immersed in suffering… and not be touched by it is as unrealistic as expecting to be able to walk through water without getting wet."

Conceptualizing Compassion Fatigue

Compassion fatigue is not a pathology, but rather a natural consequence of caring (Figley, 1995). It has traditionally been thought of as the manifestation of secondary traumatic stress and burnout (Stamm, 2010), but more recently, with the advent of advanced neuroimaging technologies within social neurosciences research, it has been proposed not as fatigue related to the expression of compassion but as the manifestation of chronic empathic distress (Klimecki & Singer, 2012).

Compassion Fatigue as Secondary Traumatic Stress and Burnout

According to Beth Hudnall Stamm, celebrated researcher in the field of traumatic stress, compassion fatigue is conceptualized as the manifestation of two components: secondary traumatic stress and burnout (Stamm, 2005, 2010). The first component, secondary traumatic stress – also known as compassion stress – is the stress experienced as a helper when exposed to the trauma, pain, and suffering of others (Figley, 1995). It is both natural and unavoidable, derived from a sense of duty together with the desire to alleviate the suffering (Newsome et al., 2019). The second component, burnout, is a psychological syndrome characterized by three features: (1) feelings of energy depletion or exhaustion; (2) feelings of negativism or cynicism related to (or increased mental distance from) one's job; and (3) reduced professional efficacy (WHO, 2019; Maslach et al., 1996). It is the consequence of a chronic imbalance between the demands of the job (too high) and the resources available to carry out the job (too low) (Mastenbroek et al., 2012), causing chronic work-related stress (Freudenberger, 1974). Chronic workplace stress together with compassion stress sets the stage for compassion fatigue. Bearing in mind the additive effect of *all* forms of stress, other stresses, such as those within one's personal life, can contribute to, and increase the risk of, compassion fatigue.

Compassion fatigue can be further understood in relation to Stamm's *Professional Quality of Life Measure* (ProQOL), the most employed measure of the positive and negative aspects of working as a caregiver, helping those who experience trauma, pain, and suffering (Stamm, Proqol.org, 2021; CVMA ProQOL, 2021). Compassion satisfaction is seen as a positive aspect, bolstering quality of life, while compassion fatigue is seen as a negative aspect, undermining quality of life (Stamm, 2010). The relationships between these parts are shown in the model below (Fig. 3.1).

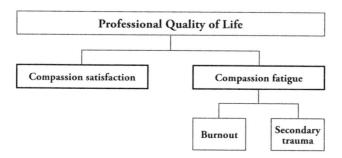

Fig. 3.1 Model of professional quality of life. (Adapted from Stamm (2010) with permission from ProQOL)

Compassion Fatigue as Chronic Empathic Distress

Another way of understanding compassion fatigue has arisen with the evidence drawn from the social neurosciences research of Dr. Tania Singer and colleagues of the Max Planck Institute for Human Cognitive and Brain Sciences (Klimecki & Singer, 2012). Through research employing advanced neuroimaging technologies, Klimecki and Singer (2012) have postulated that compassion fatigue might not really be "compassion" fatigue, but rather "empathic distress" fatigue (Klimecki & Singer, 2012).

Compassion entails three capacities: noticing, feeling, and responding (Kanov et al., 2004). "Feeling" refers to empathy, that innate and learned ability to resonate with the feelings of others, regardless of valence (positive/negative) and awareness that the other is the source of this emotion (de Vignemont & Singer, 2006). The sharing of *positive* emotions is typically enjoyable, and thus easy, but the sharing of *negative* emotions can be difficult, and may not always lead to sympathy, concern, and compassion. In fact, research has shown that exposure to the suffering of others can lead to two different empathic reactions: (1) empathic concern (with sympathy and compassion) and (2) empathic distress (Singer & Klimecki, 2014). Whether a caregiver responds with empathic concern or empathic distress depends on several factors, including the person's disposition, personality, and ability to regulate emotions, and the characteristics of the situation (Klimecki & Singer, 2012). It also depends on the capacity for "self-other" differentiation – a critical factor. This is the ability to distinguish between one's own emotional states and the states shared with others (Lamm et al., 2007; Preckel et al., 2018). If the distinction between the "self" and "other" is somehow blurred, the caregiver will not *feel with* the other – and respond with empathic concern – but instead *take on* the emotional pain of the other as their own, and respond with empathic distress, withdrawing from the situation to protect the self from the pain rather than moving toward the situation and attempting to relieve the pain (Preckel et al., 2018). Over-identification with the suffering of others will induce empathic distress (Klimecki & Singer, 2012) (Fig. 3.2).

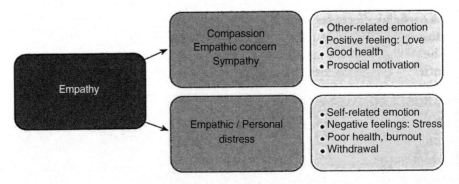

Fig. 3.2 A schematic model depicting two different forms an empathic reaction can take. (Adapted from Klimecki and Singer (2012) Fig. 28.2. With permission from Oxford University Press)

Neuroimaging studies have shown that a "self" orientation with empathic distress and an "other" orientation with empathic concern (compassion) activate different areas of the brain. A "self" orientation (with empathic distress) activates the areas of the brain involved in the processing of threat or pain (Lamm et al., 2007) and over time will cause a depletion of brain dopamine levels (Borsook et al., 2016). This will eventually lead to burnout (McCray et al., 2008). An "other" orientation (empathic concern, i.e., compassion) activates the areas of the brain associated with reward, love, and affiliation (Klimecki et al., 2013). It facilitates the production of opioids, oxytocin, and dopamine (Panksepp, 2011), which generate positive emotions toward suffering and motivate helping behavior. Interestingly, through the generation of positive emotions, compassion may even be viewed as capable of buffering or counteracting negative emotions (Preckel et al., 2018). Overall, Klimecki and Singer (2012) offer that it is not "compassion" that fatigues (indeed, quite the opposite!), but "empathic distress," and propose that compassion fatigue be more aptly called empathic distress fatigue (Klimecki & Singer, 2012). Research in both veterinary medicine (McArthur et al., 2017b) and social work (Thomas, 2013) has found that empathic (personal) distress was positively associated with secondary traumatic stress. With empathic distress *also* associated with burnout – in other words, with *both* of the traditional components of compassion fatigue – it seems opportune to embrace both conceptualizations of compassion fatigue, traditionally, as the manifestation of secondary traumatic stress and burnout (Stamm, 2010) and, more recently, as the manifestation of chronic empathic distress (Klimecki & Singer, 2012). Each conceptualization understands compassion fatigue to be the result of exposure to occupational stress as a caregiver within a caregiving environment.

Causes of Compassion Fatigue

Any aspects of work that can induce compassion stress (secondary traumatic stress) and general stress (particularly chronic, unresolvable stress) can contribute to compassion fatigue, compassion stress being the necessary precursor. The sources of stress vary in relation to the field of care – animal health, animal welfare, and biomedical research – and nature of the work. Within all three fields, workers need to contend with their emotional responses to the suffering of those in their care as well as the usual stresses and dissatisfactions of work (Scotney et al., 2015).

Veterinary Practices

The provision of companion animal veterinary services (caring for dogs, cats, small mammals, birds, and exotics) and certain large animal veterinary services (caring for pleasure horses and hobby farm animals) has shifted from the delivery of care solely to animals (i.e., patients) to attending to the needs of both patients and their owners. The HAB has evolved over recent decades, with animals increasingly being seen not only for their instrumental value but as members of the family (Shaw et al., 2012). With pets of all sorts often viewed as children, veterinarians have taken on the role of pediatrician (Figley & Roop, 2006), providing medical care to the patient and empathetic care to the family (Polachek & Wallace, 2018; Holcombe et al., 2016; Hanrahan et al., 2018). Although this dual caring role, characterized by greater emotional complexity, can increase the likelihood of compassion satisfaction, it can also increase the risk of compassion fatigue (Polachek & Wallace, 2018; Cohen, 2007; Mitchener & Ogilvie, 2002). As Polachek and Wallace (2018) aptly state, "Performing compassionate work can, paradoxically, be both satisfying and stressful such that the same types of interactions may relate to both greater compassion satisfaction and greater compassion fatigue" (pp. 239–240).

Beyond the provision of preventive care, the very nature of practice, caring for sick, injured, and dying animals exposes veterinary caregivers to the suffering of patients and distress of clients, inherently incurring compassion stress (Figley & Roop, 2006). Emergency work can be particularly taxing, with the treatment of life-threatening injuries, adverse reactions, and chronic disease downturns. The multi-faceted care of patients with complex medical conditions, the long-term care of patients with chronic diseases, and terminal or end-of-life care can also be taxing (Polachek & Wallace, 2018; Gardner & Hini, 2006; Figley, 1995; Figley & Roop, 2006; Foster & Maples, 2014). Managing client expectations, dealing with difficult and noncompliant clients, working with clients who are unable or unwilling to pay for appropriate care, managing client disputes with fees and billing, delivering bad news, discussing euthanasia, and consoling traumatized and grieving clients can all negatively affect well-being (Figley & Roop, 2006; Bartram et al., 2009; Gardner & Hini, 2006; Polachek & Wallace, 2018; Platt et al., 2012).

When making patient care decisions, veterinarians will routinely take into account a variety of contextual factors. Such factors include the client's financial status, the client's bond to their pet, their own level of expertise, the availability of specialists, and the workplace environment, including the economics of the practice (Stoewen et al., 2013; Springer et al., 2019; Kippermann et al., 2017; Kondrup et al., 2016; Hartnack et al., 2016; Batchelor & McKeegan, 2012; Coe et al., 2007; Martin & Taunton, 2006). The complexity of medical care decision-making can make patient care challenging – especially morally (Springer et al., 2019). Veterinarians can find themselves torn between patients' interests, clients' interests, and medical feasibility and have to make decisions that collide with their patient advocacy role: to keep the patient's best interests in mind (Springer et al., 2019). This can lead to ethical conflict and moral "di/stress" (Springer et al., 2019; Mullan & Fawcett, 2017). Moral di/stress, as coined by Andrew Jameton (1984), is "the experience of knowing the right thing to do while being in a situation in which it is nearly impossible to do it" (Jameton, 1984, 2017, p. 617). An increasingly recognized cause of compassion fatigue is the moral di/stress that veterinarians *routinely* face in day-to-day practice (Moses et al., 2018; Scotney et al., 2015; Perry et al., 2011; Kahler, 2015).

Euthanasia, which, as a treatment option, can be riddled with moral dilemmas, is a major stressor for veterinary caregivers (Rollin, 2011; Foster & Maples, 2014). Veterinarians can be faced with the extremes of being asked to end pets' lives prematurely when there is no health or behavioral reason for it (i.e., "convenience euthanasia") and prolonging pets' lives beyond what is in their best interest (Rollin, 2011; Chur-Hansen, 2010; Fogle & Abrahamson, 1990; Morris, 2012). Beyond inciting moral di/stress, euthanasia can create a sense of having failed the patient, the client, or both and having betrayed the contract of care (Rohlf & Bennett, 2005). Euthanasia is also a source of grief, which can deeply affect veterinary caregivers (Fogle & Abrahamson, 1990; Dow et al., 2019), especially as there is typically little time to debrief, reflect, or process the grief, having to resume regular duties immediately afterward (Hewson, 2014). Exposure to death has both short- and long-term emotional impacts (Fogle & Abrahamson, 1990). As death is experienced with frequency (e.g., veterinarians face death five times more often than physicians) (Mitchener & Ogilvie, 2002), it is considered a high-risk factor for compassion fatigue (Shearer, 2018).

The risk of compassion fatigue has also been linked to the concern about adequate educational preparedness and the need to keep up with advancements and new technologies (Figley & Roop, 2006; Dicks & Bain, 2016). This is a significant source of stress in veterinarians (Gardner & Hini, 2006), related to the escalating pace of sophistication and specialization in healthcare, increasing job complexity and necessitating changes in professional regulatory standards that too need to be kept up with. Compounding the pressure to keep up, veterinarians commonly practice in relative social and professional isolation (Bartram & Baldwin, 2008), working within self-reliant and self-contained hospitals with little access to supervision and mentorship. This is vastly different from physicians, who are intricately networked with residents, peers, specialists, and other caregivers working within multi-tiered systems of healthcare. Isolation in practice not only is a source of stress but increases the risk of medical errors, which can have considerable emotional impact on caregivers (Mellanby & Herrtage, 2004; West et al., 2006; Shanafelt et al., 2010) as well as harm patients and clients (Wallis et al., 2019). This impact is further exacerbated by the risk of complaints or litigation, which significantly contributes to stress (Bartram et al., 2009).

There are several other sources of work-related stress that can take their toll on veterinary caregivers. These include long work hours, work-home interference, emergency on-call, time demands, understaffing, limited resources, low remuneration, low profit margins, financial pressures, and administrative duties (Holcombe et al., 2016; Volk et al., 2018; Rohlf, 2018; Platt et al., 2012). Difficult relationships with coworkers or supervisors and conflict in the workplace can add to the burden of stress (Holcombe et al., 2016). All these factors contribute to burnout, increasing the risk of compassion fatigue (Dicks & Bain, 2016).

Humane Societies, Animal Shelters, Animal Control Services, and Animal Rescues and Rehabilitation Services

Work in humane societies, animal shelters, and animal control inherently involves working with vulnerable populations, helping those at risk and in need. As such, the work is often emotionally demanding (Figley & Roop, 2006). Workers in these settings are routinely exposed to animals that are no longer – or never were – wanted or that require rehoming due to unforeseen, difficult, or changing life circumstances. They are exposed to animals that suffer from suboptimal care, inattention, behavioral issues, neglect, abuse, and illness (Schneider & Roberts, 2016). In all of this, they need to work with the people whose challenges have led to the need for services, which can pose its own challenges, as some can be deeply grieving, uncooperative, or abusive (Figley & Roop, 2006; Schneider & Roberts, 2016; Dunn et al., 2019). Certainly, shelter workers hold a variety of roles with various responsibilities, implying varying exposures, yet directly and indirectly these types of exposures can induce stress that can culminate in compassion fatigue, especially for those who are drawn to the work with a strong sense of responsibility to animals and dedication to animal welfare.

Shelter workers commonly experience guilt, grief, and frustration with euthanasia (Frommer & Arluke, 1999). Although the statistics in recent years have been improving, approximately one in four dogs and cats that enter shelters in the United States is euthanized (American Society for the Prevention of Cruelty to Animals, 2021; Animal Euthanasia Statistics, 2021). These animals are not necessarily sick, injured, or aggressive (Reeve et al., 2004). In fact, most (close to 90%) are healthy and potentially adoptable (Animal Euthanasia Statistics, 2021). The stress (i.e., moral di/stress) associated with what Arluke (1994) calls the "caring-killing paradox" – simultaneously providing care and protection to animals while also being called to euthanize them – can put shelter workers at risk for compassion fatigue (Arluke, 1994; Andrukonis & Protopopova, 2020). Likewise, the stress felt with the social stigma attached to the killing of companion animals (Reeve et al., 2005) and the stress of euthanasia itself, known as "euthanasia stress," add to this risk (Hill et al., 2020; Schneider & Roberts, 2016; Andrukonis & Protopopova, 2020).

As in the veterinary community, euthanasia stress is a well-recognized form of occupational stress in animal welfare (Frommer & Arluke, 1999; White & Shawhan, 1996; Baran et al., 2009; Scotney et al., 2015; Rohlf & Bennett, 2005). It is conceptualized as the experience of "being aware and psychologically challenged when faced with the task of euthanizing animals" (Newsome et al., 2019, p. 290). The degree to which it affects workers varies in relation to the euthanasia decision, specifically whether it is (1) a shared decision, (2) supported by protocol, and (3) felt to be what ought to be done (Rollin, 2011; Von Dietze & Gardner, 2014). It also varies with the extent of concern over animal death and the availability of training and support (Rohlf & Bennett, 2005; Von Dietze & Gardner, 2014). Thus, the degree to which it is experienced depends on both individual and organizational factors.

Less emotionally demanding, yet also taxing, are the many workplace stressors that humane society, animal shelter, and animal control personnel are exposed to. These include the workload, the physicality of the labor, animal attacks and bites, and working in less-than-optimal environmental conditions, with exposure to noxious odors, loud noises, bright/dim lights, wetness and humidity, pathogenic organisms, hazardous materials, weather, and traffic hazards (Roberts, 2015; Figley & Roop, 2006; Dunn et al., 2019). These stressors are made worse in workplaces with limited resources, lack of training, systemic communication problems, strained work relationships, feelings of isolation, and lack of access to employee assistance programs (EAPs) (Roberts, 2015; Schabram & Maitlis, 2017; Figley & Roop, 2006; Dunn et al., 2019). These conditions, individually and together, are considered to make humane society, animal shelter, and animal control personnel susceptible to compassion fatigue (Figley & Roop, 2006).

Animal rescue workers are also susceptible to compassion fatigue, yet to date, this subspecialty of animal care remains under-researched. A recent study of feral cat rescuers and caregivers identified several sources of stress associated with compassion fatigue (Young & Thompson, 2019). According to this study, these workers, in their efforts, have to deal with a myriad of obstacles in the face of scarce resources and lack of organizational support. Despite this, they tend to be dedicated, rarely taking a day off (and at times working round-the-clock). To make matters worse, their dedication is not always met with understanding from otherwise sympathetic family and friends. They often experience stigmatization, in the form of accusations (e.g., "You obviously care more about animals than people") and negative stereotyping (e.g., the "crazy cat lady"). Altogether, despite the rewards of animal rescue and caregiving, the realities of the work – exposure to injury, suffering, and euthanasia, limited resources, frequent setbacks, and lack of social and organizational support – can take its toll, making these workers vulnerable to compassion fatigue (Young & Thompson, 2019).

Biomedical Research Laboratories

Compassion fatigue in the biomedical research laboratory may be understood as "the natural emotional distress, fatigue, or apathy that develops from caring for, investing in the wellbeing of, and bonding with, animals whose health or lives may be sacrificed for the good of discovery through research" (Hurley, 2015). As appreciated through this definition, the "cost of caring" in the laboratory setting is largely influenced by the complexity of the human-animal relationship (Rabinowitz et al., 2015).

Generally, those who are drawn to caregiving in laboratory animal research have a strong interest in animals (Chang & Hart, 2002). As such, they are naturally inclined to develop an emotional connection with those in their care (Arluke, 1999; Coleman, 2011). This connection is further forged through the provision of high-quality care (Coleman, 2011). High-quality care – an ethical and moral responsibility as well as necessity for high-quality research – is exemplified by positive interactions (e.g., providing enrichment) (Bayne et al., 1993), positive reinforcement training (Bayne, 2002; Bloomsmith et al., 1997), and spontaneous exchanges (e.g., play) (Baker, 2004; Manciocco et al., 2009). Through such care, an exchange of affection often occurs between caregivers and animals, reinforcing the bond (AALAS, 2013; Stephens, 1996; Coleman, 2011). Most lab animal personnel develop some form of emotional connection with the animals in their care (Arluke, 1999; Coleman, 2011). Their work goes far beyond the essentials of providing food, water, and clean bedding.

Despite recognizing the need for animals in research, lab animal personnel may, at times, feel morally conflicted about their role (Coleman, 2011). On the one hand, they provide humane care, and on the other, they regularly witness or induce disease, participate in invasive studies, or are exposed to or involved in the perpetuation of pain and distress (Arluke, 1999; Coleman, 2011; LaFollette et al., 2020). Likewise, they are often expected to euthanize the animals in their care, sometimes for reasons other than alleviating pain or distress (Gluckman & Rosenbaum, 2017a). This contradictory role, with animals with whom they have formed emotional bonds, creates substantial moral di/stress. To complicate matters, the di/stress experienced within the workplace is exacerbated by society's perception of their work *outside* of the workplace – with the occupational stigma of scientific research with animals (Gluckman & Rosenbaum, 2017a). The negative perceptions of family, friends, and the community can lead to anxiety and feelings of guilt, shame, and sadness (Gluckman & Rosenbaum, 2017a). It can also limit the ability to feel social support and make social connections outside of the workplace (Pavan et al., 2020). The dearth of surrounding support can be a profound *additional* moral stressor for those who work with, care for, and support the animals (Overhulse, 2002; Rohlf & Bennett, 2005; Davies & Lewis, 2010; Baran et al., 2012). According to Newsome et al. (2019), "Comparatively, very few of the human or animal care providers that experience compassion fatigue may be as affected by the degree of compounding moral stress as the laboratory animal community" (Newsome et al., 2019, p. 290).

As it relates to moral di/stress, one might assume that lab animal personnel could turn to one another for support, yet the fear of marginalization can prevent many from raising the topic (Arluke, 1994). Feeling unable or unsupported to express their feelings, especially those that arise with performing stressful tasks, leads to emotional dissonance (LaFollette et al., 2020). Emotional dissonance is the discrepancy between required (expected) emotions and felt (actual) emotions (Morris & Feldman, 1996; Zapf & Holz, 2006; Davies & Lewis, 2010). The regulation of emotions to convey a desired display is a form of emotional labor (Zapf, 2002). It drains mental resources (Grandey, 2003; Coté, 2005) and increases the risk of mental distress (Diestel & Schmidt, 2011; Indregard et al., 2018) and feelings of exhaustion (Zapf, 2002; Hülsheger & Schewe, 2011), which together can increase the risk of compassion fatigue.

Performing and/or witnessing the euthanasia of animals, especially under conditions of moral di/stress, has been associated with compassion fatigue (Kahler, 2015;

Scotney et al., 2015). Just as those who work in animal health and animal welfare, those who work in research can also experience euthanasia stress (Newsome et al., 2019). Euthanasia in the laboratory, however, is distinctively, qualitatively different from euthanasia in a veterinary hospital or animal shelter (LaFollette et al., 2020). In the laboratory, euthanasia is considered the expected, necessary outcome, conducted after the animal has made a contribution to research (LaFollette et al., 2020). Typically, the decisions as to timing and method are clearly standardized and determined before the animals arrive at the facilities. Even with these differences, which are in some ways protective, the stress of euthanasia and the grief associated with the losses can make laboratory animal personnel vulnerable to compassion fatigue (Coleman, 2011). Laboratory animal research necessitates a constant making and breaking of human-animal bonds (LaFollette et al., 2020).

Overall, laboratory animal research is emotionally demanding and exposes caregiving personnel to layers of moral stressors (Pavan et al., 2020) which together makes them uniquely susceptible to compassion fatigue (LaFollette et al., 2020; Gluckman & Rosenbaum, 2017a; Coleman, 2011). Although those who work directly with the animals are the most susceptible, anyone in laboratory animal research programs, including researchers, facility management support, members of institutional animal care and use committees (IACUCs) and compliance committees, institutional officials, board members, vendors, security personnel, and administrative staff, can experience compassion fatigue (Newsome et al., 2019; Gluckman & Rosenbaum, 2017a). Such is the emotionality and moral complexity in the biomedical research context.

Personal Aspects of the Caregiver

From the person-in-environment perspective (Kondrat, 2008), it is not just the aspects of the workplace (i.e., environment) that can put a person at risk of compassion fatigue but the aspects of the person too. Although there has been little research on the personal factors that increase the risk of compassion fatigue (Figley & Roop, 2006), a person's age (younger), gender (female), personality, attitudes, motivations, coping strategies, social relations, compassion satisfaction, and number of years in the field may play a role (Figley & Roop, 2006; McArthur et al., 2017b; Pavan et al., 2020; Dow et al., 2019; Sprang et al., 2007; Stamm, 2010; Thompson et al., 2014). Likewise, a history of traumatic experiences and current unresolved trauma may also play a role (Newsome et al., 2019). Many personal variables may come into play. As Figley and Roop (2006) allegorize, "Some workers are like a cork in a turbulent creek, sometimes going under the water or bumping into a rock, but always bobbing back to the surface. Other workers may be more like paper boats, far less resistant to the jostling of the same turbulent creek" (Figley & Roop, 2006, p. 9).

Symptoms and Consequences of Compassion Fatigue

Compassion fatigue can lead to a wide range of symptoms (i.e., changes in the person). Indeed, there are so many symptoms that compassion fatigue can appear differently from one person to the next (Mathieu, 2011). Regardless of occupation (Owen & Wanzer, 2014), anyone can have any combination and number of symptoms (ranging from few to many), and the expression and intensity thereof may vary – some may be more subtle and nonspecific, while others obvious and pointed (Gluckman & Rosenbaum, 2017a). And as the symptoms can vary day to day and over time, the appearance of compassion fatigue in any one person can likewise vary. All of this can make compassion fatigue exceedingly difficult to identify. Adding to this difficulty is the insidious nature of compassion fatigue, with the onset of symptoms often so gradual they are missed (Mathieu, 2011; Cohen, 2007). In order to address compassion fatigue, it needs to be recognized. Thus, it is imperative to become aware of the symptoms – and the many personal, professional, and organizational consequences of compassion fatigue.

Symptoms

The classic symptom of compassion fatigue is a reduced ability to feel sympathy and empathy for others and, subsequently, act from a place of compassion (Mathieu, 2011). Sympathy, empathy, and compassion are fundamental to caregiving. With compassion fatigue, sympathy's "I care about your suffering," empathy's "I feel your suffering," and compassion's "I want to relieve your suffering" will fade into the past, often imperceptibly. Without realizing it, the person may become more task- and less emotion-focused, concentrating on "the job to be done" to the exclusion of interactions with others, human or animal, that could draw on emotions. Sooner or later, numbness, apathy, and social isolation can become the norm (Gluckman & Rosenbaum, 2017b).

The other classic symptom of compassion fatigue is a profound exhaustion, physical as well as mental and emotional (Mathieu, 2011), aptly described as, "feeling fatigued in every cell of your being" (van Dernoot Lipsky & Burk, 2009, p. 111). As fatigue can significantly affect human functioning – most notably the keystones of feeling, thinking, and behavior – compassion fatigue can have serious implications in both the short and long term *and* in infinite directions.

Beyond the classic symptoms, compassion fatigue can alter a person's emotional spectrum, moving it toward the negative, with increasing feelings of annoyance, intolerance, anger, irritability, skepticism, cynicism, embitterment, and/or resentfulness (Mathieu, 2011; Hooper et al., 2010). These symptoms often incite interpersonal conflicts and lead to problems with intimacy, culminating in hurt feelings, disappointments, and disconnection. Anxiety, irrational fears, mood swings, tearfulness, melancholy, sadness, and despair may also be experienced and can, at times, lead to suicidal thoughts or gestures (Mathieu, 2011).

As well as alterations in emotional valence, compassion fatigue can lead to changes in cognitive functioning, with declines in the ability to think clearly, use good judgment, and make decisions. It may become increasingly difficult to concentrate and carry through on tasks. There may be lapses in memory or forgetfulness, and some may become uncharacteristically accident-prone. Eventually, with growing feelings of inadequacy and helplessness, the person may assume a negative self-image (Mathieu, 2011). Compassion fatigue can even disrupt a person's worldview.

Altogether, compassion fatigue can disturb the ability to modulate emotions, think clearly, feel successful, and maintain hope. The consequences of these changes are far-reaching.

Personal Consequences

Compassion fatigue can trigger the onset of a wide range of stress-related physical disorders, commonly referred to as psychosomatic (Mathieu, 2011). These include chronic pain and fatigue, headaches and migraines, and gastrointestinal disturbances such as nausea, vomiting, and diarrhea (Mathieu, 2011). It can also cause sleep disturbances, including trouble falling or staying asleep, as well as recurring nightmares. In the larger picture, it has been linked to a greater susceptibility to illness in general (Mathieu, 2011) and over the long term may increase the risk of several serious medical conditions, including cardiovascular disease, obesity, and diabetes (Warshaw, 1989; Kakiashvili et al., 2013; Melamed et al., 2006), all related to the physiology of chronic stress (Rohleder, 2016). Compassion fatigue can also trigger a range of stress-related psychiatric disorders, including mood disorders (e.g., anxiety and clinical depression), addictions (e.g., smoking, alcohol, drugs, and gambling), eating disorders, dissociative disorders, hypochondria, and personality disorders (Mathieu, 2011). Altogether, compassion fatigue can significantly impact physical and mental health. While some will struggle with their physical health, others will struggle with their mental health, while others will struggle with both. And as physical and mental health is impacted, so is the ability to perform well at work. There are professional as well as personal consequences with compassion fatigue.

Professional Consequences

Being less able to effectively sympathize, empathize, and "engage with care," the ability to connect with – and care for and about – others, human and animal, will decline, negatively impacting work performance and outcomes (Mathieu, 2011; Stebnicki, 2000). Being less caring and conscientious, the risk of mix-ups, oversights, and mistakes will increase, quality of care decrease, and work become shoddy. With reluctance to engage emotionally, some may dread – and thus try to avoid – working with certain individuals (e.g., patients, clients, or coworkers) or within certain situations (e.g., euthanasias) (Mathieu, 2011).

Alterations in cognition, attitude, and mental health can lead to indecision, misjudgments, and memory loss that further impact work performance. Troubled by exhaustion and psychosomatic illness, some will become less efficient and reliable. Work habits and patterns may become unpredictable. Some will take sick days or a leave of absence, spending *less* time at work, while others will worriedly try to keep up, spending *more* time at work. Some will take work home with them. Over time, it can become increasingly difficult to separate work life from personal life, and those afflicted with compassion fatigue can lose touch with the people and activities they used to enjoy (Mathieu, 2011).

Some people may eventually find their work and career unfulfilling. Disappointed, disheartened, and disillusioned, they may turn to alcohol or prescription/recreational drugs to ease the pain (Mathieu, 2011; Remen, 1996). Alternatively, they may move from job to job, believing the problem to be specific to the place, or type, of employment, not the actual work that they do (Mathieu, 2011). In time, they may give up their career altogether. Compassion fatigue has driven both promising and seasoned professionals out of their occupations entirely, permanently altering the direction of career paths (Mitchener & Ogilvie, 2002).

Organizational Consequences

The symptoms of compassion fatigue, along with the personal and professional consequences, can culminate in a wide array of organizational consequences. These systemic effects may include, but are not limited to, the adverse impacts noted in Table 3.1.

Compassion fatigue is a serious occupational hazard negatively impacting individuals to entire organizations all over the world. As Francoise Mathieu, leading expert on compassion fatigue, believes, there is no such thing as prevention. Instead compassion fatigue can be mitigated, transformed, and treated to enable optimal caregiving and service outcomes, long and rewarding careers, and successful organizations (Mathieu, 2011).

Mitigating, Transforming, and Treating Compassion Fatigue

> Resilience is not all or nothing. It comes in amounts. You can be a little resilient, a lot resilient; resilient in some situations but not others. And no matter how resilient you are today, you can become more resilient tomorrow. — Karen Reivich (2008, updated 2010).

The mitigation, transformation, and treatment of compassion fatigue is centered in the concept of resilience. Resilience is the capacity, process, and outcome of

Table 3.1 Potential organizational consequences of compassion fatigue

Domain	Potential consequences
Animal and human health and welfare	Compromised animal care; needless animal stress, injury, suffering, and death; inferior medical outcomes; reduced adoption rates; higher euthanasia rates; substandard client/customer care; and greater client/customer dissatisfaction and/or grief
Employment	High absenteeism, high turnover, excessive occupational health reports and workers' compensation claims, and higher than average dismissals
Coworker relationships	Inability to work well together, lack of team cohesion, unhealthy competition, gossip, incivility, conflict, difficulties reaching shared goals, outbreaks of aggressive behavior, and negativity toward management
Organizational culture	Low moral, noncompliance with standards and protocols, safety breaches, rule challenging or breaking, failure to complete tasks or respect and meet deadlines, inflexibility, workplace toxicity, reluctance to change, inability to believe that improvement is possible, and lack of a vision for the future
Organizational outcomes	Operational and financial instability; inability to realize growth potential, innovate, or meet financial goals; complaints and litigation; and less opportunity for advances in science and medicine to protect human and animal health

Sources: Figley and Roop (2006), Gluckman and Rosenbaum (2017b), Mathieu (2011), Newsome et al. (2019)

adapting well in the face of adversity, being able to "bounce back" from negative experiences and move on despite the difficulties (Reyes et al., 2015; Tugade & Fredrickson, 2004). It is not simply a personality trait, natural tendency, or learned competency (OpenLearn, 2017), but instead, a dynamic and multifaceted process whereby individuals draw on personal and contextual resources and use specific strategies, to navigate challenges and work toward adaptive outcomes (Mansfield et al., 2016).

There are several kinds of personal resources (i.e., qualities or traits), including a sense of purpose, vocation, and efficacy; a proactive attitude, enabling self-beliefs, optimism, motivation, reflective skills, self-compassion, and social and emotional competence, among others (McArthur et al., 2017a; Tempski et al., 2012; Wendt et al., 2011; Thomas et al., 2012; Mastenbroek et al., 2012; Cake et al., 2017). Likewise, there are various contextual resources (i.e., aspects of the social and physical environment), including, for example, supportive family, friends, mentors, colleagues, supervisors, and an amenable workplace (Ungar, 2011; Beltman et al., 2011; Broussard & Myers, 2010; Cake et al., 2017). Some strategies include self-care, maintaining work-life balance, goal setting, problem-solving, help-seeking, reflection, and mindfulness, among others (McArthur et al., 2017a; Tempski et al., 2012; Wendt et al., 2011; Thomas et al., 2012; Cake et al., 2017). These resources and strategies can facilitate resilience, empowering animal care providers to remain engaged, committed, and fulfilled in their careers (McArthur et al., 2017a). Resilience does not just happen. It develops over time, built on awareness, enabled by intention, and strengthened through lived experience (McArthur et al., 2017a).

Resilience in the animal care community can be built on the back of veterinary social work. Veterinary social work is an area of social work practice that supports and strengthens interdisciplinary partnerships that attend to the intersection of humans and animals (International Association of Veterinary Social Work, 2021). The role of veterinary social workers is to attend to the human needs that arise in the relationship between humans and animals (International Association of Veterinary Social Work, 2021). One of the four key competencies of this area of social work is compassion fatigue (Holcombe et al., 2016; Compassion Fatigue & Conflict Management, 2021). By being able to attend to the causes, signs, and consequences of compassion fatigue, veterinary social workers are able to support the health and well-being of those who work in animal care (Compassion Fatigue & Conflict Management, 2021). While it is not possible to *eliminate* the sources of stress, it *is* possible to preserve and enhance the resilience required to cope with stress and reduce the consequences of being exposed to these stressors (Ivancevich et al., 1990). As professionals, veterinary social workers are well positioned to promote awareness of compassion fatigue, elevate wellness to foster health and well-being, and advocate for systemic change to build personal, interpersonal, and organizational resilience.

In the animal care community, resilience starts with compassion fatigue awareness, and, through a person-in-environment perspective (Kondrat, 2008), grows with implementing personal and organizational approaches, strategies, and practices.

Compassion Fatigue Awareness

As a significant stress-related occupational hazard, it is imperative for those in the animal care community – whether in veterinary practices, humane societies, animal shelters, animal control services, animal rescues and rehabilitation services, or biomedical research laboratories – to become aware of compassion fatigue. While acknowledging the efficacy of individuals, as an occupational hazard, the responsibility for compassion fatigue awareness inherently falls within the purview of the organization to protect and support its people. According to the Centers for Disease Control and Prevention (CDC), organizations have the responsibility to provide safe and hazard-free workplaces and the opportunity to promote worker health and foster healthy work environments (Centers for Disease Control and Prevention, 2021). *Healthy* organizations provide both health protection and health promotion, preventing occupational injury and improving health and well-being (Centers for Disease Control and Prevention, 2021).

The animal care community is in the midst of a significant cultural shift, with a burgeoning awareness of the phenomenon of compassion fatigue. Integral in this shift is the impetus for education, for initiatives to foster understanding of compassion fatigue and how to cope with it (Polachek & Wallace, 2018; Newsome et al., 2019; Pavan et al., 2020; Gluckman & Rosenbaum, 2017b; Figley, 1995; Dow et al., 2019; Brannick et al., 2015; Hill et al., 2020; Hurley, 2015; Lloyd & Campion,

2017; Rank et al., 2009; Hanrahan et al., 2018). Such initiatives can include educational campaigns, education and training programs, lectures, seminars, workshops, round-table discussions, webinars, podcasts, and articles (Polachek & Wallace, 2018; Newsome et al., 2019; Pavan et al., 2020; Gluckman & Rosenbaum, 2017b). Remarkably, participating in these initiatives may not only raise awareness but also reduce stress, reduce compassion fatigue-related symptoms, and increase compassion satisfaction (Meadors & Lamson, 2008; Gentry et al., 2004; Rank et al., 2009). Simply learning about compassion fatigue can improve health and well-being, meaning training can be offered as treatment (Rank et al., 2009). The key to success with these initiatives is longevity (Gluckman & Rosenbaum, 2017b). Longevity can be ensured by talking about compassion fatigue more often and more openly, ensuring ongoing availability of educational opportunities, and incorporating awareness training into on-boarding and safety training programs (Gluckman & Rosenbaum, 2017b; Newsome et al., 2019; Pavan et al., 2020). All of these efforts not only convey recognition of compassion fatigue as a significant issue but, more importantly, that the organization cares about its people (Gluckman & Rosenbaum, 2017b).

Veterinary social workers can play a major role in delivering compassion fatigue education (Rank et al., 2009). They can work locally or travel widely to provide onsite consultation and training services or be employed on a part- or full-time basis, at veterinary colleges, veterinary hospitals, humane societies, animal shelters, and laboratory facilities (Rank et al., 2009).

Personal Approaches, Strategies, and Practices

There are a number of personal approaches, strategies, and practices that can enhance resilience, thereby reducing the risk of compassion fatigue. Although these can be pursued independently, they can also be acknowledged, substantiated, and incorporated within the organization as part of a wellness culture. When personal resiliencies are upheld within the community, the entire community benefits - and exponentially.

Engage in Self-Care Self-care is the cornerstone for the mitigation of compassion fatigue (Mathieu, 2007a). As a caregiver, the self can be likened to an instrument. To remain effective, the instrument needs to be continuously monitored, tuned, and assessed to keep it in first-class working condition (Showalter, 2010). It is a professional, ethical responsibility. In essence, to care for others, one has to first care for the self (Lama & Chan, 2014; Sanchez-Reilly et al., 2013). Knowing the cost of caring, to *not* engage in self-care can almost be seen as a form of intra-iatrogenic harm (Egan et al., 2017).

Self-care can be envisioned as a systematic discipline of refueling and rejuvenating – physically, emotionally, psychologically, spiritually, relationally, and professionally (Gentry & Baranowsky, 2013). There are many creative and personally meaningful ways to soothe the senses and feel alive, relaxed, and well, sustaining energy, buoyancy, and hope. In and through this, self-care promotes optimism, self-confidence, level headedness, hardiness, and the ability to be resourceful in the face of adversity (Lloyd & Campion, 2017; Moffett et al., 2015).

Inherent to self-care is setting healthy boundaries to maintain life balance. This necessitates taking stock of one's duties, rebalancing workload, delegating, and placing limits on availability, involvement, and personal investment in work (Mitchener & Ogilvie, 2002; Mathieu, 2007b). There needs to be balance between activities that nourish and activities that deplete.

Although self-care is ultimately an individual responsibility, as the cornerstone of resilience, given the benefits, the argument could be made to incorporate self-care into the culture of the workplace, creating a wellness culture that promotes self-care (Egan et al., 2017). Veterinary social workers are adept at facilitating cultures that strive to optimize employee health and well-being – and within this, normalizing the need for, and providing practical training in, self-care (Moses et al., 2018). Social workers can play vital roles with helping animal care providers develop individualized self-care plans and achieve their self-care goals (Holcombe et al., 2016).

Practice Mindfulness and Self-Compassion Two key factors that have been identified in the literature as enhancing resilience are mindfulness and self-compassion, both drawn from Buddhist philosophy (Williams & Kabat-Zinn, 2011). They are especially important in the realm of caregiving as they promote compassion toward others (Egan et al., 2017). As compared to mindlessness – which prompts thinking of the past and the future – mindfulness has been described as the experience of centering attention and awareness on what is taking place in the present moment, without judgment (Brown & Ryan, 2003). It is an accepting yet detached attitude.

Mindfulness can be enhanced through mindfulness training, practices that train the mind to stay focused in the moment. The usefulness of mindfulness training has been well documented (Fortney et al., 2013; Hassed et al., 2009; Flook et al., 2013). Mindfulness directly contributes to reducing anxiety, depression, and burnout (Montero-Marin et al., 2015; Atanes et al., 2015; Rushton et al., 2015; Thomas, 2011), is associated with less emotional exhaustion (Olson et al., 2015; McArthur et al., 2017a), and may significantly predict compassion fatigue and compassion satisfaction (Thomas, 2011; McArthur et al., 2017b). As an effective means of managing everyday anxieties, worries, and suffering, mindfulness could be introduced into the workplace, formally, through establishing a training program or, informally, through offering a seminar or workshop and/or incorporating mindfulness practices into the workplace as a manner of practice (e.g., taking a mindful moment prior to a meeting).

Self-compassion is a related but different construct. Self-compassion can be understood as compassion directed inward toward the self (Neff, 2003a). It consists of three components: (a) self-kindness, being kind and understanding toward oneself in instances of pain or failure rather than being harshly self-critical; (b) common humanity, seeing one's experiences as part of the human condition rather than as separating and isolating; and (c) mindfulness, holding painful thoughts and feelings in balanced awareness rather than over-identifying with them (Neff, 2003a). Self-compassion involves extending understanding and kindness to the self in response to perceptions of pain, inadequacy, or failure (Neff, 2003b). It offers the benefits of mindfulness *plus* compassion for self, an added protection when compassion from others may not always be evident or readily displayed.

Self-compassion is associated with less anxiety, burnout, and depression (Neff, 2003b; Körner et al., 2015; Wong & Mak, 2013; Rees et al., 2015; Van Dam et al., 2011; Neff et al., 2007), improvements in well-being (Neff & Germer, 2013; Barnard & Curry, 2011), and greater social connectedness (Raes, 2010) and life satisfaction (Neff, 2003b; Raes, 2010). There are many ways to develop self-compassion (Neff, 2021). As with self-care, given the benefits, it seems judicious to incorporate the principles and practices of mindfulness and self-compassion into the workplace (Egan et al., 2017). Although any one person can foster them on their own, the benefits could be manifold when fostered together within a wellness culture. A veterinary social worker can offer the leadership necessary to successfully integrate mindfulness and self-compassion into the workplace.

Cultivate Compassion As a social emotion that "informs and motivates our duties towards others" (O'Connell, 2009, p. 3), compassion is a key motivator of altruistic (e.g., helping) behavior. Compassion is not only the property of a person or situation – it can be learned (Singer & Klimecki, 2014). It is a skill that can be cultivated through training (Weng et al., 2013).

Compassion training makes use of Buddhist-derived meditative techniques that focus on cultivating affective empathy for the suffering of others (referred to as *compassion* meditation) (Shamay-Tsoory, 2011) or a feeling of love for all beings (called *loving kindness* meditation) (Lee et al., 2012). The empirical evidence suggests that compassion training can reduce psychological distress, loneliness, and depression (Shonin et al., 2015; Mascaro et al., 2018), enhance positive emotions (Klimecki et al., 2013; Singer & Klimecki, 2014; Shonin et al., 2015; Zeng et al., 2015; Klimecki et al., 2013), and foster emotional well-being (Fredrickson et al., 2008), all of which strengthen resilience. It also suggests that training reinforces caregivers' ability to care. Compassion training has been found to deepen compassion (Mascaro et al., 2018), improve empathic accuracy (Shonin et al., 2015), and buffer against empathic erosion (Mascaro et al., 2018). Furthermore, it has been shown to increase prosocial motivation (Singer & Klimecki, 2014) and promote both prosocial and altruistic behavior (Leiberg et al., 2011; Singer & Klimecki, 2014; Weng et al., 2013). Compassion training can offer wide benefits, from strengthening resilience to reinforcing the ability to provide compassionate care, benefitting care givers and receivers alike (Singer & Klimecki, 2014). Although training can be pursued independently, through many available resources, it could also be introduced into the workplace, formally, via a professional organizational training program (e.g., Compassion It) (Compassion It, 2021), or informally, with a self- or team-developed program. A veterinary social worker can provide the initiative and guidance necessary to procure, develop, and/or maintain a compassion training program.

Grow Compassion Satisfaction Compassion satisfaction can be described as the positive feelings and sense of reward, fulfillment, and accomplishment experienced when attending to the needs of others (Gluckman & Rosenbaum, 2017b) and the pleasure derived from being able to do one's work well as a professional caregiver (Stamm, 2010). In a sense, it can be thought of as an emotional counterbalance to compassion fatigue (Gluckman & Rosenbaum, 2017b).

The notion of "making a difference" to those in need is recognized as a key predictor of compassion satisfaction (Polachek & Wallace, 2018; Alkema et al., 2008; Wendt et al., 2011; Figley & Roop, 2006; Dasan et al., 2015). Building rapport, relationships, and partnerships with others, human or animal, can also be satisfying (Polachek & Wallace, 2018). The more one can stay connected to the hope, joys, rewards, and sense of purpose and meaning within caregiving, the less the risk of compassion fatigue. Thus, as a strategy to counter compassion fatigue, it may be worthwhile to focus on increasing feelings of compassion satisfaction (Pavan et al., 2020; Gluckman & Rosenbaum, 2017b). This requires being mindful of how and when compassion satisfaction is experienced and intentionally savoring these experiences – necessitating a shift from dwelling on the negative (the natural human tendency) to focusing on the positive (Gluckman & Rosenbaum, 2017b).

From another perspective, through the lens of positive psychology, Melissa Radey and Charles Figley (2007) posited a conceptual model of how to create compassion satisfaction and, in this, counter compassion fatigue. According Radey and Figley (2007), one can create the positivity necessary to experience compassion satisfaction by using "good discernment and judgment" to focus on three things, (1) affect, (2) resources, and (3) self-care (Radey & Figley, 2007). Affect refers to one's emotions and ways of looking at things, i.e., one's perspective or interpretation of life. Resources refers to one's intellectual, social, and physical capital, meaning assets and abilities. And self-care refers to caring for the whole self, the balance of body, mind, and spirit.

These three things are reciprocally related, one influencing the other. Positivity is "the ratio of pleasant feelings and sentiments (or positive affect) to unpleasant feelings and sentiments (or negative affect) over time" (Radey & Figley, 2007, p. 210) and needs to be at least 3:1, meaning a person needs to experience at least three *positive* experiences to one *negative* experience to experience compassion satisfaction and avoid becoming compassion fatigued. Aside from the mathematics of it, the take-home messages are to sustain a positive attitude (i.e., be optimistic), participate in lifelong learning (i.e., keep "sharpening the saw"), maintain social connectedness, and attend to one's physical health; and, as it relates to self-care, to engage in creative and personally meaningful ways to feel alive, relaxed, and well. By doing these things, one may protect the heart from giving out and instead continue to feel the joys and flourish (Radey & Figley, 2007). Taking these as tips or calls to action, compassion fatigue can be transformed into compassion satisfaction (Mathieu, 2007b). The benefits of compassion satisfaction and how to grow it can be pursued independently or instilled within a workplace culture that celebrates successes (Newsome et al., 2019) and reveres positivity, continuing education, collegiality, good health, and self-care. As wellness leaders, veterinary social workers are well equipped to support both individual and collective efforts to grow compassion satisfaction.

Organizational Approaches, Strategies, and Practices

Animal care organizations can only benefit from acknowledging the existence of compassion fatigue and promoting sustainable organizational approaches, strategies, and practices to reduce the risk and build resilience. Managing compassion fatigue and its consequences is an ongoing challenge, but one wherein great gains can be made through the deliberate, purposeful creation of a supportive work environment – also an ongoing challenge, but one well worth pursuing. A supportive work environment enables workers to thrive despite the challenges. As environments vary, with differences in institutional structure and function, the policies and practices will also vary. Yet at the same time, there are many ways to create a supportive work environment, whether in the animal health, animal welfare, or biomedical research community.

Reduce Workplace Stress There are a number of strategies that can reduce the level and sources of stress in the workplace that contribute to burnout and, in turn, compassion fatigue. Anything that eases adjustment to the job, improves work performance, and enhances job satisfaction and morale is likely to reduce the risk of compassion fatigue (Yakl & Van Fleet, 1992). Starting with the basics, it is important to attend to workloads, working hours, and work processes (Bartram & Boniwell, 2007; Gardner & Hini, 2006; O'Driscoll & Cooper, 2002; Warr, 2007; Mathieu, 2007a). This necessitates reviewing scheduling, staffing, hours worked, breaks taken, overtime policy, on-call duties, administrative support, and vacation. As *excess* demands reduce well-being, it is critical to ensure that they are reasonable and manageable (Schaufeli & Bakker, 2004). Workers can be offered the opportunity to "opt out" of emotionally challenging tasks, as needed, by offering rotational scheduling (Gluckman & Rosenbaum, 2017b). Job rotations are recommended as a way to mitigate compassion fatigue (Hooper et al., 2010; Smart et al., 2014; Rogelberg et al., 2007; Rhoades, 2002; Pavan et al., 2020; Gluckman & Rosenbaum, 2017b). Flexible work schedules may also be helpful as they enable greater work-life balance and reduce work-home interference.

The work environments and technologies should be appropriate and the necessary resources available (Gardner & Hini, 2006; O'Driscoll & Cooper, 2002; Wallace, 2014; Reeve et al., 2004). Priorities, workflow, equipment needs, ergonomics, and other safety concerns should be reviewed on a regular basis to identify ways in which the work may be done with greater ease. Opportunities can be created for variety in routines, as it relates to tasks, skills, and caseload, and prospects for novel experiences (Pavan et al., 2020). The promotion of continuing education is important, especially in job-related skills where the lack thereof may be generating stress (Gardner & Hini, 2006; Mathieu, 2007a; Cake et al., 2017); professional development is integral to job endurance.

Supportive and considerate supervision is essential. How management interacts with workers can ease or exacerbate compassion fatigue (Hill et al., 2020). A participative management style (McMillan, 2021), giving workers a voice in their workplace, increasing their control over their work, and widening their decision latitude (professional autonomy) suitable to their roles and responsibilities, may reduce stress (Bartram & Boniwell, 2007; Gardner & Hini, 2006; O'Driscoll & Cooper, 2002; Warr, 2007; Cake et al., 2017; Reeve et al., 2004). The provision of mentorship, coaching, and guidance, blended with positive feedback with appropriate levels of challenge (Bartram & Boniwell, 2007; Gardner & Hini, 2006; O'Driscoll & Cooper, 2002; Warr, 2007), will promote job satisfaction and create additional opportunities. Clear job expectations, a sense of job security, and equitable reward systems (Bartram & Boniwell, 2007; Gardner & Hini, 2006; O'Driscoll & Cooper, 2002; Warr, 2007) are also essential, as are regular performance appraisals. Building cohesive teams is a priority; research demonstrates that a more cohesive group at work reduces the effects of stress and trauma, helping to prevent burnout and compassion fatigue (Li et al., 2014).

Communication practices should be assessed to identify problematic areas and make concerted efforts to reduce the problems (Warr, 2007). Methods can be developed or training offered to better manage the conversations that prove to be difficult over and over again. Safeguarding good interpersonal communication can reduce compassion fatigue (Reeve et al., 2004).

Veterinary social workers can help reduce workplace stress by attending to the systemic relationship-based issues of supervision, teamwork, and communication. Social workers are interaction experts, schooled in relationship dynamics and advanced communication techniques. They can use their knowledge, skills, and attitudes to inspire supportive supervision, encourage participative management, and buoy up cohesive teams, contributing to a healthy workplace environment. They can provide training in communication, social support skills, and recognizing, naming, and navigating ethical conflict. They can even take on certain communications to reduce the staff workload (Moses et al., 2018), such as co-facilitating complicated healthcare decisions and resolving conflicts with clients. Beyond this, they can be called upon in critical circumstances, when stress can be at its highest, and later provide critical incident debriefing.

Minimize Euthanasia Stress Euthanasia is generally a significant source of stress for those working in the animal care community. As the circumstances particular to euthanasia differ for those working within (1) veterinary practices; (2) humane societies, animal shelters, animal control services, and animal rescues and rehabilitation services; and (3) biomedical research laboratories, the options to reduce the stress associated with it also differ.

*[I] **Veterinary Practices*** Euthanasia is typically requested by the animal owner/ guardian or recommended by the veterinarian in relation to health or behavioral problems that significantly impact the quality of life of the animal and/or family or

are untreatable due to financial limitations. At times, veterinarians are asked to euthanize an animal for reasons beyond this, what is referred to as "convenience" euthanasia. Convenience euthanasia (i.e., euthanasia of a physically and psychologically healthy animal) is recognized as one of the most difficult situations in practice (Rathwell-Deault et al., 2017).

To reduce the stress of euthanasia, veterinarians and their teams can create criteria under which they do or do not recommend euthanasia and identify (in advance) the situations within which they would refuse to euthanize (Hill et al., 2020). As well, they can develop a set of resources for pet owners to treat behavioral or relatively minor medical issues (Hill et al., 2020) and identify the avenues of care from which families of limited income might access veterinary care, in these ways avoiding unnecessary euthanasia. They can also divide the euthanasia workload among themselves, thereby apportioning the stress, distress, and grief (Hill et al., 2020).

The stress of euthanasia can further be divided (i.e., lessened) through conversations with colleagues or trusted others who "understand." As informal sharing can help reduce the emotional load, it is important to foster an environment that encourages open dialogue (Newsome et al., 2019). It may also be helpful to create a safe place or "sanctuary" within the workplace where employees can decompress, particularly after intensely emotional experiences (Cohen, 2007; Gardner & Hini, 2006; Mitchener & Ogilvie, 2002).

Veterinary social workers can do much to help veterinary personnel manage the stress of euthanasia. They can reduce the staff workload by co-facilitating euthanasia decision-making – helping clients with quality of life assessments, navigating the available options, and making difficult decisions (Arkow, 2020). With training in grief and loss, they can provide clients with emotional support during and after euthanasia, and if needed, grief counseling, preserving both staff time and emotions (Rank et al., 2009). Being present for the staff, social workers can create a safe space for expressions of distress, guilt, and grief and facilitate "the ties that bind" to sustain a supportive cohesive team (Arkow, 2020; Rank et al., 2009). They can also promote a nonjudgmental culture of help-seeking and be a resource for individual or group consultation (Arkow, 2020; Rank et al., 2009; Compassion Fatigue & Conflict Management, 2021).

[II] Humane Societies, Animal Shelters, Animal Control Services, and Animal Rescues and Rehabilitation Services The most proactive way to reduce euthanasia stress in humane societies and shelters is to reduce the need for euthanasia. This can be achieved through a variety of policies and practices that enable optimal management of the animals within the shelter, shelter systems, and community at large. The need can be reduced in several ways, including (1) by employing diversion programs to keep animals from being relinquished, (2) by developing foster care programs, (3) by establishing a robust transfer network to move animals from shelters at capacity to others with space, (4) by offering spay/neuter programs to reduce the number of unwanted animals in the community, (5) by increasing adoptions (e.g., hosting adoption promotion events), and (6) by incorporating socialization and behavior enrichment programs to address aggression and kennel neurosis (Hill et al., 2020). In reducing the need for, and thus incidence of, euthanasia, the risk of compassion fatigue likewise is reduced (Reese, 2018; Reeve et al., 2004).

When euthanasia *is* necessary, the stress can be reduced if decisions are made using codified criteria and through a communal process wherein the responsibility is shared (Hill et al., 2020). Codified criteria help bring clarity and predictability to the decision-making process (Hill et al., 2020). A communal (or multi-level) approach reduces the decision-making burden on any one person, providing a protective buffer for those involved in the process (Andrukonis & Protopopova, 2020; Hill et al., 2020). Making decisions together also, albeit inadvertently, creates a support group that understands the stress (Hill et al., 2020). Despite the difficulty of engaging in these decisions, some shelter personnel express feeling *less* occupational stress when management seeks their opinions (Rogelberg et al., 2007). In other words, inclusion in the decision-making process may be important in reducing stress (Andrukonis & Protopopova, 2020).

For those who perform or are affected by euthanasia, job rotations help reduce the stress (Reeve et al., 2004; Rogelberg et al., 2007). Permitting workers to engage in other shelter activities, such as working in adoptions, delivering humane education, and being responsible for animal enrichment can provide enough of a break to reduce the stress and remember the broader functions of the shelter beyond euthanization (Irvine, 2002; Reeve et al., 2004, 2005). Break times and time off can also be helpful (Reeve et al., 2004; Rogelberg et al., 2007).

Animal control and animal rescues and rehabilitation services can also reduce the stress of euthanasia, by finding ways to reduce the need for euthanasia, using codified criteria for making decisions, sharing the burden of decision-making (e.g., creating a committee), and engaging in pursuits that revitalize the passion for animal welfare and the differences that can be made.

As within animal health, social workers can do much to support personnel in animal welfare manage the stress of euthanasia, whether the euthanasia is in-person (i.e., with the family) or otherwise. Veterinary social workers can facilitate the emotionality of in-person euthanasias (Arkow, 2020), reducing the emotional labor required by the staff, and in this, the risk of emotional depletion. They can encourage dialogue and camaraderie within an open workplace atmosphere, engendering the safety needed for personnel to reach out for support to help manage the guilt and grief that accompany euthanasia (Compassion Fatigue & Conflict Management, 2021). In recent years, social work services have been introduced into community animal shelters with social work field placements (Hoy-Gerlach et al., 2019).

[III] Biomedical Research Laboratories As euthanasia in the laboratory is considered the expected necessary outcome, and the decisions as to timing and method of euthanasia are clearly standardized and determined before the animals even arrive at the facilities, the awareness of, and stress associated with, euthanasia is tied into the entire research process from inception onward. Thus, within the research setting, whatever can be done to reduce the overall burden of stress and build resilience along the entire research process will contribute to reducing euthanasia stress. *Exemplary* animal care and use programs engage in initiatives to reduce stress and

build resilience to keep their personnel well. They endorse compassion and respect for both the laboratory animals and the people who work with them (Brown et al., 2018). They endorse what is called a "culture of care" (Brown et al., 2018). In a culture of care, institutions celebrate the compassion, caring, and respect their staff exhibit toward animals and likewise address the consequences that may arise thereof as it relates to animal morbidity and mortality.

Perhaps the most significant source of stress in the biomedical laboratory is the moral conflict that arises with using animals in research. There are a number of strategies that may be taken to reduce this and the associated di/stress that may be experienced. At the institute level, to address the occupational stigma of research with animals, institutions can commit to engaging in public outreach to increase awareness of the benefits of scientific research and, too, public trust in the care and use of research animals (Brown et al., 2018). Likewise, to counter the misconceptions that lead to stigma, they can prioritize awareness of the positive impact that research personnel have in their work (Scotney et al., 2015; Newsome et al., 2019). Resource materials are available from various organizations to support such efforts in public outreach (Brown et al., 2018). Furthermore, since the use of animals in research can be a sensitive topic, institutions can benefit their research and animal care personnel by offering training to help them talk about the work that they do (with friends, family, and neighbors) and the impact that it has on both human and animal health and welfare (Brown et al., 2018; LaFollette et al., 2020). Such training widens their understanding of the issues and encourages pride in their contributions to biomedical research (Brown et al., 2018). Training can also be offered to help employees understand why animals are necessary in research, the ethics of such use, and the importance of animal welfare (Brown et al., 2018). It can be delivered by way of in-person lectures, online offerings, or self-learning materials. Veterinary social workers can play an integral part both in public outreach and employee training.

At the research planning level, studies can be designed in ways that recognize the intrinsic value of animals, endorse the humane care and use of animals, and treat animals according to high ethical and scientific standards (Brown et al., 2018). Giving animal welfare the highest priority, each use can be carefully evaluated and the principles of replacement, reduction, and refinement (the 3Rs) applied. Giving animal care personnel a voice in the ethical decisions, enabling their expert opinion and moral concerns to be considered is helpful (Herzog, 2002). It enables different perspectives to be heard and engenders empowerment within a sense of ownership in the decisions being made about animal care and use (Brown et al., 2018).

At the research implementation level, researchers can share with animal care personnel the importance of their studies, the reasons for procedures, the expected clinical signs, and the humane endpoints (and rationale for those endpoints), openly acknowledging the moral conflicts therein and resultant emotions that may naturally arise (Brown et al., 2018; LaFollette et al., 2020; Herzog, 2002). Helping personnel understand the nature and importance of the research may help them better cope with the morality, morbidity, and mortality (Brown et al., 2018).

Also at the implementation level is the ability for personnel to be able to raise concerns about animal welfare (Brown et al., 2018), assured that reporting is expected. Reporting should include the option for anonymity as well as guaranteed protection from retribution (Brown et al., 2018). To then have the opportunity to collaborate on the solutions to improve animal welfare may improve not only animal welfare but morale as well (Brown et al., 2018). The ability to report concerns and identify solutions is empowering (Brown et al., 2018).

As in the animal health and welfare settings, the option for personnel to opt out of circumstances that may cause angst should be available (Brown et al., 2018). This includes the euthanasia of an animal to which the caregiver has become especially bonded. In such situations, the option of having a trusted colleague perform the euthanasia should always be provided when requested (Newsome et al., 2019; LaFollette et al., 2020). In a study by LaFollette et al. (2020), laboratory animal personnel with less control over euthanasia reported having higher compassion fatigue, suggesting that "it may be important for laboratory animal personnel to be able to make the decision concerning whether they are the one to euthanize the animals they have cared for" (LaFollette et al., 2020, p. 9). A veterinary social worker could provide guidance with the decision-making and follow-up with grief counseling should it be desired.

The consequences of caring for laboratory animals, both moral and emotional, should not be ignored, minimized, or dismissed (Coleman, 2011). When the grief associated with the euthanasia of animals is openly acknowledged and supported, both caregivers and institutions benefit (Coleman, 2011). Some institutions provide access to counseling resources (Gluckman & Rosenbaum, 2017b; Newsome et al., 2019; Brown et al., 2018). With expertise in euthanasia stress, grief and loss, and compassion fatigue, as well as the human-animal bond, veterinary social workers are uniquely positioned to provide such counseling. To be effective, counselors need to be knowledgeable in these areas (Newsome et al., 2019), and when they are, their guidance and support can be invaluable. Social workers can also be instrumental in helping to identify those with greater emotional vulnerability, fewer adaptive coping strategies, an intensified connection with the animals in their care, and/or a deeper desire to relieve suffering, as these individuals may be at greater risk of experiencing difficulties (Newsome et al., 2019). They can also foster an environment that encourages open dialogue about euthanasia and its effects on health and well-being to broaden social support (Newsome et al., 2019). For institutions desiring counseling resources, innovative partnerships with institutions of higher education and with students training in social work, psychology, or psychiatry may be an option (Gluckman & Rosenbaum, 2017b).

Increasingly institutions are developing programs of remembrance to honor the "animal heroes" that have contributed their lives for scientific advancement and bettering human and animal health (Herzog, 2002; Iliff, 2002; Brown et al., 2018; Newsome et al., 2019). Some hold organized "ceremonies," such as monthly or annual memorial or recognition services, which publicly acknowledge the debt owed to the animals and legitimize the relationship bonds and grief felt by the personnel (Newsome et al., 2019; Iliff, 2002). Others create a dedicated quiet place, such as a garden, often with a plaque or monument, where personnel can take the time to reflect (Brown et al., 2018; Nishikawa & Morishita, 2012; Dickens, 2013; Wenting, 2016). Opportunities to remember and reflect not only acknowledge and support the grief associated with euthanasia but also provide the chance to share feelings in a supportive environment (Lynch & Slaughter, 2001; Iliff, 2002; Coleman, 2011).

Although most studies necessitate euthanasia (for final tissue or data collection, etc.), not all do. A proactive way to help personnel cope is to have programs for rehoming animals (Brown et al., 2018). Such programs can engage employees who are not caregivers to assist in the steps needed before adoption (e.g., socialization), making rehoming a high-profile aspect of an institution's animal care and use program (Bratcher, 2014; Bratcher et al., 2012; Carbone et al., 2003). Such programs improve not only the welfare of laboratory animals but also the professional quality of life of laboratory personnel (LaFollette et al., 2020).

Provide Therapeutic Interventions for Occupational Stress Therapeutic interventions for occupational stress tend to focus on psychoeducation and improving resources and coping skills through the development of self-awareness, reflection, relational skills, and relaxation techniques (Rank et al., 2009; Soni et al., 2015; Unsworth et al., 2010; Regehr et al., 2014; Ruotsalainen et al., 2008). The predominant form of intervention for compassion fatigue is psychoeducation (Flarity et al., 2013; Meadors & Lamson, 2008; Potter et al., 2013). While there is little research documenting the effectiveness of occupational stress interventions in the animal care community, preliminary evidence suggests that these interventions are beneficial, with reports of reduced stress, anxiety, and burnout (Rohlf, 2018). Until such interventions gain ground, and the efficacy is established, it seems appropriate to follow the programming in other occupational sectors, where the efficacy is better understood (Rohlf, 2018).

A program for human care providers that was proven to be effective in reducing stress and anxiety, improving quality of life, and building resilience was the Stress Management and Resiliency Training program (Sood et al., 2014). It consisted of one 90-min group session intervention. Based on what is known and offered in other occupational sectors, it is "programs that incorporate psychoeducation, coping skills training, and relaxation methods within a cognitive-behavioral orientation with possible mindfulness-based approaches" that offer the animal care community a useful starting point from which to base future interventions (Rohlf, 2018). When workers are provided the knowledge, skills, and attitudes to better manage the many sources and types of occupational stress to which they are exposed, they will be better prepared and enabled to mitigate euthanasia stress and compassion fatigue – and sustain well-being (Dunn et al., 2019).

With expertise in stress management from a person-in-environment perspective, veterinary social workers are well positioned to broaden awareness of occupational stress and its detrimental effects and teach stress management and coping skills to support employee resilience. A social worker could develop a customized intervention program or subcontract specialized services, incorporating the learnings into the organization. Professional associations may also offer resources to help animal care providers cope with the demands of compassionate work. Recognizing the need for greater awareness, many associations (e.g., American Veterinary Medical Association, Humane Society of the U.S., American Association for Laboratory Animal Science) are doing their part with educational campaigns, online resources, and continuing education opportunities. For example, the American Veterinary Medical Association offers a variety of online resources, including self-assessment tools, recommendations on how and when to seek assistance, and information on self-care and stress management (see avma.org/wellness) (American Veterinary Medical Association, 2021). Professional associations are increasingly aware of the mental health challenges faced with occupational stress (Polachek & Wallace, 2018).

Enhance Social Support Social support is essential for good physical and mental health (Ozbay et al., 2007; Southwick et al., 2005). Low social support has been strongly associated with stress, anxiety, depression, and posttraumatic stress disorder (PTSD), as well as medical morbidity and mortality (Southwick et al., 2005). High social support, on the other hand, plays a key role in reducing stress and appears to have protective and buffering effects on mental and physical illness (Ozbay et al., 2007; Southwick et al., 2005). Though both are important, the *quality* of relationships is a better predictor of good health than the *quantity* of relationships (Southwick et al., 2005).

Research has demonstrated that workplace environments that build strong, supportive social networks can help reduce the risk of secondary traumatic stress and burnout (Lakey & Cohen, 2000; Choi, 2011). When workers feel supported, heard, and cared about, they tend to exhibit fewer stress-related symptoms (such as distress, fatigue, and burnout) (van der Ploeg & Kleber, 2003). Hence, interventions that promote connectedness, social support, and strong working relationships have the potential to enhance resilience (Dunn et al., 2019; Southwick et al., 2005).

A key intervention is to encourage peer support, debriefing, and regular check-ins, enabling workers to safely discuss the impact of their work on their personal and professional lives (Mathieu, 2007a). Being able to share narratives of the painful and difficult experiences permits workers to put these experiences behind them and, in this, ameliorate the stressful effects (Baranowsky et al., 2011). It also gives rise to normalization, strengthening the connections with one another and reducing isolation (McArthur et al., 2017a; Coleman, 2011; American Association for Laboratory Animal Science, 2013). Beyond this, and importantly, it enables workers to exchange ideas on how they personally manage the day-to-day difficulties as well as the more significant challenges of moral di/stress, burnout, and compassion fatigue (Newsome et al., 2019; Pavan et al., 2020). Social support can also be accessed through in-person and online support groups, also known as self-help or mutual aid groups, focused on stress, mental health, and wellness (Dunn et al., 2019; Rogelberg et al., 2007; Rhoades, 2002; LaFollette et al., 2020). Online support groups are cost-effective and have been shown to help enhance self-efficacy

(Barak et al., 2008; Rains & Young, 2009). Workers can also be encouraged to identify their natural social support systems, such as family, trusted friends, personal mentors, and pets, also key to resilience (Newsome et al., 2019; Cake et al., 2017; LaFollette et al., 2020).

Many workers do not understand that being a care provider necessitates the responsibility to develop and maintain a support network (Gentry & Baranowsky, 2013). Most unconsciously assume that others will spontaneously provide the support that they need when they need it. Thus, it is important to highlight this and help workers recruit, train, maintain, and utilize their own personal social support system (e.g., peers, supervisors, mentors, family, friends, and pets) (Gentry & Baranowsky, 2013; Newsome et al., 2019). Veterinary social workers can play an integral role with this, as well as skillfully facilitating peer support, debriefing, and check-ins (LaFollette et al., 2020; Dunn et al., 2019).

In a systematic review of workplace stress in animal care workers, social support was identified as crucial to minimizing workplace stress (Scotney et al., 2015). In fact, social support is one of the key predictors of whether a worker will stay well or suffer (Fisher & Abrahamson, 2002). Intentionally building a community from which workers can draw support is an essential element of resilience (Gentry & Baranowsky, 2013).

Develop a Wellness Culture and Program Wellness is defined as "an *active process* through which people become aware of, and make choices toward, a more successful existence" (National Wellness Institute, 2020). Wellness is about being responsible and accountable and living consciously (Ardell, 1999). It is a choice. *And* it is about potential – about moving toward the highest state of health and well-being of which one is capable. Wellness is not just a matter of individual responsibility, but also social responsibility, because, for better or worse, through mutual influence, health behaviors spread from person to person (Christakis & Fowler, 2009). A person's social environment can enable or limit their wellness (McLeroy et al., 1988). (For a detailed discussion of veterinary wellness and well-being, see Volk's discussion in Chap. 11 of this volume.)

In recent years, as organizations have increasingly recognized the role that the workplace can play in supporting worker health, wellness has moved into the workplace. In organizations with a wellness culture, having healthy people is a top priority. Although occupational stress cannot be eliminated, wellness initiatives can be introduced to reduce the stress and prevent the stressors from wearing workers down. Wellness programs make collective resilience possible.

Wellness programs can incorporate anything that supports worker health and well-being. From increasing awareness of occupational stress and its consequences to focusing on strategies to enhance resilience, including attention to personal resources and coping strategies (Cake et al., 2017), self-care, mindfulness, self-compassion, compassion, and compassion satisfaction, and reducing workplace and euthanasia stress, offering therapeutic interventions, and enhancing social support, each component can make a difference. Workplace wellness can also include an employee assistance program (EAP) (Newsome et al., 2019; Pavan et al., 2020; Polachek & Wallace, 2018). EAPs assist workers and their family members with personal and/or work-related problems that may impact their job performance, physical health, and mental and emotional well-being (Wikipedia, 2021; Azzone et al., 2009). They generally offer confidential assessments, short-term counseling, referrals, and follow-up services, although some offer health promotion education on health, fitness, nutrition, and mental health as well (Kotschessa, 1995).

Wellness initiatives within a wellness culture create healthy organizations with healthy people who can meet their mandate and achieve their goals. Social workers can play a vital role in establishing and supporting a wellness culture and program, built on strengths and customized to the needs and interests of the organization.

Summary

Compassion is a core value and ethical imperative within any helping profession and the essential quality in caring for others. Compassionate work can be greatly rewarding yet also costly. It can incur a cost, "the cost of caring" commonly known as compassion fatigue. For those in the animal care community, compassion fatigue has come to be recognized as a significant stress-related occupational hazard.

Compassion fatigue arises in relation to the stress associated with the nature of the work and the field of care – in the animal care community, the fields of animal health, animal welfare, and biomedical research. The symptoms and consequences can vary from person to person and within different contexts. In order to address compassion fatigue, it needs to be recognized. Thus, it is imperative to become aware of the symptoms – and the personal, professional, and organizational consequences.

Although compassion fatigue cannot be prevented, it can be mitigated, transformed, and treated. This is centered in the concept of resilience, which starts with compassion fatigue awareness, and grows with implementing personal and organizational approaches, strategies, and practices. Importantly, resilience in the animal care community can be built on the back of veterinary social work. Compassion fatigue is one of the key competencies of veterinary social work. By attending to the causes, signs, and consequences of compassion fatigue, veterinary social workers can support the health and well-being of those who work in animal care and promote personal, interpersonal, and organizational resilience.

The animal care community can only benefit from acknowledging the existence of compassion fatigue and promoting sustainable personal and organizational approaches, strategies, and practices to reduce the risk and build resilience. Confronting compassion fatigue and its consequences is an ongoing challenge, but one wherein great gains can be made, especially with the expertise, guidance, and support of veterinary social work.

References

Alkema, K., Linton, J. M., & Davies, R. (2008). A study of the relationship between self-care, compassion satisfaction, compassion fatigue, and burnout among hospice professionals. *Journal of Social Work in End-of-Life & Palliative Care, 4*(2), 101–119. https://doi.org/10.1080/15524250802353934

American Association for Laboratory Animal Science (AALAS). (2013). *Cost of caring: Recognizing human emotions in the care of laboratory animals.* AALAS.

American Society for the Prevention of Cruelty to Animals. (2021). *Pet statistics.* https://www.aspca.org/animal-homelessness/shelter-intake-and-surrender/pet-statistics. Accessed 19 Feb 2021.

American Veterinary Medical Association. (2021). *Wellbeing resources for veterinary professionals | American Veterinary Medical Association* (avma.org) or https://www.avma.org/resources-tools/wellbeing. Accessed 2 May 2021.

Andrukonis, A., & Protopopova, A. (2020). Occupational health of animal shelter employees by live release rate, shelter type, and euthanasia-related decision. *Anthrozoös, 33*(1), 119–131. https://doi.org/10.1080/08927936.2020.1694316

Animal Euthanasia Statistics. (2021). *Animal euthanasia statistics [2021]: Shelter data by year (spots.com).* https://spots.com/animal-euthanasia-statistics/. Accessed 19 Feb 2021.

Ardell, D. B. (1999). *14 days to wellness: The easy, effective, and fun way to optimum health.* New World Library.

Arkow, P. (2020). Human-animal relationships and social work: Opportunities beyond the veterinary environment. *Child & Adolescent Social Work Journal, 37*, 573–588. https://doi.org/10.1007/s10560-020-00697-x

Arluke, A. (1994). Managing emotions in an animal shelter. In A. Manning & J. Serpell (Eds.), *Animals and human society* (pp. 145–165). Routledge.

Arluke, A. (1999). Uneasiness among laboratory technicians. *Occupational Medicine (Philadelphia, Pa.), 14*(2), 305–316. PMID: 10329907.

Atanes, A. C., Andreoni, S., Hirayama, M. S., Montero-Marin, J., Barros, V. V., Ronzani, T. M., et al. (2015). Mindfulness, perceived stress, and subjective well-being: A correlational study in primary care health professionals. *BMC Complementary and Alternative Medicine, 15*, 303. https://doi.org/10.1186/s12906-015-0823-0

Azzone, V., McCann, B., Merrick, E., Hiatt, D., Hodgkin, D., & Horgan, C. (2009). Workplace stress, organizational factors and EAP utilization. *Journal of Workplace Behavioral Health, 24*(3), 344–356. https://doi.org/10.1080/15555240903188380

Baker, K. (2004). Benefits of positive human interaction for socially housed chimpanzees. *Animal Welfare, 13*, 239–245. https://doi.org/10.1016/j.applanim.2009.05.007

Barak, A., Boniel-Nissim, M., & Suler, J. (2008). Fostering empowerment in online support groups. *Computers in Human Behavior, 24*(5), 1867–1883. https://doi.org/10.1016/j.chb.2008.02.004

Baran, B. E., Allen, J. A., Rogelberg, S. G., Spitzmüller, C., DiGiacomo, N. A., Webb, J. B., et al. (2009). Euthanasia-related strain and coping strategies in animal shelter employees. *Journal of the American Veterinary Medical Association, 235*(1), 83–88.

Baran, B. E., Rogelberg, S. G., Lopina, E. C., Allen, J. A., Spitzmüller, C., & Bergman, M. (2012). Shouldering a silent burden: The toll of dirty tasks. *Human Relations, 65*, 597–626. https://doi.org/10.1177/0018726712438063

Baranowsky, A. B., Gentry, J. E., & Schultz, F. (2011). *Trauma practice: Tools for stabilization & recovery* (2nd ed.). Hogrefe.

Barnard, L. K., & Curry, J. F. (2011). Self-compassion: Conceptualizations, correlates, & interventions. *Review of General Psychology, 15*(4), 289–303. https://doi.org/10.1037/a0025754

Bartram, D. J., & Baldwin, D. S. (2008). Veterinary surgeons and suicide: Influences, opportunities and research directions. *Veterinary Record, 162*, 36–40. https://doi.org/10.1136/vr.162.2.36

Bartram, D., & Boniwell, I. (2007). The science of happiness: Achieving sustained psychological well-being. *In Practice, 29*(8), 478–482. https://doi.org/10.1136/inpract.29.8.478

Bartram, D. J., Yadegarfar, G., & Baldwin, D. S. (2009). Psychosocial working conditions and work-related stressors among UK veterinary surgeons. *Occupational Medicine, 59*(5), 334–341.

Batchelor, C. E., & McKeegan, D. E. (2012). Survey of the frequency and perceived stressfulness of ethical dilemmas encountered in UK veterinary practice. *Veterinary Record, 170*, 19. https://doi.org/10.1136/vr.100262

Bayne, K. (2002). Development of the human-research animal bond and its impact on animal well-being. *ILAR Journal, 43*(1), 4–9. https://doi.org/10.1093/ilar.43.1.4

Bayne, K., Dexter, S. L., & Strange, G. M. (1993). The effects of food treat provisioning and human interaction on the behavioral well-being of rhesus monkeys (*Macaca mulatta*). *Contemporary Topics in Laboratory Animal Science, 33*(2), 6–9. PMID: 16471479.

Beltman, S., Mansfield, C., & Price, A. (2011). Thriving not just surviving: A review of research on teacher resilience. *Educational Research Review, 6*(3), 185–207. https://doi.org/10.1016/j.edurev.2011.09.001

Bloomsmith, M. A., Lambeth, S. P., Stone, A. M., & Laule, G. E. (1997). Comparing two types of human interaction as enrichment for chimpanzees. *American Journal of Primatology, 42*, 96.

Borsook, D., Linnman, C., Faria, V., Strassman, A. M., Becerra, L., & Elman, I. (2016). Reward deficiency and anti-reward in pain chronification. *Neuroscience & Biobehavioral Reviews, 68*, 282–297.

Brannick, E. M., DeWilde, C. A., Frey, E., Gluckman, T. L., Keen, J. L., Larsen, M. R., et al. (2015). Taking stock and making strides toward wellness in the veterinary workplace. *Journal of the American Veterinary Medical Association, 247*(7), 739–742. https://doi.org/10.2460/javma.247.7.739

Bratcher, N.A. (2014). *Adoption of research beagles: Considerations for creating a successful adoption program.* Presented at MSMR Enrichment Symposium, Newton, MA.

Bratcher, N., Cohan, J., Von Sande, T., Morgan, S., & Medina, S. (2012). Enhanced dog socialization and adoption program: Improved animal welfare and improved employee morale. *Journal of the American Association for Laboratory Animal Science: JAALAS, 51*(5), 680–680.

Broussard, L., & Myers, R. (2010). School nurse resilience: Experiences after multiple natural disasters. *The Journal of School Nursing, 26*(3), 203–211. https://doi.org/10.1177/1059840509358412

Brown, K. W., & Ryan, R. M. (2003). The benefits of being present: Mindfulness and its role in psychological Well-being. *Journal of Personality and Social Psychology, 84*(4), 822–848. https://doi.org/10.1037/0022-3514.84.4.822

Brown, M. J., Symonowicz, C., Medina, L. V., Bratcher, N. A., Buckmaster, C. A., Klein, H., et al. (2018). Culture of care: Organizational responsibilities. In R. H. Weichbrod, G. A. H. Thompson, & J. N. Norton (Eds.), *Management of animal care and use programs in research, education, and testing* (2nd ed.). CRC Press/Taylor & Francis. https://doi.org/10.1201/9781315152189-2. https://www.ncbi.nlm.nih.gov/books/NBK500402/. Accessed 21 Apr 2021.

Cake, M. A., McArthur, M. M., Matthew, S. M., & Mansfield, C. F. (2017). Finding the balance: Uncovering resilience in the veterinary literature. *Journal of Veterinary Medical Education, 44*(1), 95–105. https://doi.org/10.3138/jvme.0116-025R

Canadian Veterinary Medical Association. *ProQOL.* https://www.canadianveterinarians.net/documents/ProQOL-assessment-EN OR Microsoft Word - ProQOL_5_English_Self-Score_3_2012 (canadianveterinarians.net). Accessed 30 Apr 2021.

Carbone, L., Guanzini, L., & McDonald, C. (2003). Adoption options for laboratory animals. *Lab Animal, 32*(11), 37–41. https://doi.org/10.1038/laban1003-37

Centers for Disease Control and Prevention (CDC). *Workplace health model.* https://www.cdc.gov/workplacehealthpromotion/model/index.html. Accessed 28 Jan 2021.

Chang, F. T., & Hart, L. H. (2002). Human-animal bonds in the laboratory: How animal behavior affects the perspectives of caregivers. *ILAR Journal, 43*(1), 10–18. https://doi.org/10.1093/ilar.43.1.10

Choi, G.-Y. (2011). Organizational impacts on the secondary traumatic stress of social workers assisting family violence or sexual assault survivors. *Administration in Social Work, 35*(3), 225–242. https://doi.org/10.1080/03643107.2011.575333

Christakis, N. A., & Fowler, J. H. (2009). *Connected: The surprising power of our social networks and how they shape our lives*. Little Brown and Company.

Chur-Hansen, A. (2010). Grief and bereavement issues and the loss of a companion animal: People living with a companion animal, owners of livestock, and animal support workers. *Clinical Psychologist, 14*(1), 14–21. https://doi.org/10.1080/13284201003662800

Coe, J. B., Adams, C. L., & Bonnett, B. N. (2007). A focus group study of veterinarians' and pet owners' perceptions of the monetary aspects of veterinary care. *Journal of the American Veterinary Medical Association, 231*(10), 1510–1518. https://doi.org/10.2460/javma.231.10.1510

Cohen, S. P. (2007). Compassion fatigue and the veterinary health team. *Veterinary Clinics of North America: Small Animal Practice, 37*(1), 123–134. https://doi.org/10.1016/j.cvsm.2006.09.006

Coleman, K. (2011). Caring for nonhuman primates in biomedical research facilities: Scientific, moral and emotional considerations. *American Journal of Primatology, 73*(3), 220–225. https://doi.org/10.1002/ajp.20855

Compassion Fatigue & Conflict Management. (2021). *Veterinary Social Work*. http://vetsocialwork.utk.edu/about-us/compassion-fatigue-management/. Accessed 21 Apr 2021.

Compassion It. *About Us - Compassion It*. https://compassionit.com/about-us/. Accessed 21 Apr 2021.

Coté, S. (2005). A social interaction model of the effects of emotion regulation on work strain. *Academy of Management Review, 30*(3), 509–530. https://doi.org/10.5465/amr.2005.17293692

Dasan, S., Gohil, P., Cornelius, V., & Taylor, C. (2015). Prevalence, causes and consequences of compassion satisfaction and compassion fatigue in emergency care: A mixed-methods study of UK NHS consultants. *Emergency Medicine Journal, 32*(8), 588–594. https://doi.org/10.1136/emermed-2014-203671

Davies, K., & Lewis, D. (2010). Can caring for laboratory animals be classified as emotional labour? *Animal Technology and Welfare, 9*(1), 1–6.

de Vignemont, F., & Singer, T. (2006). The empathic brain: How, when and why? *Trends in Cognitive Science, 10*, 435–441.

Dickens, D. (2013). Russian scientists build monument to honor lab rats. *BuzzFeed*. http://www.buzzfeed.com/donnad/russian-scientists-build-monument-to-honor-lab-rats#.jhOvwr60GL. Accessed 21 Apr 2021.

Dicks, M., & Bain, B. (2016). Chipping away of the soul: New data on compassion fatigue—and compassion satisfaction—in veterinary medicine. *DVM360 Magazine*. https://www.avma.org/PracticeManagement/BusinessIssues/Documents/2016-Nov-29_Chipping-away-of-the-soul_New-data-on-compassion-fatigue_and-compassion-satisfaction_in-veterinary-medicine.pdf. Accessed 19 Feb 2021.

Diestel, S., & Schmidt, K. H. (2011). Costs of simultaneous coping with emotional dissonance and self-control demands at work: Results from two German samples. *Journal of Applied Psychology, 96*(3), 643–653. https://doi.org/10.1037/a0022134

Dow, M. Q., Chur-Hansen, A., Hamood, W., & Edwards, S. (2019). Impact of dealing with bereaved clients on the psychological wellbeing of veterinarians. *Australian Veterinary Journal, 97*, 382–389. https://doi.org/10.1111/avj.12842

Dunn, J., Best, C., Pearl, D. L., & Jones-Bitton, A. (2019). Occupational stressors and desired changes for wellness amongst employees at a Canadian animal welfare organization. *The Canadian Veterinary Journal, 60*(4), 405–413.

Egan, H., Mantzios, M., & Jackson, C. (2017). Health practitioners and the directive towards compassionate healthcare in the UK: Exploring the need to educate health practitioners on how to be self-compassionate and mindful alongside mandating compassion towards patients. *Health Professions Education, 3*(2), 61–63. https://doi.org/10.1016/j.hpe.2016.09.002

Employee assistance program. Wikipedia. (2021). *Employee assistance program – Wikipedia*. Accessed 2 May 2021.

Fernando, A. T., Arroll, B., & Consedine, N. S. (2016). Enhancing compassion in general practice: it's not all about the doctor. *British Journal of General Practice, 66*(648), 340–341.

Figley, C. R. (1982). Traumatization and comfort: Close relationships may be hazardous to your health. In *Keynote presentation at the conference, families and close relationships: Individuals in social interaction*. Texas Tech University, Lubbock.

Figley, C. R. (1995). *Compassion fatigue: Coping with secondary traumatic stress disorder*. Brunner/Mazel.

Figley, C. R. (Ed.). (2002). *Treating compassion fatigue*. Brunner/Routledge.

Figley, C. R., & Roop, R. G. (2006). *Compassion fatigue in the animal care community*. The Humane Society of the United States.

Fisher, P., & Abrahamson, K. (2002). *When working hurts: Stress, burnout and trauma in human, emergency and health services*. Spectrum Press.

Flarity, K., Gentry, J. E., & Mesnikoff, N. (2013). The effectiveness of an educational program on preventing and treating compassion fatigue in emergency nurses. *Advanced Emergency Nursing Journal, 35*(3), 247–258. https://doi.org/10.1097/TME.0b013e31829b726f

Flook, L., Goldberg, S., Pinger, L., Bonus, K., & Davidson, R. (2013). Mindfulness for teachers: A pilot study to assess effects on stress, burnout, and teaching efficacy. *Mind, Brain, and Education, 7*(3), 182–195. https://doi.org/10.1111/mbe.12026

Fogle, B., & Abrahamson, D. (1990). Pet loss: A survey of the attitudes and feelings of practicing veterinarians. *Anthrozoös, 3*(3), 143–150. https://doi.org/10.2752/089279390787057568

Fortney, L., Luchterhand, C., Zakletskaia, L., Zgierska, A., & Rakel, D. (2013). Abbreviated mindfulness intervention for job satisfaction, quality of life, and compassion in primary care clinicians: A pilot study. *Annals of Family Medicine, 11*(5), 412–420.

Foster, S. M., & Maples, E. H. (2014). Occupational stress in veterinary support staff. *Journal of Veterinary Medical Education, 41*(1), 102–110.

Fredrickson, B. L., Cohn, M. A., Coffey, K. A., Pek, J., & Finkel, S. M. (2008). Open hearts build lives: Positive emotions, induced through loving-kindness meditation, build consequential personal resources. *Journal of Personal and Social Psychology, 95*(5), 1045–1062. https://doi.org/10.1037/a0013262

Freudenberger, H. J. (1974). Staff burnout. *Journal of Social Issues, 30*, 159–165.

Frommer, S. S., & Arluke, A. (1999). Loving them to death: Blame-displacing strategies of animal shelter workers and surrenderers. *Society and Animals, 7*(1), 1–16. https://doi.org/10.1163/156853099X00121

Gardner, D. H., & Hini, D. (2006). Work-related stress in the veterinary profession in New Zealand. *New Zealand Veterinary Journal, 54*, 119–124.

Gentry, J. E., & Baranowsky, A. B. (2013). *Compassion fatigue resiliency – A new attitude*. https://www.psychink.com/ti2012/wp-content/uploads/2013/10/Compassion-Resiliency-A-New-Attitude.pdf. Accessed 28 Apr 2021.

Gentry, J. E., Baggerly, J. J., & Baranowsky, A. B. (2004). Training-as-treatment: The effectiveness of the certified compassion fatigue specialist training. *International Journal of Emergency Mental Health, 6*(3), 147–155.

Geppert, C. M. A., & Pies, R. W. (2019). Compassion in clinical care. *OBM Integrative and Complementary Medicine, 4*(1), 8. https://doi.org/10.21926/obm.icm.1901016

Gluckman, T., & Rosenbaum, M. (2017a). Compassion fatigue in our community. *Laboratory Animal Science Professional*, March, (Part I), 15–16.

Gluckman, T., & Rosenbaum, M. (2017b). Compassion fatigue in our community. *Laboratory Animal Science Professional*, May issue (Part II), (no page numbers).

Grandey, A. A. (2003). When "the show must go on": Surface acting and deep acting as determinants of emotional exhaustion and peer-rated service delivery. *Academy of Management Journal, 46*(1), 86–96. https://doi.org/10.5465/30040678

Hanrahan, C., Sabo, B. M., & Robb, P. (2018). Secondary traumatic stress and veterinarians: Human-animal bonds as psychosocial determinants of health. *Traumatology, 24*(1), 73–82.

Hartnack, S., Springer, S., Pittavino, M., & Grimm, H. (2016). Attitudes of Austrian veterinarians towards euthanasia in small animal practice: Impacts of age and gender on views on euthanasia. *BMC Veterinary Research, 12*, 26. https://doi.org/10.1186/s12917-016-0649-0

Hassed, C., de Lisle, S., Sullivan, G., & Pier, C. (2009). Enhancing the health of medical students: Outcomes of an integrated mindfulness and lifestyle program. *Advances in Health Sciences Education: Theory and Practice, 14*(3), 387–398. https://doi.org/10.1007/s10459-008-9125-3

Herzog, H. (2002). Ethical aspects of relationships between humans and research animals. *Institute for Laboratory Animal Research – ILAR Journal, 43*(1), 27–32. https://doi.org/10.1093/ilar.43.1.27

Hewson, C. (2014). Grief for pets – Part 2: Avoiding compassion fatigue. *Veterinary Nursing Journal, 29*, 388–391. https://doi.org/10.1111/vnj.12199

Hill, E. M., LaLonde, C. M., & Reese, L. A. (2020). Compassion fatigue in animal care workers. *Traumatology, 26*(1), 96–108. https://doi.org/10.1037/trm0000218

Hoad, T. (Ed.). (1996). *Oxford concise dictionary of English etymology.* Oxford University Press. http://www.oxfordreference.com/view/10.1093/acref/9780192830982.001.0001/acref-9780192830982-e-3125?rskey=iHDCC9 & result=1. Accessed 28 Jan 2021.

Holcombe, T. M., Strand, E., Nugent, W. R., & Ng, Z. Y. (2016). Veterinary social work: Practice within veterinary settings. *Journal of Human Behavior in the Social Environment, 26*, 69–80.

Hooper, C., Craig, J., Janvrin, D. R., Wetsel, M. A., & Reimels, E. (2010). Compassion satisfaction, burnout, and compassion fatigue among emergency nurses compared with nurses in other selected inpatient specialties. *Journal of Emergency Nursing, 36*(5), 420–427. https://doi.org/10.1016/j.jen.2009.11.027

Hoy-Gerlach, J., Delgado, M., Sloane, H., & Arkow, P. (2019). Rediscovering connections between animal welfare and human welfare: Creating social work internships at a humane society. *Journal of Social Work, 19*(2), 216–232. https://doi.org/10.1177/1468017318760775

Hülsheger, U. R., & Schewe, A. F. (2011). On the costs and benefits of emotional labor: A meta-analysis of three decades of research. *Journal of Occupational Health Psychology, 16*(3), 361–389. https://doi.org/10.1037/a0022876

Hurley, E. A. (2015). *From the director: Shedding light on compassion fatigue.* https://blog.primr.org/from-director-shedding-light-on/. Accessed 19 Feb 2021.

Iliff, S. A. (2002). An additional "R": Remembering the animals. *Institute for Laboratory Animal Research – ILAR Journal, 43*(1), 38–47. https://doi.org/10.1093/ilar.43.1.38

Indregard, A.-M. R., Knardahl, S., & Nielsen, M. B. (2018). Emotional dissonance, mental health complaints, and sickness absence among health- and social workers. The moderating role of self-efficacy. *Frontiers in Psychology, 9*, 592. https://doi.org/10.3389/fpsyg.2018.00592

International Association of Veterinary Social Work. (2021). https://veterinarysocialwork.org/. Accessed 21 Apr 2021.

Irvine, L. (2002). Animal problems/people skills: Emotional and interactional strategies in humane education. *Society and Animals, 10*(1), 63–91. https://doi.org/10.1163/156853002760030888

Ivancevich, J. M., Matteson, M. T., Freedman, S. M., & Phillips, J. S. (1990). Worksite stress management interventions. *American Psychologist, 45*(2), 252–261. https://doi.org/10.1037/0003-066X.45.2.252

Jameton, A. (1984). *Nursing practice, the ethical issues.* Prentice-Hall.

Jameton, A. (2017). What moral distress in nursing history could suggest about the future of health care. *AMA Journal of Ethics, 19*(6), 617–628. https://doi.org/10.1001/journalofethics.2017.19.6.mhst1-1706

Joinson, C. (1992). Coping with compassion fatigue. *Nursing, 22*(4), 116–122, 118–119, 120. https://doi.org/10.1097/00152193-199204000-00035

Kahler, S. C. (2015). Moral stress the top trigger in veterinarians' compassion fatigue: Veterinary social worker suggests redefining veterinarians' ethical responsibility. *Journal of the American Veterinary Medical Association News, 246*, 16–18.

Kakiashvili, T., Leszek, J., & Rutkowski, K. (2013). The medical perspective on burnout. *International Journal of Occupational Medicine and Environmental Health, 26*(3), 401–412. https://doi.org/10.2478/s13382-013-0093-3

Kanov, J. M., Maitlis, S., Worline, M. C., Dutton, J. E., Frost, P. J., & Lilius, J. M. (2004). Compassion in organizational life. *American Behavioral Scientist, 47*(6), 808–827.

Kippermann, B. S., Kass, P. H., & Rishniw, M. (2017). Factors that influence small animal veterinarians' opinions and actions regarding cost of care and effects of economic limitations on patient care and outcome and professional career satisfaction and burnout. *Journal of the American Veterinary Medical Association, 250*(7), 785–794. https://doi.org/10.2460/javma.250.7.785

Klimecki, O., & Singer, T. (2012). Empathic distress fatigue rather than compassion fatigue? Integrating findings from empathy research in psychology and social neuroscience. In B. Oakley, A. Knafo, G. Madhavan, & D. S. Wilson (Eds.), *Pathological altruism* (pp. 1–23). Oxford University Press.

Klimecki, O. M., Leiberg, S., Lamm, C., & Singer, T. (2013). Functional neural plasticity and associated changes in positive affect after compassion training. *Cerebral Cortex, 23*(7), 1552–1561. https://doi.org/10.1093/cercor/bhs142

Kondrat, M. E. (2008). Person-in-environment. In T. Mizrahi & L. E. Davis (Eds.), *Encyclopedia of social work* (20th ed.). Oxford University Press. https://doi.org/10.1093/acrefore/9780199975839.013.285

Kondrup, S. V., Anhøj, K. P., Rødsgaard-Rosenbeck, C., Lund, T. B., Nissen, M. H., & Sandøe, P. (2016). Veterinarian's dilemma: A study of how Danish small animal practitioners handle financially limited clients. *Veterinary Record, 179*(23), 596. https://doi.org/10.1136/vr.103725

Körner, A., Coroiu, A., Copeland, L., Gomez-Garibello, C., Albani, C., Zenger, M., et al. (2015). The role of self-compassion in buffering symptoms of depression in the general population. *PLoS One, 10*(10), e0136598. https://doi.org/10.1371/journal.pone.0136598

Kotschessa, B. (1995). EAP research: The state of the art. *Employee Assistance Quarterly, 10*(2), 63–72. https://doi.org/10.1300/J022v10n02_05

LaFollette, M. R., Riley, M. C., Cloutier, S., Brady, C. M., O'Haire, M. E., & Gaskill, B. N. (2020). Laboratory animal welfare meets human welfare: A cross-sectional study of professional quality of life, including compassion fatigue in laboratory animal personnel. *Frontiers in Veterinary Science, 7*, 114. https://doi.org/10.3389/fvets.2020.00114

Lakey, B., & Cohen, S. (2000). Social support theory and measurement. In S. Cohen, L. G. Underwood, & B. H. Gottlieb (Eds.), *Social support measurement and intervention: A guide for health and social scientists* (pp. 29–52). Oxford University Press.

Lama, D., & Chan, V. (2014). *The wisdom of compassion: Stories of remarkable encounters and timeless insights.* Penguin Group.

Lamm, C., Batson, C. D., & Decety, J. (2007). The neural substrate of human empathy: Effects of perspective-taking and cognitive appraisal. *Journal of Cognitive Neuroscience, 19*, 42–58.

Lee, T. M., Leung, M.-K., Hou, W.-K., Tang, J. C., Yin, J., So, K.-F., et al. (2012). Distinct neural activity associated with focused-attention meditation and loving-kindness meditation. *PLoS One, 7*(8), e40054. https://doi.org/10.1371/journal.pone.0040054

Leiberg, S., Klimecki, O., & Singer, T. (2011). Short-term compassion training increases prosocial behavior in a newly developed prosocial game. *PLoS One, 6*(3), e17798. https://doi.org/10.1371/journal.pone.0017798

Li, A., Early, S. F., Mahrer, N. E., Klaristenfeld, J. L., & Gold, J. I. (2014). Group cohesion and organizational commitment: Protective factors for nurse residents' job satisfaction, compassion fatigue, compassion satisfaction, and burnout. *Journal of Professional Nursing, 30*(1), 89–99. https://doi.org/10.1016/j.profnurs.2013.04.004

Lloyd, C., & Campion, D. P. (2017). Occupational stress and the importance of self-care and resilience: Focus on veterinary nursing. *Irish Veterinary Journal, 70*, 30. https://doi.org/10.1186/s13620-017-0108-7

Lynch, J., & Slaughter, B. (2001). Recognizing animal suffering and death in medicine. *The Western Journal of Medicine, 175*(2), 131–132. https://doi.org/10.1136/ewjm.175.2.131-a

Manciocco, A., Chiarotti, F., & Vitale, A. (2009). Effects of positive interaction with caretakers on the behaviour of socially housed common marmosets (*Callithrix jacchus*). *Applied Animal Behaviour Science, 120*(1–2), 100–107. https://doi.org/10.1016/j.applanim.2009.05.007

Mansfield, C. F., Beltman, S., Broadley, T., & Weatherby-Fell, N. (2016). Building resilience in teacher education: An evidenced informed framework. *Teaching and Teacher Education, 54,* 77–87. https://doi.org/10.1016/j.tate.2015.11.016

Martin, F., & Taunton, A. (2006). Perceived importance and integration of the human-animal bond in private veterinary practice. *Journal of the American Veterinary Medical Association, 228*(4), 522–527. https://doi.org/10.2460/javma.228.4.522

Mascaro, J. S., Kelley, S., Darcher, A., Negi, L. T., Worthman, C., Miller, A., et al. (2018). Meditation buffers medical student compassion from the deleterious effects of depression. *The Journal of Positive Psychology, 13*(2), 133–142. https://doi.org/10.1080/17439760.2016.1233348

Maslach, C., Jackson, S., & Leiter, M. (1996). *Maslach burnout inventory manual* (3rd ed.). Consulting Psychologists Press.

Mastenbroek, N. J. J. M., Jaarsma, A. D. C., Scherpbier, A. J. J. A., van Beukelen, P., & Demerouti, E. (2012). The role of personal resources in explaining well-being and performance: A study among young veterinary professionals. *European Journal of Work and Organizational Psychology, 23*(2), 190–202. https://doi.org/10.1080/1359432X.2012.728040

Mathieu, F. (2007a). Running on empty: Compassion fatigue in health professionals. *Rehabilitation & Community Care Medicine.* http://www.compassionfatigue.org/pages/RunningOnEmpty. pdf. Accessed 28 Apr 2021.

Mathieu, F. (2007b). *Transforming compassion fatigue into compassion satisfaction: Top 12 self-care tips for helpers.* Top 12 self care tips for helpers updated 2016 (tendacademy.ca) or https://www.tendacademy.ca/wp-content/uploads/2018/11/Top-12-self-care-tips-for-helpers-updated-2016.pdf. Accessed 21 Apr 2021.

Mathieu, F. (2011). *The compassion fatigue workbook: Creative tools for transforming compassion fatigue and vicarious traumatization.* Routledge.

McArthur, M., Mansfield, C., Matthew, S., Zaki, S., Brand, C., Andrews, J., et al. (2017a). Resilience in veterinary students and the predictive role of mindfulness and self-compassion. *Journal of Veterinary Medical Education, 44*(1), 106–115. https://doi.org/10.3138/jvme.0116-027R1

McArthur, M. L., Andrews, J. R., Brand, C., & Hazel, S. J. (2017b). The prevalence of compassion fatigue among veterinary students in Australia and the associated psychological factors. *Journal of Veterinary Medical Education, 44*(1), 9–21. https://doi.org/10.3138/jvme.0116-016R3

McCray, L. W., Cronholm, P. F., Bogner, H. R., Gallo, J. J., & Neill, R. A. (2008). Resident physician burnout: Is there hope? *Family Medicine, 40,* 626–632.

McLeroy, K. R., Bibeau, D., Steckler, A., & Glanz, K. (1988). An ecological perspective on health promotion programs. *Health Education & Behavior, 15*(4), 351–377. https://doi. org/10.1177/109019818801500401

McMillan, A. (2021). *Participative management.* Participative Management – organization, levels, style, manager, company, business (referenceforbusiness.com) or https://www.referenceforbusiness.com/management/Or-Pr/Participative-Management.html

Meadors, P., & Lamson, A. (2008). Compassion fatigue and secondary traumatization: Provider self care on intensive care units for children. *Journal of Pediatric Health Care, 22*(1), 24–34. https://doi.org/10.1016/j.pedhc.2007.01.006

Melamed, S., Shirom, A., Toker, S., Berliner, S., & Shapira, I. (2006). Burnout and risk of cardiovascular disease: Evidence, possible causal paths, and promising research directions. *Psychological Bulletin, 132*(3), 327–353. https://doi.org/10.1037/0033-2909.132.3.327

Mellanby, R. J., & Herrtage, M. E. (2004). Survey of mistakes made by recent veterinary graduates. *Veterinary Record, 155,* 761–765. http://veterinaryrecord.bmj.com/content/155/24/761

Mitchener, K. L., & Ogilvie, G. K. (2002). Understanding compassion fatigue: Keys for the caring veterinary healthcare team. *Journal of the American Animal Hospital Association, 38*(4), 307–310. https://doi.org/10.5326/0380307

Moffett, J., Matthew, S., & Fawcett, A. (2015). Building career resilience. *In Practice, 37*(1), 38–41. https://doi.org/10.1136/inp.g3958

Monk, L. (2021). *5 pathways for healing compassion fatigue*. CTRI Crisis & Trauma Resource Institute. https://ca.ctrinstitute.com/blog/5-pathways-healing-compassion-fatigue/. Accessed 28 Apr 2021.

Montero-Marin, J., Tops, M., Manzanera, R., Piva Demarzo, M. M., Álvarez de Mon, M., & García-Campayo, J. (2015). Mindfulness, resilience, and burnout subtypes in primary care physicians: The possible mediating role of positive and negative affect. *Frontiers in Psychology, 6*, 1895. https://doi.org/10.3389/fpsyg.2015.01895

Morris, P. (2012). Managing pet owners' guilt and grief in veterinary euthanasia encounters. *Journal of Contemporary Ethnography, 41*, 337–365. https://doi.org/10.1177/0891241611435099

Morris, J. A., & Feldman, D. C. (1996). The dimensions, antecedents, and consequences of emotional labor. *Academy of Management Review, 21*(4), 986–1010. https://doi.org/10.2307/259161

Moses, L., Malowney, M. J., & Boyd, J. W. (2018). Ethical conflict and moral distress in veterinary practice: A survey of North American veterinarians. *Journal of Veterinary Internal Medicine, 32*, 2115–2122. https://doi.org/10.1111/jvim.15315

Mullan, S., & Fawcett, A. (2017). Veterinary ethics and why it matters. In S. Mullan & A. Fawcett (Eds.), *Veterinary ethics: Navigation tough cases* (pp. 26–30). 5m Publishing.

National Wellness Institute (NWI). (2020). *Six dimensions of wellness*. https://nationalwellness.org/resources/six-dimensions-of-wellness/. Accessed 2 May 2021.

Neff, K. D. (2003a). Self-compassion: An alternative conceptualization of a healthy attitude toward oneself. *Self and Identity, 2*(2), 85–101. https://doi.org/10.1080/15298860309032

Neff, K. D. (2003b). The development and validation of a scale to measure self-compassion. *Self and Identity, 2*(3), 223–250. https://doi.org/10.1080/15298860309027

Neff, K. (2021). *Self-compassion*. self-compassion.org. Accessed 14 Apr 2021.

Neff, K. D., & Germer, C. K. (2013). A pilot study and randomized controlled trial of the mindful self-compassion program. *Journal of Clinical Psychology, 69*(1), 28–44. https://doi.org/10.1002/jclp.21923

Neff, K. D., Kirkpatrick, K. L., & Rude, S. S. (2007). Self-compassion and adaptive psychological functioning. *Journal of Research in Personality, 41*(1), 139–154. https://doi.org/10.1016/j.jrp.2006.03.004

Newsome, J. T., Clemmons, E. A., Fitzhugh, D. C., Gluckman, T. L., Creamer-Hente, M. A., Tambrallo, L. J., et al. (2019). Compassion fatigue, euthanasia stress, and their management in laboratory animal research. *Journal of the American Association for Laboratory Animal Science, 58*(3), 289–292. https://doi.org/10.30802/AALAS-JAALAS-18-000092

Nishikawa, T., & Morishita, N. (2012). Current status of memorial services for laboratory animals in Japan: A questionnaire survey. *Experimental Animals, 61*(2), 177–181. https://doi.org/10.1538/expanim.61.177

Nunberg, G., & Newman, E. (Eds.). (2000). *The American heritage dictionary of the English language*. Houghton Mifflin. https://www.thefreedictionary.com/compassion. Accessed 28 Jan 2021.

O'Connell, M. (2009). *Compassion: Loving our neighbor in an age of globalization*. Orbis Books.

O'Driscoll, M. P., & Cooper, C. L. (2002). Job-related stress and burnout. In P. Warr (Ed.), *Psychology at work* (5th ed., pp. 203–228). Penguin.

Olson, K., Kemper, K. J., & Mahan, J. D. (2015). What factors promote resilience and protect against burnout in first-year pediatric and medicine-pediatric residents? *Journal of Evidence-Based Complementary & Alternative Medicine, 20*(3), 192–198. https://doi.org/10.1177/2156587214568894

OpenLearn. (2017). *Supporting and developing resilience in social work*. The Open University. Social work and resilience - Google Search.

Overhulse, K. A. (2002). Coping with lab animal morbidity and mortality: A trainer's role. *Lab Animal, 31*(6), 39–42.

Owen, R. P., & Wanzer, L. (2014). Compassion fatigue in military healthcare teams. *Archives of Psychiatric Nursing, 28*(1), 2–9. https://doi.org/10.1016/j.apnu.2013.09.007

Ozbay, F., Johnson, D. C., Dimoulas, E., Morgan, C. A., Charney, D., & Southwick, S. (2007). Social support and resilience to stress: From neurobiology to clinical practice. *Psychiatry (Edgmont), 4*(5), 3540.

Panksepp, J. (2011). Cross-species affective neuroscience decoding of the primal affective experiences of humans and related animals. *PLoS One, 6*(9), e21236. https://doi.org/10.1371/journal.pone.0021236

Pavan, A. D., O'Quin, J., Roberts, M. E., & Freed, C. L. (2020). Using a staff survey to customize burnout and compassion fatigue mitigation recommendations in a lab animal facility. *Journal of the American Association for Laboratory Animal Science, JAALAS, 59*(2), 139–147. https://doi.org/10.30802/AALAS-JAALAS-19-000080

Perry, B., Toffner, G., Merrick, T., & Dalton, J. (2011). An exploration of the experience of compassion fatigue in clinical oncology nurses. *Canadian Oncology Nursing Journal, 21*(2), 91–105. https://doi.org/10.5737/1181912x2129197

Platt, B., Hawton, K., Simkin, S., & Mellanby, R. J. (2012). Suicidal behaviour and psychosocial problems in veterinary surgeons: A systematic review. *Social Psychiatry and Psychiatric Epidemiology, 47*, 223–240.

Polachek, A. J., & Wallace, J. E. (2018). The paradox of compassionate work: A mixed-methods study of satisfying and fatiguing experiences of animal health care providers. *Anxiety, Stress, and Coping, 31*(2), 228–243. https://doi.org/10.1080/10615806.2017.1392224

Potter, P., Deshields, T., Berger, J. A., Clarke, M., Olsen, S., & Chen, L. (2013). Evaluation of a compassion fatigue resiliency program for oncology nurses. *Oncology Nursing Forum, 40*(2), 180–187. https://doi.org/10.1188/13.ONF.180-187

Preckel, K., Kanske, P., & Singer, T. (2018). On the interaction of social affect and cognition: Empathy, compassion and theory of mind. *Current Opinion in Behavioral Sciences, 19*, 1–6.

Rabinowitz, P. M., Lefkowitz, R. Y., Conti, L. A., Redlich, C. A., & Weigler, B. J. (2015). Occupational health of laboratory animal workers. In J. G. Fox, G. M. Otto, M. T. Whary, L. C. Anderson, & K. R. Pritchett-Corning (Eds.), *Laboratory animal medicine* (3rd ed., pp. 1382–1401). Academic Press.

Radey, M., & Figley, C. R. (2007). The social psychology of compassion. *Clinical Social Work Journal, 35*(3), 207–214. https://doi.org/10.1007/s10615-007-0087-3

Raes, F. (2010). Rumination and worry as mediators of the relationship between self-compassion and depression and anxiety. *Personality and Individual Differences, 48*(6), 757–761. https://doi.org/10.1016/j.paid.2010.01.023

Rains, S. A., & Young, V. (2009). A meta-analysis of research on formal computer mediated support groups: Examining group characteristics and health outcomes. *Human Communication Research, 35*(3), 309–336. https://doi.org/10.1111/j.1468-2958.2009.01353.x

Rank, M., Zaparanick, T., & Gentry, J. (2009). Non-human animal care compassion fatigue: Training as treatment. *Best Practices in Mental Health, 5*(2), 40–61.

Rathwell-Deault, D., Godard, B., Frank, D., & Doizé, B. (2017). Expected consequences of convenience euthanasia perceived by veterinarians in Quebec. *The Canadian Veterinary Journal, 58*(7), 723–728.

Rees, C. S., Breen, L. J., Cusack, L., & Hegney, D. (2015). Understanding individual resilience in the workplace: The international collaboration of workforce resilience model. *Frontiers in Psychology, 6*, 73. https://doi.org/10.3389/fpsyg.2015.00073

Reese, L. A. (2018). *Strategies for successful animal shelters*. Elsevier.

Reeve, C. L., Spitzmuller, C., Rogelberg, S. G., Walker, A., Schultz, L., & Clark, O. (2004). Employee reactions and adjustment to euthanasia-related work: Identifying turning-point events through retrospective narratives. *Journal of Applied Animal Welfare Science, 7*(1), 1–25. https://doi.org/10.1207/s15327604jaws0701_1

Reeve, C. L., Rogelberg, S. G., Spitzmuller, C., & Digiacomo, N. (2005). The caring-killing paradox: Euthanasia-related strain among animal-shelter workers. *Journal of Applied Social Psychology, 35*(1), 119–143. https://doi.org/10.1111/j.1559-1816.2005.tb02096.x

Regehr, C., Glancy, D., Pitts, A., & LeBlanc, V. R. (2014). Interventions to reduce the consequences of stress in physicians: A review and meta-analysis. *Journal of Nervous and Mental Disease, 202*(5), 353–359. https://doi.org/10.1097/NMD.0000000000000130

Reivich, K. (2008, updated 2010). *The resilience ingredient list*. https://www.cnbc.com/id/25464528/. Accessed 21 June 2021.

Remen, R. N. (1996). *Kitchen table wisdom: Stories that heal*. Penguin.

Reyes, A. T., Andrusyszyn, M., Iwasiw, C., Forchuk, C., & Babenko-Mould, Y. B. (2015). Resilience in nursing education: An integrative review. *The Journal of Nursing Education, 54*(8), 438–444. https://doi.org/10.3928/01484834-20150717-03

Rhoades, R. H. (2002). *The humane Society of the United States euthanasia training manual*. Humane Society Press.

Roberts, J. S. (2015). *Occupational stress in animal shelter workers*. Dissertation, University of Toronto. https://tspace.library.utoronto.ca/bitstream/1807/69236/3/Roberts_Jesse_201506_MA_thesis.pdf. Accessed 19 Feb 2021.

Rogelberg, S. G., DiGiacomo, N., Reeve, C. L., Spitzmuller, C., Clark, O. L., Teeter, L., et al. (2007). What shelters can do about euthanasia-related stress: An examination of recommendations from those on the front line. *Journal of Applied Animal Welfare Science, 10*(4), 331–347. https://doi.org/10.1080/10888700701353865

Rohleder, N. (2016). Chronic stress and disease. In I. Berczi (Ed.), *Insights to neuroimmune biology* (2nd ed., pp. 201–214). Elsevier. https://doi.org/10.1016/B978-0-12-801770-8.00009-4

Rohlf, V. I. (2018). Interventions for occupational stress and compassion fatigue in animal care professionals – a systematic review. *Traumatology, 24*, 186–192. https://doi.org/10.1037/trm0000144

Rohlf, V., & Bennett, P. (2005). Perpetration-induced traumatic stress in persons who euthanize nonhuman animals in surgeries, animal shelters, and laboratories. *Society and Animals, 13*, 201–220. http://dx.doi.org/10 .1163/1568530054927753

Rollin, B. E. (2011). Euthanasia, moral stress, and chronic illness in veterinary medicine. *Veterinary Clinics of North America: Small Animal Practice, 41*, 651–659. https://doi.org/10.1016/j.cvsm.2011.03.005

Ruotsalainen, J., Serra, C., Marine, A., & Verbeek, J. (2008). Systematic review of interventions for reducing occupational stress in health care workers. *Scandinavian Journal of Work, Environment & Health, 34*(3), 169–178. https://doi.org/10.5271/sjweh.1240

Rushton, C. H., Batcheller, J., Schroeder, K., & Donohue, P. (2015). Burnout and resilience among nurses practicing in high-intensity settings. *American Journal of Critical Care, 24*(5), 412–420. https://doi.org/10.4037/ajcc2015291

Sanchez-Reilly, S., Morrison, L. J., Carey, E., Bernacki, R., O'Neill, L., Kapo, J., et al. (2013). Caring for oneself to care for others: Physicians and their self-care. *The Journal of Supportive Oncology, 11*(2), 75–81. https://doi.org/10.12788/j.suponc.0003

Schabram, K., & Maitlis, S. (2017). Negotiating the challenges of a calling: Emotion and enacted sensemaking in animal shelter work. *Academy of Management Journal, 60*, 584–609. https://doi.org/10.5465/amj.2013.0665

Schaufeli, W. B., & Bakker, A. B. (2004). Job demands, job resources, and their relationship with burnout and engagement: A multi-sample study. *Journal of Organizational Behavior, 25*(3), 293–315. https://www.jstor.org/stable/4093692

Schneider, M., & Roberts, J. (2016). Shelter-specific occupational stress among employees in animal shelters. *Human-Animal Interaction Bulletin, 4*(1), 19–38. HABRI Central - Resources: Shelter-specific occupational stress among employees in animal shelters: Supporting Docs. Accessed 19 Feb 2021.

Scotney, R. L., McLaughlin, D., & Keates, H. L. (2015). A systematic review of the effects of euthanasia and occupational stress in personnel working with animals in animal shelters, veterinary clinics, and biomedical research facilities. *Journal of the American Veterinary Medical Association, 247*, 1121–1130. https://doi.org/10.2460/javma.247.10.1121

Shamay-Tsoory, S. G. (2011). The neural bases for empathy. *The Neuroscientist, 17*(1), 18–24. https://doi.org/10.1177/1073858410379268

Shanafelt, T. D., Balch, C. M., Bechamps, G., Russell, T., Dyrbye, L., Satele, D., et al. (2010). Burnout and medical errors among American surgeons. *Annals of Surgery, 251*(6), 995–1000. https://doi.org/10.1097/SLA.0b013e3181bfdab3

Shaw, J. R., Adams, C. L., Bonnett, B. N., Larson, S., & Roter, D. L. (2012). Veterinarian satisfaction with companion animal visits. *Journal of the American Veterinary Medical Association, 240*, 832–841. https://doi.org/10.2460/javma.240.7.832

Shearer, J. K. (2018). Euthanasia of cattle: Practical considerations and application. *Animals, 8*(4), 57. https://doi.org/10.3390/ani8040057

Shonin, E., Van Gordon, W., Compare, A., Zangeneh, M., & Griffiths, M. D. (2015). Buddhist-derived loving-kindness and compassion meditation for the treatment of psychopathology: A systematic review. *Mindfulness, 6*, 1161–1180. https://doi.org/10.1007/s12671-014-0368-1

Showalter, S. E. (2010). Compassion fatigue: What is it? Why does it matter? Recognizing the symptoms, acknowledging the impact, developing the tools to prevent compassion fatigue, and strengthen the professional already suffering from the effects. *American Journal of Hospice & Palliative Medicine, 27*(4), 239–242.

Singer, T., & Klimecki, O. M. (2014). Empathy and compassion. *Current Biology, 24*(18), R875–R878. https://doi.org/10.1016/j.cub.2014.06.054

Smart, D., English, A., James, J., Wilson, M., Daratha, K. B., Childers, B., et al. (2014). Compassion fatigue and satisfaction: A cross-sectional survey among U.S. healthcare workers. *Nursing and Health Sciences, 16*(1), 3–10. https://doi.org/10.1111/nhs.12068

Soni, S. R., Vyas, J. M., Pestonjee, D. M., Kher, H. N., Thakker, K. A., & Vijaya, L. Y. (2015). Impact of the art of living programme on burnout and organizational role stress among animal husbandry personnel. *Journal of Psychiatry, 18*(4), 288.

Sood, A., Sharma, V., Schroeder, D. R., & Gorman, B. (2014). Stress management and resiliency training (SMART) program among department of radiology faculty: A pilot randomized clinical trial. *Explore (New York, N.Y.), 10*(6), 358–363. https://doi.org/10.1016/j.explore.2014.08.002

Southwick, S. M., Vythilingam, M., & Charney, D. S. (2005). The psychobiology of depression and resilience to stress: Implications for prevention and treatment. *Annual Review of Clinical Psychology, 1*, 255–291. https://doi.org/10.1146/annurev.clinpsy.1.102803.143948

Sprang, G., Clark, J. J., & Whitt-Woosley, A. (2007). Compassion fatigue, compassion satisfaction, and burnout: Factors impacting professional's quality of life. *Journal of Loss and Trauma, 12*, 259–280. https://doi.org/10.1080/15325020701238093

Springer, S., Sandoe, P., Lund, T. B., & Grimm, H. (2019). "Patients' interests first, but…"– Austrian veterinarians' attitudes to moral challenges in modern small animal practice. *Animals, 9*(5), 241. https://doi.org/10.3390/ani9050241

Stamm, B. H. (2002). Measuring compassion satisfaction as well as fatigue: Developmental history of the compassion satisfaction and fatigue test. In C. R. Figley (Ed.), *Treating compassion fatigue* (pp. 107–119). Brunner-Routledge.

Stamm, B. H. (2005). *The ProQOL manual.* The professional quality of life scale: Compassion satisfaction, burnout & compassion fatigue/secondary trauma scales. http://www.compassion-fatigue.org/pages/ProQOLManualOct05.pdf. Accessed 28 Jan 2021.

Stamm, B. H. (2010). *The concise ProQOL manual* (2nd ed.). ProQOL.org. https://proqol.org/uploads/ProQOLManual.pdf. Accessed 28 Jan 2021.

Stamm, B. H. *Professional quality of life measure.* https://proqol.org/. Accessed 30 Jan 2021.

Stebnicki, M. A. (2000). Stress and grief reactions among rehabilitation professionals: Dealing effectively with empathy fatigue. *Journal of Rehabilitation, 66*(1), 23–29.

Stephens, U. K. (1996). Human/research animal relationships: Animal staff perspectives. In L. Krulisch, S. Mayer, & R. C. Simmonds (Eds.), *The human/research animal relationship* (pp. 61–65). Scientists Center for Animal Welfare.

Stoewen, D. L. (2019). Moving from compassion fatigue to compassion resilience part 1: Compassion — A health care priority, core value, and ethical imperative. *Canadian Veterinary Journal, 60*, 783–784.

Stoewen, D. L., Coe, J. B., MacMartin, C., Stone, E. A., & Dewey, C. E. (2013). Factors influencing veterinarian referrals to oncology specialists for treatment of dogs with lymphoma and osteosarcoma in Ontario, Canada. *Journal of the American Veterinary Medical Association, 243*(10), 1415–1425.

Tempski, P., Martins, M. A., & Paro, H. B. M. S. (2012). Teaching and learning resilience: A new agenda in medical education. *Medical Education, 46*(4), 345–346. https://doi.org/10.1111/j.1365-2923.2011.04207.x

Thomas, J. T. (2011). *Intrapsychic predictors of professional quality of life: Mindfulness, empathy, and emotional separation [dissertation]*. University of Kentucky.

Thomas, J. (2013). Association of personal distress with burnout, compassion fatigue, and compassion satisfaction among clinical social workers. *Journal of Social Service Research, 39*(3), 365–379. https://doi.org/10.1080/01488376.2013.771596

Thomas, J., Jack, B. A., & Jinks, A. M. (2012). Resilience to care: A systematic review and meta-synthesis of the qualitative literature concerning the experiences of student nurses in adult hospital settings in the UK. *Nurse Education Today, 32*(6), 657–664. https://doi.org/10.1016/j.nedt.2011.09.005

Thompson, I., Amatea, E., & Thompson, E. (2014). Personal and contextual predictors of mental health counselors' compassion fatigue and burnout. *Journal of Mental Health Counseling, 36*(1), 58–77. https://doi.org/10.17744/mehc.36.1.p61m73373m4617r3

Tugade, M. M., & Fredrickson, B. L. (2004). Resilient individuals use positive emotions to bounce back from negative emotional experiences. *Journal of Personality and Social Psychology, 86*(2), 320–333. https://doi.org/10.1037/0022-3514.86.2.320

Ungar, M. (2011). The social ecology of resilience: Addressing contextual and cultural ambiguity of a nascent construct. *American Journal of Orthopsychiatry, 81*(1), 1–17. https://doi.org/10.1111/j.1939-0025.2010.01067.x

Unsworth, K. L., Rogelberg, S. G., & Bonilla, D. (2010). Emotional expressive writing to alleviate euthanasia-related stress. *The Canadian Veterinary Journal, 51*(7), 775–777.

Van Dam, N. T., Sheppard, S. C., Forsyth, J. P., & Earlywine, M. (2011). Self-compassion is a better predictor than mindfulness of symptom severity and quality of life in mixed anxiety and depression. *Journal of Anxiety Disorders, 25*, 123–130. https://doi.org/10.1016/j.janxdis.2010.08.011

van der Ploeg, E., & Kleber, R. J. (2003). Acute and chronic job stressors among ambulance personnel: Predictors of health symptoms. *Occupational and Environmental Medicine, 60*(Suppl), i40–i46. https://doi.org/10.1136/oem.60.suppl_1.i40

van Dernoot Lipsky, L., & Burk, C. (2009). *Trauma stewardship: An everyday guide to caring for self while caring for others*. Berrett-Koehler.

Volk, J. O., Schimmack, U., Strand, E. B., Lord, L. K., & Siren, C. W. (2018). Executive summary of the Merck animal health veterinary wellbeing study. *Journal of the American Veterinary Medical Association, 252*(10), 1231–1238. https://doi.org/10.2460/javma.252.10.1231

Von Dietze, E., & Gardner, D. (2014). Euthanizing wildlife: Experiences and coping strategies among people who conduct euthanasia. *Pacific Conservation Biology, 20*(1), 28–36. https://doi.org/10.1071/PC140028

Wallace J. E. (2014). *Maintaining momentum: How veterinarians and technicians cope*. https://www.canadianveterinarians.net/documents/veterinarian-and-aht-wellness-2014-cvma-convention-presentation. Accessed 21 Apr 2021.

Wallis, J., Fletcher, D., Bentley, A., & Ludders, J. (2019). Medical errors cause harm in veterinary hospitals. *Frontiers in Veterinary Science, 6*, 12. https://doi.org/10.3389/fvets.2019.00012

Warr, P. (2007). *Work, happiness and unhappiness*. Psychology Press.

Warshaw, L. J. (1989). *Stress, anxiety and depression in the workplace* (pp. 1–21). Presented at the conference on stress and anxiety and depression in the workplace, October 18, New York.

Wendt, S., Tuckey, M. R., & Prosser, B. (2011). Thriving, not just surviving, in emotionally demanding fields of practice. *Health and Social Care in the Community, 19*(3), 317–325. https://doi.org/10.1111/j.1365-2524.2010.00983.x

Weng, H. Y., Fox, A. S., Shackman, A. J., Stodola, D. E., Caldwell, J. Z., Olson, M. C., et al. (2013). Compassion training alters altruism and neural responses to suffering. *Psychological Science, 24*(7), 1171–1180. https://doi.org/10.1177/0956797612469537

Wenting, Z. (2016). We have a responsibility to be kind' to lab animals: Expert. *China Daily.* http://usa.chinadaily.com.cn/china/2016-01/17/content_23122942.htm. Accessed 21 Apr 2021.

West, C. P., Huschka, M. M., Novotny, P. J., Sloan, J. A., Kolars, J. C., Habermann, T. M., et al. (2006). Association of perceived medical errors with resident distress and empathy. *Journal of the American Medical Association, 296*(9), 1071–1078. https://doi.org/10.1001/jama.296.9.1071

White, D. J., & Shawhan, R. (1996). Emotional responses of animal shelter workers to euthanasia. *Journal of the American Veterinary Medical Association, 208*(6), 846–849. https://doi.org/10.2460/javma.235.1.83

Williams, J. M. G., & Kabat-Zinn, J. (2011). Mindfulness: Diverse perspectives on its meaning, origins, and multiple applications at the intersection of science and dharma. *Contemporary Buddhism, 12*(1), 1–18. https://doi.org/10.1080/14639947.2011.564811

Wong, C. C. Y., & Mak, W. W. S. (2013). Differentiating the role of three self-compassion components in buffering cognitive-personality vulnerability to depression among Chinese in Hong Kong. *Journal of Counseling Psychology, 60*(1), 162–169. https://doi.org/10.1037/a0030451

World Health Organization (WHO). (2019). *Burn-out an "occupational phenomenon": International Classification of Diseases.* https://www.who.int/news/item/28-05-2019-burn-out-an-occupational-phenomenon-international-classification-of-diseases. Accessed 30 Jan 2021.

Yakl, G., & Van Fleet, D. D. (1992). Theory and research on leadership in organizations. In M. D. Dunnett & L. Hough (Eds.), *Handbook of industrial and organizational psychology* (Vol. 3, pp. 147–197). Consulting Psychologists.

Young, R. L., & Thompson, C. Y. (2019). Exploring empathy, compassion fatigue, and burnout among feral cat caregivers. *Society & Animals, 28*(2), 151–170. https://doi.org/10.1163/15685306-00001704

Zapf, D. (2002). Emotion work and psychological Well-being: A review of the literature and some conceptual considerations. *Human Resource Management Review, 12*(2), 237–268. https://doi.org/10.1016/S1053-4822(02)00048-7

Zapf, D., & Holz, M. (2006). On the positive and negative effects of emotion work in organizations. *European Journal of Work and Organizational Psychology, 15*(1), 1–28. https://doi.org/10.1080/13594320500412199

Zeng, X., Chiu, C. P. K., Wang, R., Oei, T. P. S., & Leung, F. Y. K. (2015). The effect of loving-kindness meditation on positive emotions: A meta-analytic review. *Frontiers in Psychology, 6*, 1693. https://doi.org/10.3389/fpsyg.2015.01693

Chapter 4
The LINK: Violence Toward People and Animals

Susan Hatters Friedman, Renee M. Sorrentino, John Allgire, and Joshua B. Friedman

Introduction

More American homes have pets than children (Vincent et al., 2019). Over two-thirds of American households include a pet (National Pet Owners Survey, 2014). Well-cared-for pets may be protective for human mental health (Arkow, 2015). Most pets are cherished members of the family; however, some people consider animals to be their property. Violence at home can be directed at both pets and family members, and animal cruelty has been described as being a sentinel for family violence (Arkow, 2015).

Amalgamated Case

At your veterinary practice, a Good Samaritan brings in a German shepherd who was loose. The dog appears to be injured and underweight. The dog is limping and has anal abrasions. X-rays reveal healing fractures of various ages. He eats ravenously at your practice.

S. H. Friedman (✉)
Case Western Reserve University School of Medicine, Psychiatry, Cleveland, OH, USA
e-mail: sjh8@case.edu

R. M. Sorrentino
Institute for Sexual Wellness, Weymouth, MA, USA

J. Allgire
Whatcom County Sheriff's Office, Bellingham, WA, USA

J. B. Friedman
Case Western Reserve University School of Medicine, Cleveland, OH, USA

Ownership is eventually established, but it was difficult since the owner did not actively attempt to find the dog. You get a strange feeling when the owner comes in to pick up the dog. He smells of alcohol and is quite irritable, snapping at the front desk staff. You suspect that the owner is the person who has harmed the dog. You start to worry about the future safety of the German shepherd, as well as the home environment in general.

Should you call the police? Should you call the Humane Society? Are you a mandatory reporter? Is a report confidential?

Animal Abuse

"Battered pet syndrome" was initially described in 1996 (Arkow, 2015). Animal abuse may include physical abuse or sexual abuse (described below). Intentional cruelty may include torturing, maiming, mutilating, or killing of an animal (Humane Society, n.d.). Animals may present with unexplained or repetitive injuries, low body weight, unexplained burns, bruises, poisoning, or wounds, for example (Arkow, 2015). Like violence toward humans, animals may suffer various types of non-accidental injuries. Legal definitions of animal cruelty vary by jurisdiction, but tend to include intentional injury or death, and lack of appropriate shelter and nutrition (Vincent et al., 2019).

Animal Neglect

Animal neglect may be more ambiguous in definition than abuse. This may include abandoned pets, animal hoarding, and chained dogs (Humane Society, n.d.). Findings in cases of animal neglect may include a lack of attending to the pet's basic needs (such as food and water, sanitation, shelter, and space) or their medical needs when they are symptomatic or in pain. Various motives for neglect include the owner being lazy or overwhelmed, experiencing a family emergency, or lack of understanding of the animal's needs, but may also include purposeful neglect. Neglect may exist on its own, or may occur together with animal abuse. Animal neglect may, however, be more difficult to prove.

Animal Sexual Abuse

Bestial acts have been described as early as Biblical times and throughout ancient civilization. Despite the long history of bestiality and representation in many cultures, bestiality is an often ignored area in both the legal and scientific literature. One explanation for why the behavior is poorly understood is the overwhelming societal disgust regarding the topic. Learning more about the behavior, however, informs strategies for assessment and intervention.

The term bestiality refers to sexual behavior between humans and animals. Bestiality is considered a criminal behavior in most states and in many countries. The definition of what constitutes the illegal behavior and the punishment varies by jurisdiction. The range of behaviors includes penetrating animals, receiving oral or genital contact from an animal, or the production of animal pornography. The term bestiality itself does not convey information about the motivation, sexual orientation, or clinical features of the individual engaged in the behavior.

A portion of individuals who engage in bestiality are further defined as zoophiles. Zoophilia is defined as sexual attraction to human-animal contact. A zoophile may be diagnosed with the psychiatric disorder of zoophilic disorder if they experience marked distress or impairment in functioning.

The prevalence of bestiality and zoophilia is difficult to determine due to the few studies performed. Early studies by Alfred Kinsey found that 8% of men and 3.6% of women engaged in human-animal sex (Kinsey et al., 1948, 1953). A study in the 1970s found the prevalence of bestial acts in men to be 4.9% and 1.9% in women (Hunt, 1974). Prevalence in specialized populations such as sexual offenders found higher rates of bestial acts ranging from 18% to 43% (Gephard et al., 1965; English et al., 2003; Simons et al., 2008). Among the incarcerated male population, 15% reported bestial acts compared to 8% of the control group (Gephard et al., 1965). The prevalence of zoophilia is not known.

Dogs and cows are the most common animals involved in human-animal sex (Miletski, 2002). Miletski surveyed a group of self-identified zoophiles and found the most common reason for engaging in the behavior to be sexual attraction to animals, affection or "love" for the animal, and curiosity (Miletski, 2002). The range of sexual behaviors include fondling, masturbating, and oral, vaginal, and anal sex.

Beirne (1997) noted that bestiality should be reconceptualized as interspecies sexual assault and that the situation of abused animals actually parallels the situation of abused children and partners. Beirne also noted that coercion often exists, and bestiality can lead to pain or animal death. Further, animals are not able to speak out regarding their own maltreatment (Beirne, 1997). In a typology of interspecies sexual assault, Beirne (1997) noted various types including sexual fixation or zoophilia, commodification of animals, sexual experimentation with animals as an adolescent, and aggravated cruelty.

Parallels between bestiality and pedophilia include the pedophile claiming that the child assented to the behavior, the power differential, and the fact that animals or children are not peers of adults. Adams noted, "Silence is a major problem. Unlike most forms of sexual contact, in which either partner can report the experience, only one of the participants in bestiality can talk." Adams also noted "Relationships of unequal power cannot be consensual. In human-animal relationships, the human being has control of many—if not all—of the aspects of the animal's wellbeing."

Connections

Intersection with Child Maltreatment

The Link between child maltreatment and animal cruelty has been studied for decades since the establishment of a childhood triad of animal cruelty, fire-setting, and enuresis. Yet in practice, abuse of family pets is often an unrecognized part of a more complex web of child abuse, exposure to family violence, and the development of violent interpersonal relationships. Three interacting elements of this link are apparent: co-occurrence of abusive acts toward animals and people in the child's environment, brain chemistry and structure alterations for children raised with traumatic experiences such as exposure to animal cruelty and interpersonal violence, and appearance of different manifestations of modelling, social learning, and innate callous-unemotional traits over the lifespan (Bright et al., 2018; McEwan et al., 2014).

Abuse and threats of abuse to animals in the home may have the purpose to upset or coerce other family members, including children. Adults in the home may have a low frustration tolerance and exhaustion, with a household of dependents such as children and animals. They may have unrealistic expectations of the children and pets—especially with regard to stressful times such as feeding, bathing, crying, and toileting. These similar situations may incite violence toward both the children and the pets. Children may get between abusers and animals to try to protect the animals, and sentient animals may get between abusers and children, and thereby suffer direct physical harm. Out of concern to protect pets and with a widespread lack of refuge options that accept pets, family members who would otherwise leave the abuser and take the children and pets for protection instead stay and risk repeated animal and child abuse.

Research of general, mental health treatment and correctional populations demonstrate that childhood rates of exposure to animal maltreatment vary from 29% to 62% (Monsalve et al., 2017). Among children with exposure to violence between adults in the home, two out of three report abuse of the pets in the home (Monsalve et al., 2017). Nearly all of these children report being upset by this animal abuse. Between one-half and three-quarters of children in such circumstances risk their own safety to intervene in the abuse of pets. Among homes with child abuse substantiated by child protective services, up to four out of five with pets also have animal abuse. Children may then as part of their own survival develop decreased empathy and desensitization to animal suffering and grow to accept—as well as be traumatized by— such an environment. While in rare instances a child may kill their pet in order for the animal's suffering to stop, children who are exposed to animal maltreatment have a three to eight times likelihood of abusing animals themselves (Monsalve et al., 2017).

Conversely, 3–44% of children who have abused animals have themselves been abused (Lee-Kelland & Finlay, 2018). In a UK birth cohort study of several thousand twins, according to parent report, the rate of abusing animals ranged from 6% in young children and 1.5% for children older than 10 years (McEwen et al., 2014).

Children abusing animals were approximately three times more likely to be abused themselves compared to children who did not abuse animals. However, children who abused animals only accounted for one-fifth of all maltreated children in this sample. Animal abuse by children uncovering child maltreatment is more common than the reverse of child abuse uncovering animal abuse by children (McEwen et al., 2014). The overall incidence of any household member abusing animals in these households is not reported; however, studies based on self and parent reports likely underreport the true incidence.

Furthermore, in several studies, there is a gender differential with regard to children abusing animals since the majority of children who abuse animals—up to a three to one ratio—are boys. Yet, the likelihood of co-occurring or past child abuse for girls who abuse animals is higher than that for boys. Children with developmental delay, attention problems, or conduct disorder may have higher rates of both perpetrating animal abuse and being victimized by child abuse, although the relationships are unclear. Studies suggest that environments fraught with ongoing violence contribute to children's development of a reactive brain chemistry and structure desensitized to violence that promotes internalizing and externalizing symptoms. If left untreated, these may persist into adolescence and likely adulthood (Bright et al., 2018).

Structured interviews of children suggest motives for abusing animals along a spectrum of "non-pathological" to "pathological" (Lee-Kelland & Finlay, 2018). These include curiosity, exploration, peer pressure, imitation, as well as re-enacting, rehearsing, and regaining a sense of power from being a victim of beatings, punishment, bullying, sexual assaults, emotional conflicts, or neglect that they themselves receive by abusing animals. Among all ages, chief motivations for animal maltreatment include anger, fun, fear, dislike, control, revenge, imitation, and sexual satisfaction (Monsalve et al., 2017). However, "has been physically cruel to animals" is one of the diagnostic criteria for conduct disorder in the DSM-5, and conduct disorder is often a precursor to antisocial personality disorder (American Psychiatric Association, 2013).

Innate genetic predisposition and temperament, along with family environment and societal mores and culture, are postulated to contribute to animal cruelty traits in the childhoods of individuals who go on to possess premeditating criminality and psychopathology as adults (Johnson, 2018). Results of studies in this area are mixed, likely due to inconsistent definitions and small samples (Monsalve et al., 2017). Some have shown that individuals who had a history of abusing animals were three times more likely to have other criminality including murder, rape, robbery, assault, harassment, threats of violence, and substance abuse.

Detection and intervention are required to stop the abuse and prevent further steps down the path of delinquency and trauma in childhood, as well as psychopathy and criminality in later adulthood for these individuals. Medical professionals caring for children should screen for abuse of pets and understand local animal welfare reporting. When there is concern that animal abuse has occurred due to a child's actions, a differential response includes holding the child accountable, helping them develop empathy for the animal's feelings, and, in more severe occurrences, counseling, referral to animal care and social services, or filing a complaint with local law enforcement.

Similarly, animal care professionals should have heightened awareness for signs of child abuse among their client families for whom they suspect animal abuse. Screening tools for animal abuse include the FINISH mnemonic (food adequacy, injury past history, number of pets, intimidation, shelter adequacy, how did this injury happen) (Lee-Kelland & Finlay, 2018) and TEN4 FACES for child abuse (injuries to the torso, ears, and neck for children who are 4 years old and younger; any bruise for infant 4 months and younger, injuries to the frena, angle of jaw, chin, or eye sclera) (Pierce et al., 2010). Animal and human medicine professionals should familiarize themselves with their state's reporting requirements to their local public children's services agency and animal welfare services.

By being aware of the Link, professionals for both animal and human health and welfare, as well as law enforcement and animal control, can be prepared to screen vulnerable animals and children they encounter for abuse as well as cross-reporting their concerns. More and more communities recognizing the Link are establishing networks of professionals to facilitate transdisciplinary approaches of information and resource sharing to provide thorough investigations, identification of violent offenses, and safe disposition for surviving victims (Bright et al., 2018; Johnson, 2018; Lee-Kelland & Finlay, 2018; Monsalve et al., 2017).

Intersection with Intimate Partner Violence

If the veterinarian or veterinary social worker suspects animal abuse, then not only child abuse but also other subtypes of family violence may be linked. Intimate partner violence (IPV) in humans has multiple domains, including physical violence, sexual violence, threats of such violence, and psychological or emotional abuse. For example, physical abuse may include hitting, punching, pushing or choking, beating, or using a weapon. There are various theories of intimate partner violence, including whether one is part of a subculture which has developed norms permitting the use of violence, violence being related to the lack of power in the relationship, and use of violence to obtain goals when benefits of that violence appear to outweigh the costs (Friedman et al., 2008). Those who are victimized by IPV may stay in the relationship for various reasons including traumatic bonding.

Four patterns of IPV have been described, including coercive controlling violence, violent resistance, situational couple violence, and separation-instigated violence. Depending on the research sample studied, men or women may be more likely to be perpetrators. Situational couple violence is the most common type of IPV. In situational couple violence, an argument escalates into violence as a result of poor coping skills and anger. In general, men and women perpetrate similar rates of situational couple violence, while men tend to be the perpetrators of coercive controlling violence (Kelly & Johnson, 2008). Coercive controlling violence tends to involve more severe violence and more frequent acts on average. Violent resistance is akin to a self-defense response, and more severe victimization may subsequently occur.

Techniques to maintain power and control in coercive controlling relationships may include intimidation and threats, financial abuse, isolating the partner from their support system, and using children against the victim. In some IPV cases, threats against animals may be part of abusive power and control. Abusers may exploit the bond between their human victims and their pets, in order to control, manipulate, frighten, and punish their victims (Arkow, 2015). A "cycle of violence" occurs in many violent relationships, in which the tension builds in the relationship, until the abuse takes place. Subsequent apologies and excuses and promises that the violence will not occur again may serve to keep the victim in the relationship.

One must consider that IPV does not only occur in heterosexual marriages. IPV also occurs in dating relationships. IPV also occurs in gay couples. As noted above, IPV is not only perpetrated by men. IPV may be bidirectional rather than unidirectional (Straus, 2008). By being aware of the many ways that IPV can manifest and the various motives, the provider may better comprehend cases.

A strong link has been described between animal abuse and abuse of humans (Long & Kulkarni, 2013; Walters, 2014). Intimate partner violence and animal abuse may co-occur in 25–86% of cases of women at domestic violence shelters (Monsalve et al., 2017). Actual rates are difficult to ascertain since animal abuse is not routinely or systematically queried. Women living at a domestic violence shelter were almost 11 times more likely to report that their partner had either purposely hurt or killed pets than were women who reported they had not been victims of intimate partner violence (Ascione et al., 2007). Severe physical violence was a predictor of animal abuse. Women also reported that they had not sought help for themselves sooner because of concern for their pets. In fact, pets may remain under the care of the abusive partner if the maltreated partner leaves (Monsalve et al., 2017). Pets have been described as "pawns" to secure obedience of family members to the abuser (Arkow, 2015). A recent study of 42 male incarcerated IPV perpetrators found that 81% reported perpetrating animal cruelty in their lifetime (Haden et al., 2018). Finally, in cases of familicide (killing of the entire family) (Friedman et al., 2005), the family pet may be killed as well as the partner and the children.

The veterinary provider should be aware that while laws about child abuse reporting are fairly similar across the country, laws vary by location regarding reporting of IPV and elder abuse. The American College of Obstetricians and Gynecologists has recommended screening questions that may similarly be helpful in asking a partner about victimization. However, reporting IPV is controversial, though mandated in some locales and some circumstances. It is important to reference your local reporting requirements. Providing information about domestic violence hotlines and shelters could be of great help to sufferers.

Intersection with Elder Abuse/Neglect

Many of the elderly are strongly attached to their pets. Similar to the relationships between child abuse, IPV, and animal abuse, a link is seen between animal abuse and the abuse of vulnerable adults and elders. Over one-third of respondents from Adult Protective Services noted that their clients had talked about pets being injured, threatened, killed, or denied veterinary care by a caregiver (Lockwood, 2002). Thus, threats against animals or actual harm used, similarly to in cases of IPV, may be used to harm vulnerable victims.

Alternatively, a vulnerable adult themselves may lack understanding of their pet's needs or lack the ability to fulfil these needs. As such, animal neglect may be a visible warning sign which prompts consideration of self-neglect among the elderly (Lockwood, 2002).

Intersection of Bestiality and Family Violence

The relationship between bestiality and violence is not well understood, though some studies have suggested a link. Hensley et al. (2006) found that male offenders with less education and those who had been convicted of committing crimes against people were more likely to have a childhood history of bestiality. They hypothesized that in these offenders, bestiality was a form of animal cruelty associated with violence in which male offenders with a history of childhood bestiality were more likely to commit adult violent crimes (Hensley et al., 2006, 2008). A limited number of studies have found an association between bestial acts and human sexual offending. One juvenile offender study found that 96% of juveniles with a history of bestiality committed human sexual offenses (Jory et al., 2002). Abel and Harlow (2009) found that a history of bestiality was the most significant factor in predicting future child sexual abuse. More recently, Holoyda et al. (2020) found a history of bestiality in 2.6% of a sample of 1248 sexually violent predators.

Ethics and Reporting

The written policy of the American Veterinary Medical Association (AVMA) on Animal Abuse and Neglect reads, "The AVMA recognizes that veterinarians may observe cases of animal abuse or neglect as defined by federal or state laws, or local ordinances. When these situations cannot be resolved through education, the AVMA considers it the responsibility of the veterinarian to report such cases to appropriate authorities" (American Veterinary Medical Association, 2019).

The determination of whether human-animal sexual contact is unethical is largely dependent on the context of the behavior. The practice of animal husbandry frequently includes collection of semen and facilitation of breeding. Such practice is within the ethical practice of veterinarians and other individuals who share the goal of safe, humane animal breeding. In most jurisdictions, other human-animal sexual encounters are considered illegal (and unethical). The principles of veterinary medical ethics of the AVMA do not specifically address the subject of bestiality. The subject might be understood in the first principle, "a veterinarian shall be influenced only by the welfare of the patient...."

Many veterinarians (43–86%) know about the link between animal abuse and family violence (Monsalve et al., 2017). Kogan et al. (2017) surveyed veterinarians and found that 87% acknowledged encountering animal abuse in practice. More than one-half (56%) had reported at least one case. When asked reasons for not reporting, these included uncertainty about abuse being accidental versus intentional and the belief that educating the owner would be better than reporting. Similarly, from the child protection literature, some parents do discontinue care with that physician after a report is made to Child Protective Services. However, that risk is conceptualized as of less importance than is the protection of the child.

To date, 20 states require veterinarians to report suspected animal cruelty to law enforcement (Wisch, 2020). Other states include reporting suspected animal abuse as part of a professional responsibility of the veterinarian, with possible disciplinary action for failure to report (Wisch, 2020). Some jurisdictions provide the veterinarian with immunity for civil or criminal liability from reporting (Dunn, 2016). Some states, in recognition of the relationship between family violence and animal abuse, have mandated "the cross-reporting of animal and child abuse between animal health care providers, animal control agencies, child health care providers, and child protection agencies" (American Veterinary Medical Association, 2019).

When mental health professionals such as psychiatrists, psychologists, social workers, or therapists encounter cases of suspected animal abuse or neglect in the course of patient care, efforts should be made to address the problem. This should include direct questioning of the patient as well as interviews with collateral sources of information to better understand the risk posed to the animal. To date, veterinarians, animal control officers, and veterinary social workers are the most common mandated reporters of animal abuse (Montanaro et al., 2019). Mental health workers have not been identified as mandated reporters, although there has been some movement in this direction.

Strategies for Assessment and Intervention

The barriers to the assessment and appropriate intervention in suspected cases of animal abuse or neglect parallel the barriers to reporting child abuse, intimate partner violence, and elder abuse (Arkow, 2015). They include ignorance of such issues among animal professionals, ethical quandaries raised by issues such as confidentiality and the best interests of the animal client, concern about legal implications, and the absence of an infrastructure to assist in addressing these complicated, time-consuming problems (Arkow, 2015).

The first step toward addressing these barriers is to educate animal care professionals about the prevalence of the problem and the important implications of the problem, such as possible co-existing sexual, child, elder, or intimate partner violence. As discussed earlier, screening tools such as the FINISH or TEN4 FACES may be useful in guiding clinical judgment in cases of suspected abuse or neglect. Understanding the common patterns of IPV and elder abuse can help the animal health professional recognize high-risk cases. Animal sexual abuse, in particular, is not a core competency in veterinary training. As a result, the extent and prevention of such behavior are unknown. Recent enactment of laws which criminalize animal abuse has focused more attention on this matter, but to date, addressing animal sexual abuse is not a popular topic. An algorithm for evaluating animal sexual abuse proposed by Bradley and Rasile (2014) reviews pathways for managing suspected or actual sexual abuse. This includes securing a safe environment for the animal, notifying law enforcement, and when possible performing a medical-forensic examination. Veterinary pathologists may be consulted to investigate cases of suspected human-animal sexual abuse. Injuries to the genital areas, anus, and nipples provide direct evidence of abuse (Stern & Smith-Blackmore, 2016). Cases of genital or rectal injury should include consideration of human-animal sexual abuse (Bradley & Rasile, 2014). Other indications of possible human-animal sexual abuse include oversexualized behaviors in animals, recurrent urinary tract infections, or more subtle injuries such as abrasions from restraining animals. A specialized evaluation including alternative light source examination, genital and anal swabs for DNA analysis, and nail clippings to detect human seminal fluid may be critical in the detection of animals' sexual abuse (Stern and Smith-Blackmore, 2016).

Investigation and Police Perspectives

In 2015, the National Sheriffs' Association convened a panel comprised of experts in animal cruelty and domestic violence and prosecutors and judges to increase awareness of the link between animal cruelty and other violence. It has long been held that crimes involving human victims had a higher priority than crimes involving animal victims. Priorities dictate the allocation of limited investigative resources. However, the link between animal cruelty and domestic violence, elder abuse, and child abuse has been conclusively established. The recognition of this link has caused a shift in the priorities to focus on animal abuse cases because of the potential to proactively prevent crimes. With a goal of preventing crimes against persons, there is now a focus on prosecuting suspects in animal abuse crimes. Regardless of the justification, this change in allocation of resources for the investigation and prosecution of animal abuse in America is a net positive.

This change in thinking and priorities caused US lawmakers to acknowledge the link, passing the Preventing Animal Cruelty and Torture (PACT) Act in 2019. This law made specific types of animal abuse a federal felony in the United States. This law was an expansion of Animal Crush Video Prohibition Act, which was passed in 2010, that made the creation and distribution of animal crushing videos illegal. State prosecutors around the country are also recognizing the link and are taking measures to enforce animal cruelty laws in efforts to curtail potential abuse.

With this established link, there has been a move to prioritize the prosecution of animal abuse as a means to combat other forms of (human) abuse. Some judicial systems around the country are recognizing that holding people accountable for their treatment of animals may be an intervention into family violence and may even save lives. Collaborative investigation engaging with veterinarians, Child Protective Services, police, prosecutors, and animal advocates is necessary. Communities should focus on forming investigative partnerships with the goals of increasing awareness, recognition of the signs, reporting suspected abuse, and prosecution of animal abuse cases.

Law enforcement has multiple challenges when investigating animal cruelty cases. Animals, like young children, cannot verbally accuse their abusers of violent acts, and corroborating evidence is critically important to establish the occurrence of criminal acts (Holoyda et al., 2018).

The Victim

The animal victim cannot speak, so police are taking the initial information from the reporting party. The first step is determining the nature of injury or cause of death. Is the incident criminal in nature or an accident? Is it negligence (should they have known better) or reckless (they knew better and did it anyhow)? Is there obvious malice?

Ensuring a veterinarian reviews the case or details a determination as an expert witness may be important. Veterinarians can provide a voice for the victim to describe to a prosecutor and eventually to a jury what the victim may have experienced. When questioning potential expert witnesses, investigators need to consider their knowledge base. The veterinarian can describe how long a wound had been in existence, determine substantial suffering (a prong of animal cruelty in most states), and describe how slowly or quickly a wound becomes fatal. They can describe potential lifesaving efforts that could have been undertaken by suspects. Veterinarians are able to point out the location of wounds and how the wounds caused suffering or death. For example, a veterinarian may utilize an x-ray to show pooling of blood in the lungs indicating a prolonged death as a result of a shotgun blast that caused punctures in the lungs. Veterinarians can also explain how a broken claw or broken bone would affect an animal. They can describe how the wound would manifest itself and provide evidence of how animals experience and exhibit pain.

By way of case example, a suspect child acknowledged abusing family pets, having confessed to throwing a cat against the wall. The suspect was angry at his sister and so he abused her pet. The veterinarian became suspicious because of the nature of the injury when the family brought the cat in for an eye issue, and he found the retina had become detached. The prosecutor explored alternative explanations (sometimes referred to as "innocent explanations"), and they discussed what was possible and probable. They discussed a timeline which exposed a pattern of abuse with "odd injuries" and no reasonable explanations. The veterinarian had to consider whether this animal was incredibly unlucky or whether more was going on.

The police should be mindful of potential signs of torture in their investigation. Is there documentation of previous healed injuries through x-rays or other methods? Can the veterinarian complete a review of vet visits and progress of health? Are there implications from a lack of veterinarian visits? Can a veterinarian reach out to see if the pet has been treated in other vet clinics? Could this be a case of "Dr. Shopping" to hide repeated injuries (similar to what is seen in some child abuse cases)? Veterinarians can also provide insight into how an animal might still show affection to the abuser and why that may occur. This may be important for a jury to understand, similar to some cases of human abuse victims still showing affection toward their abuser.

The Suspect

Examining the details of the incident can direct the investigation and identify suspects or motive. Careful documentation of the source of information at the time of reporting and with whom the animal was in care at the time of injury is imperative. Who is the abuser? Can the identity of the abuser be established through examining a timeline of access to the animal? Is there a way to determine a motive? Does a neighbor have a standing issue with the animal?

Being cognizant of the potential motives can help shape questions to ask suspects in an investigation. There are various reasons a person would abuse an animal, and it is necessary to recognize that not everyone who abuses an animal is a sadistic animal torturer. The acts of animal abuse need to be examined with thoughtful questions to explore the individual's motivation.

What would motivate someone to abuse an animal? Could it be ignorance? In a case of neglect, is it lack of empathy by allowing an injured animal to remain injured or in pain and not seek medical treatment? Could the abuse be motivated by the owner seeing an animal as property rather than a living being? Could the suspect be acting out on feelings of rage, anger, or frustration or a sadistic desire to cause injury to an animal?

What do the mechanics of a particular injury say about the intention of the person inflicting it? Is there a cruelty of heart in that action? What does this act say about the lack of empathy?

For example, if someone wrapped tape around a dog's snout, was it to keep him quiet? Frustration? Repeated issues? Is there intention to cause harm? Correct an issue? Are they ignorant of the pain and suffering they are causing, or do they relish it? With these questions in mind, an investigator can set a "trap" for a suspect by minimizing the malicious intent and focusing on their "good intentions." An example comes from multiple cases where a suspect wrapped tape around a dog's snout to keep the dog from barking. The suspect was lulled into confessing to committing the heinous act of abuse by a savvy investigator who tapped into the theme of "just being a good and considerate neighbor" and keep the dog quiet. This distinction, while important to the suspect to make himself or herself look better, makes no difference in a court of law. The existence of the wound and a veterinarian who can testify to the pain and suffering, coupled with a suspect's "good intentions," should still result in a guilty verdict.

A Window into the Family Dynamic

In some cases, a suspect may blame children in the home for the injury to a pet. This may legitimately have occurred with the child as the suspect for this particular incident of animal abuse. However, one should still consider the possibility of whether the child is imitating what they have witnessed in the home. Does the family have a culture of animal abuse? Is there domestic violence in the home? Again, one must consider the larger picture or potential connection. A suspect may be reticent to talk about abuse of children or their partner, but they may see the animal as property.

Witnesses

Eyewitness testimony from involved family members may well prove difficult to obtain; if abuse of an animal is occurring in a home, the likelihood of family violence is increased. Speaking out against the suspect in an animal abuse case would then require the abused to speak out against their abuser on behalf of the family pet. This can cause an understandable (but regrettable) reticence to report. Understanding that reticence and the ability to break down barriers by thorough and thoughtful interviewing is imperative. Police may look to witnesses outside the home in a neighborhood canvas.

Case Discussion

Regarding the amalgamated case presented in the Introduction, various ages of fractures in a found dog who eats ravenously could signal both animal abuse and neglect, respectively. The findings of a rectal abrasion should raise a level of suspicion for animal sexual abuse. Other signs of sexual abuse should be investigated including with a genital exam. Although not definitive, asking the owner if he has observed any behavior which could result in such injuries is imperative. If the totality of the presentation is unexplainable, and you remain concerned for animal abuse, you should check with your professional licensing board to determine mandated and ethical duties and confidentiality status.

The humane society should be called, and perhaps the police, who can start the process of an investigation. Document observations: how the animal was located, observed injuries, the status of the dog, and any interaction with the owner. The veterinarian will be called upon as an expert, to explain why a call was made and what was observed related to injuries. The reporting individual should be mindful that if something cannot be done in this case, the process of simply documenting the concerns may still be part of a larger case that comes later. In addition, just making a report and having a subsequent investigation may be enough to stop abuse as the suspect may give up the animal rather than face the scrutiny of an investigation.

Conclusion: Moving Forward

In 2012, the American Society for the Prevention of Cruelty to Animals (ASPCA) created a document entitled "Toolkit for Starting a Link Coalition in Your Community" and placed it online, to assist in starting a Link Coalition. If a person feels as though there is no process and they are going to have to "blaze the trail themselves" to get things going, they are less likely to report. By having a community organized with a reporting process in place, with stakeholders supporting the witnesses, the likelihood of reporting is increased. Collaboration across disciplines is important to protect both animals and humans. A recent model put forward in Ohio includes training, legislation, and multidisciplinary task forces for cross-reporting among professions (Vincent, et al., 2019). Challenges of underreporting of animal maltreatment mirror the underreporting of maltreatment of other vulnerable populations, such as children and the elderly. Understanding the link will help improve detection and can help save both animal and human lives.

References

Abel, G. G., & Harlow, N. (2009). *What can 44,000 men and 12,000 boys with sexual behavior problems teach us about preventing sexual abuse?* Presented at the Annual Training Conference of the California Coalition on Sexual Offending, 11th Annual Training Conference, San Francisco, California, USA.

American Pet Products Association. *National pet owners survey*, 2013-2014. Retrieved from http://www.petfoodindustry.com/APPA_releases_201314_National_Pet_Owners_Survey.html

American Psychiatric Association. (2013). *Diagnostic and statistical manual of mental disorders* (5th ed.). https://doi.org/10.1176/appi.books.9780890425596

American Society for the Prevention of Cruelty to Animals. (2012). *Toolkit for starting a link coalition in your community*. Available at https://www.aspcapro.org/sites/default/files/national_link_coalition_toolkit_0.pdf

American Veterinary Medical Association. (2019). *Principles of veterinary medical ethics of AVMA, revised 2019*. https://www.michvma.org/resources/Documents/GLVC/2019%20Proceedings/Principles%20of%20Veterinary%20Medical%20Ethics%20of%20the%20AVMA%20Babcock.pdf

Animal Crush Video Prohibition Act, Pub. L. 111–294, 124 Stat. 3177. (2010, December 9).

Arkow, P. (2015). Recognizing and responding to cases of suspected animal cruelty, abuse, and neglect: What the veterinarian needs to know. *Veterinary Medicine (Auckland, N.Z.), 6*, 349–359. https://doi.org/10.2147/VMRR.S87198

Ascione, F. R., Weber, C. V., Thompson, T. M., Heath, J., Maruyama, M., & Hayashi, K. (2007). Battered pets and domestic violence: Animal abuse reported by women experiencing intimate violence and by nonabused women. *Violence Against Women, 13*(4), 354–373. https://doi.org/10.1177/1077801207299201

Beirne, P. (1997). Rethinking bestiality: Towards a concept of interspecies sexual assault. *Theoretical Criminology, 1*(3), 317–340.

Bradley, N., & Rasile, K. (2014). Recognition & management of animal sexual abuse. *Clinician's Brief, 4*, 73–75.

Bright, M. A., Huq, M. S., Spencer, T., Applebaum, J. W., & Hardt, N. (2018). Animal cruelty as an indicator of family trauma: Using adverse childhood experiences to look beyond child abuse and domestic violence. *Child Abuse & Neglect, 76*, 287–296.

Dunn, L. (2016). An animal victim's best chance: Veterinary legal duty to report cruelty in the U.S. *Animal Sentience, 6*(6), 083. https://www.wellbeingintlstudiesrepository.org/cgi/viewcontent.cgi?article=1096 & context=animsent. Accessed 24 March 2021.

English, K., Jones, L., Patrick, D., & Pasini-Hill, D. (2003). Sexual offender containment: Use of the post-conviction polygraph. *Annals of the New York Academy of Science, 989*, 411–427.

Friedman, S. H., Hrouda, D. R., Holden, C. E., Noffsinger, S. G., & Resnick, P. J. (2005). Filicide-suicide: Common factors in parents who kill their children and themselves. *Journal of the American Academy of Psychiatry and the Law Online, 33*(4), 496–504.

Friedman, S. H., Stankowski, J. E., & Loue, S. (2008). Intimate partner violence and the clinician. In R. I. Simon & K. Tardiff (Eds.), *Textbook of violence assessment and management* (pp. 483–499). American Psychiatric Publishing.

Gephard, P. H., Gagnon, J. H., Pomeroy, W. B., & Christenson, C. V. (1965). *Sex offenders: An analysis of types*. Harper & Row and Paul B. Hoeber, Medical Books.

Haden, S. C., McDonald, S. E., Booth, L. J., Ascione, F. R., & Blakelock, H. (2018). An exploratory study of domestic violence: Perpetrators' reports of violence against animals. *Anthrozoös, 31*(3), 337–352.

Hensley, C., Tallichet, S., & Singer, S. (2006). Exploring the possible link between childhood and adolescent bestiality and interpersonal violence. *Journal of Interpersonal Violence, 21*(7), 910–923.

Hensley, C., Tallichet, S. E., & Dutkiewicz, E. L. (2008). Recurrent childhood animal cruelty is there a relationship to adult recurrent interpersonal violence? *Criminal Justice Review, 34*(2), 248–257.

Holoyda, B., Sorrentino, R., Friedman, S. H., & Allgire, J. (2018). Bestiality: An introduction for legal and mental health professionals. *Behavioral Sciences & the Law, 36*(6), 687–697.

Holoyda, B. J., Gosal, R., & Welch, K. M. (2020). Bestiality among sexually violent predators. *Journal of the American Academy of Psychiatry and Law, 48*(3), 358–364.

Humane Society of the United States. *Animal cruelty and neglect FAQ*. https://www.humanesociety.org/resources/animal-cruelty-and-neglect-faq.

Hunt, M. M. (1974). *Sexual behavior in the 1970s* (1st ed.). Playboy Press.

Johnson, S. A. (2018). Animal cruelty, pet abuse & violence: The missed dangerous connection. *Forensic Research & Criminology International Journal, 6*(6), 403–415.

Jory, B., Fleming, W., & Burton, D. (2002). Characteristics of juvenile offenders admitting to sexual activity with nonhuman animals. *Society & Animals, 10*(1), 31–45.

Kelly, J. B., & Johnson, M. P. (2008). Differentiation among types of intimate partner violence: Research update and implications for interventions. *Family Court Review, 46*(3), 476–499.

Kinsey, A. C., Pomeroy, W. B., & Martin, C. E. (1948). *Sexual behavior in human male.* W.B. Saunders Company.

Kinsey, A. C., Pomeroy, W. B., Martin, C. E., & Gebhard, P. H. (1953). *Sexual behavior in human female.* W.B. Saunders Company.

Kogan, L. R., Schoenfeld-Tacher, R. M., Hellyer, P. W., Rishniw, M., & Ruch-Gallie, R. A. (2017). Survey of attitudes toward and experiences with animal abuse encounters in a convenience sample of US veterinarians. *Journal of the American Veterinary Medical Association, 250*(6), 688–696.

Lee-Kelland, R., & Finlay, F. (2018). Children who abuse animals: When should you be concerned about child abuse? A review of the literature. *Archives of Disease in Childhood, 103*(8), 801–805.

Lockwood, R. (2002). Making the connection between animal cruelty and abuse and neglect of vulnerable adults. *The Latham Letter, 23*(1), 10–11.

Long, D. D., & Kulkarni, S. J. (2013). Cross-reporting of interpersonal violence and animal cruelty: The Charlotte Project. *Journal of Sociology & Social Welfare, 40*(8), 131.

McEwen, F. S., Moffitt, T. E., & Arseneault, L. (2014). Is childhood cruelty to animals a marker for physical maltreatment in a prospective cohort study of children? *Child Abuse & Neglect, 38*(3), 533–543.

Miletski, H. (2002). *Understanding bestiality and zoophilia.* East West Publishing.

Monsalve, S., Ferreira, F., & Garcia, R. (2017). The connection between animal abuse and interpersonal violence: A review from the veterinary perspective. *Research in Veterinary Science, 114*, 18–26.

Montanaro, L., Cusick, T., & Smith-Blackmore, M. (2019). *Multi-jurisdiction laws concerning mandated reporting, immunity for reporting, and cross-reporting for animal cruelty and abuse. Compiled for "Paws II" special commission.* https://nationallinkcoalition.org/wp-content/uploads/2019/09/Cross-reporting-state-laws.pdf

Pierce, M. C., Kaczor, K., Aldridge, S., O'Flynn, J., & Lorenz, D. J. (2010). Bruising characteristics discriminating physical child abuse from accidental trauma. *Pediatrics, 125*(1), 67–74.

Simons, D. A., Wurtele, S. K., & Durham, R. L. (2008). Developmental experiences of child sexual abusers and rapists. *Child Abuse & Neglect, 32*, 548–560.

Stern, A. W., & Smith-Blackmore, M. (2016). Veterinary forensic pathology of animal sexual abuse. *Veterinary Pathology, 53*(5), 1057–1066.

Straus, M. A. (2008). Dominance and symmetry in partner violence by male and female university students in 32 nations. *Children and Youth Services Review, 30*(3), 252–275.

Vincent, A., McDonald, S., Poe, B., & Deisner, V. (2019). The link between interpersonal violence and animal abuse. *Society Register, 3*, 83–101.

Walters, G. D. (2014). Testing the direct, indirect, and moderated effects of childhood animal cruelty on future aggressive and non-aggressive offending. *Aggressive Behavior, 40*(3), 238–249. deleted

Wisch, R. F. (2020). *Table of veterinary report requirement and immunity laws.* Animal Legal and Historical Center. https://www.animallaw.info/topic/table-veterinary-reporting-requirement-and-immunity-laws.

Chapter 5
Animal-Assisted Interventions and Community Programs

Aviva Vincent, Augusta O'Reilly, and Blair McKissock

Introduction

Human-animal interaction (HAI) refers to interaction between humans and animals that is reciprocal, bi-directional, and persistent (Hosey & Melfi, 2014; Risley-Curtiss et al., 2013). HAI can be thought of as an umbrella and encompasses animal-assisted interaction (AAI), animal-assisted activities (AAA), and animal-assisted therapy (AAT). The term AAI refers to the act of engaging in HAI and denotes all types of engagement between humans and animals. Engagement may be therapeutic in nature, such as working with a physical, occupational, or mental health therapist in collaboration with an animal, or it can be non-therapeutic and strictly for enjoyment.

AAI is a structured, facilitated intervention that intentionally includes an animal(s) as a collaborator and partner through the therapeutic process. The term "use" is avoided as it is important to account for the animal's well-being and needs throughout any interaction just as one would for a coworker. Animal species selected to engage in AAI can be diverse. The choice of animal in the AAI is dependent on the animal's innate attributes (what they enjoy and do by their innate behaviors) and goals of the intervention. Attributes of the individual should be understood for considerations of species appropriateness.

The interaction is led by a professional, paraprofessional, or volunteer who has received an assessment and/or training. The required or desired training depends on various factors including familiarity with animal collaborators, the population of interest, and experience with the desired intervention. Standards for AAI delivery

A. Vincent (✉) · A. O'Reilly
University of Tennessee, Knoxville, Knoxville, TN, USA
e-mail: Avincen9@utk.edu

B. McKissock
Strides to Success, Plainfield, IN, USA

have been in motion since the mid-1900s. There are three primary considerations for the professionalization of AAI: education of practitioners, professional role, and animal training and welfare (Pet Partners, 2016). Interventions can vary based on the intended outcomes, which can include but are not limited to motivation, skills development, educational learning, or recreational enjoyment (International Association of Human-Animal Interaction Organizations, 2014). AAI can serve as a therapeutic modality across the lifespan and is designed and facilitated in a variety of settings and populations, such as schools (youth), nursing homes, assisted living (elder adults), and medical centers (all populations), issues that are explored further in this chapter.

Veterinary Social Work: The Foundation of AAI

Reliance on animals in a therapeutic capacity dates as far back as the third century and the ancient Greeks' use of horseback riding to rehabilitate soldiers (Jacobson, 2019; Morgan, 1894). During the 1800s, John Locke and Florence Nightingale relied on animals as therapeutic agents in medical clinics to support mental and physical recovery (Serpell, 2000; Matuszek, 2010). Various animals were brought in to support the recovery of wounded and disabled veterans at the York Retreat and the Bethlem Royal Hospital (McCardle et al., 2017).

As the health field advanced in the twentieth century, rehabilitation research focused on medical and pharmaceutical interventions. AAI was not included with the emergent positivist paradigm and medical model which supported the use of the *Diagnostic and Statistical Manual of Medical Disorders* (American Psychiatric Association, 2013) and treatment through pharmaceutical interventions. As a result, the therapeutic capacity of animals was considered to be a novelty rather than a strategic intervention (Serpell, 2000; Gray & Zide, 2012).

The adoption of AAI as a structured therapeutic modality in social work has been slowly increasing since the 1940s (Geist, 2011). Its integration into mental health practice was not explicit until 1962 when Dr. Boris Levinson, referred to as "the father of animal assisted therapy," began bringing his dog Jingles to his clinical practice and published a book about his observations. Levinson (in Fine, 2019) noted that Jingles served as a social lubricant and helped build rapport between him and his clients (Bekoff, 2007). Currently, lead practitioners like Tedeschi et al. (2005), Fine (2019), Chandler (2012), and others have mirrored Levenson's contribution.

AAI made its way to social work in the first peer-reviewed paper in 1975 in a case study of medical social workers and a collaborative dog (Bikales, 1975). To gain an understanding about social workers who collaborate with animals in clinical social work, Dr. Risley-Curtis (1986) surveyed social workers nationally. Her findings demonstrated that social workers were bringing animals (mostly dogs) into practice without training to do so. Over 30 years have passed, and though the survey has not been replicated to date, it appears that the demand for practitioners who provide AAI has increased.

The field of social work as a profession is aptly poised to accept AAI as a core competency and strategy for forthcoming practitioners. The success of current education models and demand for course offerings further support the need for social work to embrace AAI as a clinical tool. And yet, it is imperative to understand that AAI is one facet of veterinary social work. Although a veterinary social worker can practice without engaging in AAI, a practitioner cannot engage in AAI without being competent in veterinary social work.

Ethical Foundations

Veterinary social work follows the *Code of Ethics* of social work practice (NASW, 2021). As a modality, AAI also follows the *Code of Ethics* of social work. The values of dignity, social justice, dignity and worth of the person, integrity, and competence are upheld through VSW training. The standards of practice are directly applicable and applied. Social workers have also sought to explicitly include human-animal relationships in the *Code of Ethics* by encouraging the omission of species dignity of relationships, not only human relationships (Sterman and Bussert, 2020).

Currently, there is no requirement for certification to deliver AAI. However, the International Association of Veterinary Social Work is striving to work collaboratively with flagship institutions and experts in the field to develop best practices and standards of practice. Similarly, at this time, there is no specific certification requirement, though that too will likely change in the coming years in an effort to create a formal professionalization of our practice.

As with all licensure and professional practice, continuing education is an ethical responsibility. The *Code of Ethics* holds social workers responsible for staying abreast of new knowledge and practices. AAI content and learning is readily accessible through a variety of continuing education opportunities in-person and online.

As professionals, veterinary social workers and aligned professionals can hold a variety of positions, all of which are important to the development and delivery of AAI. Professionals can serve as direct practice clinicians, program directors, funding/development, executive director, and/or owner. Essentially, as with social work in general, an educated and trained professional can hold any position in an organization. The beauty of social work is that the core practice is grounded in person-in-environment; veterinary social work moves this practice forward to social work at the intersection of the human-animal bond, which is embodied as the practice of AAI.

Since AAI can directly (engagement) or indirectly (observation) involve animals, it is important for practitioners to be knowledgeable about the animals engaged in the practice. Social workers are not veterinarians. Rather, the role of the social worker is to maintain a standard of care for the animal's welfare (International Association of Human-Animal Interaction Organizations, 2014) and partner with a veterinarian to provide veterinary care regularly and as needed. For direct animal collaboration, it is the clinician's responsibility to ensure the animal's safety in the environment while also ensuring protection of the environment. For example, observing animals on a nature preserve also means upholding the protection of the nature preserve.

Therapeutic Collaborator Bill of Rights

The title of the following Therapeutic collaborator listing has been amended from "Therapy Dog" to "Therapeutic Collaborator" since other domesticated animals serve in therapeutic capacities. All animal partners are deserving of the same rights, in alignment with the Social Work Code of Ethics for valuing their dignity and worth.

As a therapeutic collaborator, I have the right to a handler who:

- Obtains my consent to participate in the work.
- Provides gentle training to help me understand what I am supposed to do.
- Is considerate of my perception of the world.
- Helps me adapt to the work environment.
- Guides the client, staff, and visitors to interact with me appropriately.
- Focuses on me as much as the client, staff, and visitors.
- Pays attention to my nonverbal cues.
- Takes action to reduce my stress.
- Supports me during interactions with the client.
- Protects me from overwork.
- Gives me ways to relax after sessions.
- Provides a well-rounded life with nutritious food, medical care, physical and intellectual exercise, social time, and activities beyond work
- Respects my desire to retire from work when I think it is time.

- (Howie, 2015, pg 125)

Theoretical Foundations of Veterinary Social Work

Theory serves as the foundation for VSW practice, as with all social work practices. A theoretical foundation helps explain *why* interaction with animals provides a therapeutic benefit and may also serve as a framework for the development and evaluation of specific interventions and programs.

Attachment Theory

Case Study 1

Natalie Evans is an Associate Clinical Social Worker at the Wish Fulfilling Tree, a therapeutic ranch, in June of 2020. She works to integrate her therapy dog-in-training, Balto, into her sessions with clients. Working with therapy animals provides opportunities to build relationships and connection in a safe and nonjudgmental way.

Dogs are able to tune in to how people are feeling emotionally, physically, and mentally. Oftentimes, skills and strengths cannot be built until we feel safe and accepted. Therapy animals meet people where we are in the moment, modeling trust and openness. Integrating Balto into work has allowed for opportunities to have conversations and/or do work with clients around healthy boundaries, fears, and worries, setting expectations, adjusting to new environments, emotional identification skills, problem-solving, attachment, and so much more! Clients have had opportunities to use their problem-solving skills to help Balto do what has been asked of him. This involves pausing, being clear, and slowing down so that Balto can keep up with cues and commands. Clients are often more willing to talk about their fears and challenges if we talk about Balto's fears and challenges first and have increased their confidence and self-esteem in practicing cues and commands with Balto over time. Most clients demonstrate caretaking behaviors with Balto, which can also provide opportunities to discuss and promote empathy and responsibility. Balto also helps kids in developing healthy attachment by greeting them with excitement when they arrive, being at their side in session, and walking them out at the end of session.

In the beginning, Natalie thought that Balto would need to change in order to be certified and succeed in the work. However, she has come to realize that Balto brings his own skills and strengths to work just as he is.

Natalie's experience with Balto and her clients provides an example of how attachment theory relates to AAI. Researchers have found based on their observations of human children and their caregivers that it is the quality of the emotional relationship between infant and caregiver, rather than the physical care received, that predicts the child's internal and external regulation of emotions and behavior (Bowlby, 1988; Hofer, 1995, Crittenden, 1995; Goldberg et al., 1995; Karen, 1998). Later research with macaques and rhesus monkeys revealed that, like human children, monkeys also seek physical closeness (Goldberg et al., 1995; Harlow, 1958). It was later theorized that inter-species attachment could invoke the same biological responses as those experienced between a mother and child—a pet could provide comfort, safety, and love (Zilcha-Mano et al., 2011) as could a therapy animal (Jalongo, 2018).

A modern model of attachment theory integrated the concepts of attachment, biopsychosocial framework, and physiological cascade to generate a causal pathway of AAI (Schore & Schore, 2008; Borrell-Carrio et al., 2004. See generally Handlin et al., 2012). AAI impacts children's internal mechanisms through *physical* indicators such as heart rate and blood pressure (Farhat-McHayleh et al., 2009;

Handlin et al., 2011), perception of *social* support wherein the dog provides direct support or acts as facilitator to enhance rapport in interpersonal interactions, and *emotional* functioning such as feelings of *attachment*, comfort, and amelioration of loneliness (Chandler, 2012; Matuszek, 2010).

The biological systems of emotional regulation are associated with hyperactivity of the sympathetic nervous system and hypothalamic-pituitary-adrenal axis, the brain and body's stress response that directs the reaction of *fight-freeze-flight* (Allen et al., 1991; Friedman & Tsai, 2006; Beetz et al., 2012; Cirulli et al., 2011). Another indicator of concordance between human and animal physiology is an increase in heart rate variability (HRV) (Malinowski et al., 2018; Gehrke et al., 2019). Negative internalized emotions, such as fear and anxiety, are associated with the upregulation of the sympathetic nervous system (Song et al., 2016). In AAI, the aim is for the HRV process to downregulate, which stimulates a shift to the parasympathetic nervous system. Downregulation can increase positive feelings associated with social interaction and self-regulation.

AAI is not intended to change attachment styles, nor intended to permanently change biological systems. Rather, AAI impacts the regulatory interactions for a time-bound duration to alleviate negative symptoms or intentionally invoke positive feelings (Cirulli et al., 2011; Chandler, 2012). Attachments are frequently bidirectional where an individual seeks out security of a caregiver and also gives affection to the caregiver. In this case, the caregiver can be human or animal (McConnell, 2009). An animal can provide a temporary secure base while processing and experiencing an environmental stressor (Berget & Ihlebæk, 2011). Increased positive input from the animal may increase the ability to self-regulate and decrease maladaptive coping strategies (Crittenden, 1995; Katcher et al., 1983). The relevance of attachment theory is also illustrated by the following Case Study 2.

Case Study 2
Rebecca Brit, BSW, ESMHL is the owner and founder of Stable Moments. Through the mentorship program and activities at Stable Moments, foster and adopted children develop crucial life skills. For foster children, there is great importance surrounding the development of critical life skills before reaching adulthood or "aging out" of the system. An estimated one in four children in foster care will be incarcerated within 2 years of their emancipation. Female youth who "age out" of foster care are six times more likely than the general population to give birth before the age of 21. Stable Moment's goal is to promote healing and produce practical life skills that aid a child in making healthy decisions into adulthood. Children in foster care have likely seen dozens of therapists and are often "therapied out." Face-to-face talk therapy can feel intrusive and shame inducing. The farm setting is an alternative to therapy where children often want to go, actively engage, and are proud of what they learn.Tim is a kind, engaging, 12-year-old boy who lives with his adoptive parents. Tim's goal was to develop a sense of identity and personal self-

esteem. Over the past 6 months, Tim has developed a special bond with his horse Minky. Recently, he participated in an essay and public speaking assignment at his school in which he shared how "his best brings out the best in others." Tim focused on the importance of patience, which is a fundamental life skill. Tim shared the impact of his experiences with his horse Minky. He proudly shared: "during our time together I groom her, walk her, take her through a very long obstacle course, and take her back to her stall...sometimes, Minky is very stubborn and only wants to eat grass. I have to be very patient and redirect her gently to what I am asking her to do. If you are angry and you are working with a horse, the horse will do nothing for you. Therefore, you have to be very calm when working with horses. Minky follows my instructions most of the time because I have learned to be patient and kind with her. We have developed a very special relationship." These moments with Minky have become extremely beneficial and teachable moments he applies to his own life. Tim now relates his own experiences with his parents to that of Minky. Comically, Tim will say "I am like Minky when it comes to my homework; I just constantly reach for the 'grass!' My parents have to re-direct me like I redirect Minky!" These connections made between Tim's life experiences and his horse Minky reflect the purpose behind equine assisted learning.

Biophilia Hypothesis

Farm-based residential treatment programs incorporate the objectives of AAIs into everyday life for residents. Programs often use the surrounding natural land and nature to create meaningful opportunities for residents to live, work, and engage. Utilizing the natural space in addition to the explicit interaction with animals, daily life becomes a therapeutic process. Clinical social work in varying modalities is integrated into the service delivery system. Although farm-based residential programs do not uniformly rely on the biophilia hypothesis to guide their delivery, the basic tenets of the hypothesis can be easily seen in such programs. This hypothesis suggests that humans have an innate attraction to other living things and that there is a human need or propensity to focus on and to affiliate with life and life-like systems (Wilson, 1984). Thus, humans are drawn to nature and other animals to seek out positive affiliations, such as comfort, safety, and relaxation. The following case study illustrates this framework well.

Case Study 3

Christina Goodall, MSSA, LISW-S, CDWF, Director of Outreach, Hopewell
I began working with animals as a child. I was always very attracted to anything
animal related though we only had fish in our house. At age 9, I began riding; I found
the time I spent at the barn relaxing, and that space became a place I could belong.
Professionally, I knew from a young age that I wanted to work with people and ani-
mals. The opportunity to work at Hopewell allowed me to follow this path. I was sent
to a training on the EAGALA method and quickly began working with horses and
clients in weekly groups.

Biopsychosocial Framework

The biopsychosocial framework posits that optimal health and well-being are conceived at the nexus of physical, psychological, and social functioning (Engel, 1977,
1980; Miles, 2014). The framework includes *bio*logical factors (i.e., physical ability, genetics), *psycho*logical factors (i.e., cognitive elasticity, behavior, mood), and
social factors (i.e., relationships, poverty). The biopsychosocial framework is visu-
all represented as a relationship, with a Venn diagram. Each construct, *bio-, psycho-,*
and social-, are in their own yet overlapping circle, with optimal health and well-
being located at the nexus.

AAI epitomizes the utility of the biopsychosocial framework because it associates biological functioning, social experience, and psychological processing to
understand subsequent brain response (Howe, 2009). AAI impacts children's internal mechanisms through *physical* indicators such as heart rate and blood pressure
(Farhat-McHayleh et al., 2009; Handlin et al., 2011), perception of *social* support
wherein the dog provides direct support or acts as facilitator to enhance rapport in
interpersonal interactions, and *emotional* functioning such as feelings of *attach-*
ment, comfort, and amelioration of loneliness (Chandler, 2012; Matuszek, 2010).
These various dimensions that are comprised within this framework are visible in
the two case studies immediately below.

Case Study 4

Dr. Masahiro Heima, DDS is an Associate Professor in the Department of
Global Relations and Human Sciences in Dentistry, Graduate School of
Medical and Dental Sciences, Kagoshima University, Japan. As a pediatric
dentist, his research focuses in on dental fear, and he is particularly interested
in innovative interventions, especially those that require minimal training for
dentists and do not include additional pharmaceuticals. Currently, there is
worldwide demand for dental care providers with expertise in treating patients
with dental fear. The inclusion of a therapy dog team is a minimally invasive
way to include an opportunity for grounding and relaxing without the atten-
tion and inclusion of the dental professional. Having engaged in a research
study to test the feasibility of providing AAI to children with dental fear

(Vincent, Heima, & Farkas, 2020b*), Dr. Heima noted that the dogs were specially trained to be nonreactive to their environment and potential stimuli. Patients talked to and pet the dog, either to provide a distraction or to self-sooth; they also held the leash to feel connected to the dog throughout the procedure. The therapy dogs never disturbed dental care procedures. The dental care provider can utilize the AAI in their clinic without additional training through collaboration with a certified team and/or reputable organization, such as Pet Partners. Dental professionals are encouraged to work with interdisciplinary teams (e.g., veterinary social workers) to learn about AAIs and explore if therapy dogs are an appropriate resource for their practice.*

Case Study 5
Taylor Chastain Griffin, Ph.D is the National Director of AAI Advancement for Pet Partners where she focuses on supporting research and professional development within the therapy animal arena.

> *We believe that animals can be significant attachment figures for humans and can model healthy relational skills. And, there is nothing quite like the feeling of unconditional positive regard that animals so freely offer their human counterparts. Therapy animals are the champions of this notion: they accept us as we are and share love, joy, and playfulness in a world that desperately needs more light. Therapy animals also have a way of grounding us—they keep us in the present moment and even help facilitate human-to-human connection. I've observed children in therapy who tell all of their most heartbreaking secrets to a therapy animal, opening up an opportunity for professionals to step in and provide the intervention that they need. I've witnessed young men in prison get down on the floor and snuggle my toy poodle, smiling and giggling as she cuddled into their necks. Therapy animals have a way of meeting a person where they are while somehow providing just the interaction that they need to move forward in a new way.*

AAI in Practice

Types of Interventions

Within AAA there are varying levels of interaction ranging from purely visitation (AAA) to a fully therapeutic intervention (AAT) (Pet Partners, 2016; Winkle, Rogers, Gorbing, and Vancoppernolle, 2022). The main differences lie within the nature of the interaction or intention of the interaction as well as the training and credentialing of the handler and animal partner. AAA may be a dog visiting program, such as certified therapy dogs and handlers making visits to a nursing home or a dog visiting a school to support children in the classroom. The AAA interaction is led by a professional, paraprofessional, or volunteer who has received introductory training and/or form of assessment.

The International Association of Human-Animal Interaction Organizations (IAHAIO) defines AAI, the next level of interaction, as "a goal-oriented and structured intervention that intentionally includes or incorporates animals in health, education, and human services (e.g., social work) for the purpose of therapeutic gains in humans" (Fine, 2019). The objective is to strategically incorporate an animal(s) in human health, education, and/or social service to achieve a therapeutic outcome.

AAI is similar to AAA in that animals are partnered with humans to achieve motivational, educational, and recreational benefits. An example is certified therapy dogs visiting a waiting room in a medical clinic to soothe and distract children before an appointment or a corporate group working with horses for team building. AAIs may serve various purposes, including motivation enhancement, skills development, educational learning, or recreational enjoyment (International Association of Human-Animal Interaction Organizations, 2014). Regardless of the purpose, the interaction is goal-oriented with the animal serving a specific function throughout the intervention. While an intervention differs from therapy, there may be inherent therapeutic gains made by the client through the intentional inclusion of an animal such as building rapport with the therapist, motivation to attend appointments, catharsis throughout appointments, opportunities for unstructured play and conversation, and endless opportunities for guided conversation based on the animal-collaborator (Chandler, 2012; Nimer and Lundahl, 2007).

AAI can involve an animal being present and engaged (explicit) or observational (implicit). When AAI is conducted without an animal present, the activities may include nature-based interventions. Additionally, AAI can be *about* animals, without animals present. This may include drawing animals, including animals in conversation through intake and assessment, and countless other creative activities that bring the creative spirit of animals into the therapeutic environment (Chandler, 2012). Traditional assumptions and the practice of AAI include a live animal present throughout the activity. These explicit activities are encouraged to include domesticated animals predominantly; specialized training should be obtained for specific breeds.

AAT is even more strategic than AAI in that the goal-directed intervention is facilitated by a human service professional, e.g., a social worker, with training in care, handling, and managing therapeutic interactions (Chandler, 2012; International Association of Human-Animal Interaction Organizations, 2014). (See Chap. 7 by Winston in this volume for an in-depth discussion of animal-assisted psychotherapy.) The purpose of AAT is to promote therapeutic improvements in physical, social, emotional, and/or cognitive functioning (Pet Partners, 2018). The licensed professional guides the interactions between a patient/client and an animal to reach specific goals believed to be difficult to achieve without the animal's collaboration (Chandler, 2012; International Association of Human-Animal Interaction Organizations, 2014; Nimer and Lundahl, 2007). While facilitating this interaction, the professional must also adhere to their professional code of ethics. In social work, this includes but is not limited to staying abreast of new learning and opportunities, advocating for the dignity of relationships, and referring to others when clients seek services beyond your scope of practice. As a rigorous intervention, practitioners utilizing AAT must utilize a treatment plan within the client's progress notes to guide and monitor client outcomes (International Association of Human-Animal Interaction Organizations, 2014).

Diverse Animal Roles

The essence of AAI is the feeling of safety when in the company of an animal, be it a companion animal, certified therapy animal, or service dog (Fine, 2019). Attributes of feeling safe are aligned closely with the attributes of feeling secure, e.g., non-judgement, love, support, trust, and empathy. Empirical literature has postulated that feeling safe may be associated with successful interventions (Fine, 2019; Zilcha-Mano, Mikulincer and Shaver, 2011). Thus, AAIs in the community often seek to alleviate negative internalized feelings or external behaviors caused by a negative precipitating event. Through the AAI, an individual may gain physical, mental, social, or emotional skills that may be more difficult to achieve without the collaboration with the animal. The interaction with the animal serves as a model for human interaction; a client can develop social skills while working with the animal. The experiential nature of the interaction helps facilitate the transfer of the learning from the AAI session to human-to-human interaction.

Companion animals are animals of any species that provide comfort to a specific person. Typically, this type of animal is referred to as a "pet," and the person is responsible for the care and welfare of the animal. In recent years, there has been a shift to acknowledge pets as family members. To that end, there is also a conversation about terminology of "ownership" and consideration of shifting to "guardian-ship" or "partnership" (ASPCA, n.d.)

Companion animals can become and serve as therapy animals. However, the dynamic between the person and the animal would shift from being mutually recip-rocal and internal to their relationship to being globally reciprocal and external to their relationship. A therapy animal provides a source of comfort and motivation or is part of a therapeutic intervention. Therapy animals are predominantly dogs, though other species can be certified and serve. To become certified, the animal and handler must pass a standardized test administered by an organization, such as Therapy Dogs International or Pet Partners. With the certification, teams can volun-teer in a variety of community-based organizations.

Dogs that hold a certification with Pet Partners or Therapy Dogs International may complete additional training to serve in the community following a natural disaster or interpersonal tragedy, becoming comfort animals.

Emotional support animals, commonly referred to as ESAs, move a pet to a des-ignated status as a mechanism to alleviate symptoms of mental health challenges. An ESA letter allows the indicated pet to accompany the person in their housing regardless of pet policy. Persons can request a letter from a mental health profes-sional that designates their companion animals for receipt of this enhanced status. Persons partnering with an ESA may experience a reduction of symptomatology of mental health challenges. (For best practices for writing and receiving an ESA letter, see Hoy-Gerlach et al., 2019).

The Americans with Disabilities Act (ADA) does not formally define a service animal. However, the US Department of Justice (DOJ) (2020) defines a service animal within the scope of the Americans with Disabilities Act (ADA) as working animals that is not a household pet, but rather as "any dog that is individually trained to do work or perform tasks for the benefit of an individual with a disability, including a physical, sensory, psychiatric, intellectual, or other mental disability" (Brown, 2019). Simply stated, this is a dog or miniature horse that assists only one person with a disability and function consistently in the role of service to the human. Service animals are task-trained to assist with a variety of physical and mental health challenges (ADI, 2020). Although individuals and organizations sell service animal certification or registration documents online, there are no specific training program or certification requirements for service animals. Under the ADA, persons with a service animal may access anywhere in the community that the general public can access (United States Department of Justice, Civil Rights Division, 2020). According to the DOJ, an animal whose sole function is to provide comfort or emotional support does not qualify as a service animal under the ADA. Furthermore, a service animal may be excluded from protection under Title II or Title III if the dog is out of control and the handler cannot get the animal under control. A handler may be asked to leave a public building or program if the dog is not housebroken (United States Department of Justice, Civil Rights Division, 2020). Although individuals and organizations sell service animal certification or registration documents online, there are no specific training programs or certification requirements for service animals.

The Animals

Sixty-seven percent of homes (84.9 million) in the USA have at least one pet. In 2018, this accounted for more than 89.7 million dogs and 94.2 million cats. As of 2019, the pet economy reached $95.7 billion with the average pet owner budgeting roughly $1000 to $1400 for typical purchases (i.e., food, veterinary care, boarding, groomer). Even during times of financial distress, people budget and invest in pets, financially and emotionally (American Pet Products Survey, 2020). In 2019, the American Society for the Prevention of Cruelty to Animals (ASPCA) found that 80% of pet owners consider their pet to be a family member. It is with this in mind that pets become collaborators in AAI. The most common collaborators are dogs. There is no specific breed, size, or sex that are preferred; rather it is the dog's natural ability and being that make them unique and special. As keen pets, dogs and cats join social workers in AAI to build rapport by instilling a sense of familiarity, calm, and ease. They give purpose to conversation, a mechanism for humans to connect, and inspire play. Pets step into a purposeful role of becoming a member of the care team to help humans overcome adversity and help them heal.

Horses are unique as collaborators because they typically require a specific environment and professional training. Miniature horses may very often travel into the community, to participate in therapeutic riding/driving, equine facilitated psychotherapy (EFP), or ground-based programming. However, access to the AAI may be impacted because one must travel to a farm or stable.

Case Study 6

Kathy Alm is the CEO PATH International. Kathy shared that horses have always been a part of her life...on paper.

> Growing up in the suburbs with no access to horses and no examples of how to be with horses. However, when my mom gave me a stack of drawings that I had done over the years, starting at age 5 or 6, they all included a horse or two.

She dreamt of having a horse, of riding through the fields, and spent her time playing with a "West Set" because it included horses and a ranch and teenage girls who rode and took care of their horses. She saved pennies so she could buy Breyer Horses, eventually affording five of them—which she still has today. All of that set the stage for discovering Equine-Assisted Services later in life and feeling like she'd finally found where she belonged. Spending 15 years as the Executive Director of Little Bit Therapeutic Riding Center, a PATH International Premiere Accredited Center in Redmond, Washington, afforded her the opportunity to not only have direct experience with horses but also daily interaction with the participants who attended therapy and therapeutic riding at the center. She saw firsthand the impact those activities and sessions had on the participants. Those impacts included first words, first steps, overcoming fears, strengthening muscles, learning to socialize, and building confidence to name a few. She experienced horses "knowing" what the participant needed, whether it was adjusting their gait to help balance a rider or reacting to emotions that taught participants how they impact those around them.

In equine facilitated practice (EFP), the mental health professional is the guide for the therapeutic process. Thus, it is ideal if they are comfortable with the horses as they serve as a secure base throughout the intervention.

MacLean (2011) states horses are keenly responsive and sensitive to body language because of their hypersensitivity as prey animals, making them excellent models to teach self-regulation and social skills. Horse interaction provides an experiential platform for people to practice those social skills in a live environment (McKissock et al., 2022). To many, interaction with a horse may be novel. Novelty is considered a strength in this AAI as the sense of awe, curiosity, and engagement facilitate prolonged interest through the session.

Therapy with horses may be beneficial for those who have not found healing through traditional talk therapy. The nature of EFP offers an opportunity to address key barriers to social engagement compared to other more traditional didactic interventions. For example, individuals who have prolonged stress or posttraumatic stress disorder (PTSD) typically feel internal stress and externalized anxiety as well as hyper-arousal. When anxiety is not controlled, a horse may respond by moving away from the source of the anxiety. This is referred to as an incongruence between the anticipated externalized behaviors and what is actually demonstrated. This instantaneous feedback, also known as mirroring, helps the person understand how they present to the horse. The client learns to self-regulate practicing common exercises to downregulate the nervous system; the horse will respond by reengaging with the client.

> **Case Study 7**
> *Marian Heyink, LISW-S, CTRI/ESMHL, Mental Health and Equine Specialist, and EAGALA specialist, works throughout Ohio bringing her profession of social work together with horses. She began volunteering at a therapeutic riding center as an adult and fell in love! She has held many careers including a Master's Degree in Social Work and a law degree, a medical social worker, an attorney, a compliance officer, an administrator at a residential center, and a Director of Public Policy. None of these experiences felt as fulfilling as working with the clients and the horses. She became certified as a Mental Health Practitioner and an Equine Specialist through EAGALA. Often, using metaphor, a horse will remind a client of a family member they are having a difficult relationship with, and this allows them to evaluate behaviors and reactions in a totally different setting. A client that does not thrive or feel comfortable in a traditional office setting may be more able to express themselves when they do not have to focus on the clinician.*

IAHAIO states that wild and exotic animals cannot be considered partners in direct or explicit AAI, even if they are considered tame (Fine, 2019). Nevertheless, programs such as Green Chimneys, a wildlife rehabilitation program in New York that involves clients in food preparation and care, include dolphins in therapeutic engagement for people with disabilities (Brensing et al., 2003). And, for just as long, there has been controversy about their inclusion. The therapeutic milieu is in the water of a lagoon or other environment which houses the dolphins. The goal of the session is for the dolphin to be a motivator to aid in achieving therapeutic objectives. For example, when the client exhibits a target behavior, the trainer initiates a behavior cue to the dolphin or initiates interaction between the client and the dolphin as a reward to the dolphin. The novelty of the dolphin interaction paired with the aquatic intervention can make it an attractive alternative intervention. The engagement is potentially exploitative because the dolphin is required to perform in order to receive its food as a reward, which is divergent from domesticated animal partnerships. "The Whale and Dolphin Conservation Society's statement on Dolphin Assisted Therapy is that it unlikely meets the psychological or physical welfare needs of either human participants or dolphins" (Fine, 2019, pg 417). However, AAA or AAI that is indirect or passive, such as observation of wildlife, including dolphins, is acceptable and appropriate.

AAI Venues and Contexts

This section explores the application of AAI among different community settings. Because the field of VSW and the many practices of AAI continue to expand and grow, this review is not intended to be exhaustive or exclusive.

Airports are an area of community-based AAI that is gaining momentum. Typically a stressful time for a person, running to make a flight, fears of flying, and large amounts of people can lead to an increase in anxiety and worry in some. Many airports take note from the positive benefits of AAI by having therapy dogs present throughout the airport (Alcivar & Gonzalez, 2020). Airports have experienced an increase in positive reviews and reports including a decrease in stress by travelers (Salgado, 2017).

Art comes in an abundance of forms and mediums. Individuals can experience art independently or socially, as a static or experiential moment, as a reflective moment or part of the therapeutic process. Art therapy integrates animals overtly or implicitly. There is also therapeutic benefit to creating art, and experiencing art that includes animals as collaborators of the art itself.

Case Study 8

Ruth Burke, MFA, is an Assistant Professor of Video Art in the Wonsook Kim School of Art at Illinois State University. Her focus is as a multidisciplinary artist whose practice is socially engaged with animals. Much of the "Art World" does not recognize art making with nonhuman animals as socially engaged art, yet so many people have lives that are defined and guided by our relationships with

My work provokes the paradoxical nature of human-animal relationships and portrays manifestations of interspecies kinship. 2020 marked 5 years of focused artistic research exclusively on this connection. The COVID-19 pandemic emphasized the urgency of presence in relation to interspecies relationships. Farmers, farmworkers, and animal caregivers are essential workers. During the stay-at-home lockdown in the spring, essential workers sustained and cared for my animals. I cannot connect with my equine or bovine collaborators in a meaningful way over FaceTime or Zoom. And to me, the magic is present—a synchronized breath, a shared gaze, a lean, the voluntary reduction of space between two beings. This is territory I'm careful not to over-intellectualize or too thoroughly dissect. This was difficult to do while isolated, but made much more pressing the recognition of the intangible social, and emotional benefits of being with

Art allows possibility for affective, critical, confrontational, and socially engaged responses with and for multispecies relationships. See also www. RuthKBurke.com.

The integration of dogs in the *courtroom setting* has little empirical evidence, but a large amount of support from the public. The Animals and Society Institute found that there are two models for this AAI: (1) the handler, who is also the professional in the legal system, works with their own companion dog that holds a certification from an accrediting organization, e.g., Therapy Dogs International (TDI) or Pet Partners, and (2) the legal professional which welcomes a volunteer dog-handler team from the community that has experience and training in the setting and with the population. Arkansas and Illinois have passed legislation that allows certified therapy canines to accompany children into the courtroom. Although there is limited research on the direct impact of therapy dogs in the courtroom setting, there is speculation that the dogs may sway jurors' decisions (Burd & McQuiston, 2019) and that a therapy dog may help reduce stress and anxiety and lessen the effects of retraumatization (Berget & Ihlebæk, 2011; Chandler, 2012; Walsh et al., 2018).

Educational settings are home to a host of AAIs of both passive and active engagement. Youth learn through experiential learning, including direct contact with animals, recognized as humane education (O'Hare & Montminy-Danna, 2001). Students engage in learning about animals in their community, experience caretaking of animals, and experiment in their natural work. In the classroom, animals often serve as a source of motivation, an opportunity to care (empathy), and offer a mechanism for self-soothing and calming which yields a greater readiness to learn (Beck, 2015).

Alternative schools that utilize AAI as the main academic interventions have also begun to expand in the USA. One such school is Green Chimneys in Brewster, New York. The integration of AAI with regular access to animals in the classroom has been found to reduce stress and increase motivation, focus, and task persistence (Jalongo, 2018). A variety of animals support active learning opportunities, similar to other validated models, such as the Porrer League Humane Education Program (Brelsford et al., 2017).

Many therapeutic riding centers throughout the USA work directly with private and public school systems to create therapeutic horseback riding, driving, and ground-based learning as a component of the school day (Agape, 2001; Fieldstone Farm TRC, 2020). Intervention specialists supporting children and adolescents with a variety of disabilities have found that working with therapeutic horsemanship programs aids in teaching physical, social, emotional, interpersonal, and cognitive support and growth. Centers typically enroll students to come to the farm for an 8-to-10-week session, for 2 hours, once per week. In this time, the students ride and receive a classroom- or barn-based learning (Agape, 2020; Fieldstone Farm TRC, 2020). Some school programs are purely motivational where horses become the impetus for students to accomplish academic skills, with interaction with horses as the reward (McKissock, 2003).

A different model is having the school directly on-site at the Center or stable. Gaitway High School, founded in 2006, is an alternative school founded in partnership between Fieldstone Farm Therapeutic Riding Center and the Educational Service Center of the Western Reserve (ESCWR) in northeast Ohio. The school uses a customized course of study aligned with the Ohio Learning Standards. The school has full staff through ESCWR including a principal, teachers, a job-placement coach, and a social worker. Enrollment is capped at 24 students across grades 8–12 to ensure a low student-to-teacher ratio. Integrated into their coursework, students have the opportunity to participate in animal care internships, therapeutic riding, and horse buddies. To date, all graduates have gone on to college, employment, or additional training or joined the military.

In the context of higher education, the presence of a therapy dog in the counseling center has been found to increase students' use of the counseling center (Adams et al., 2017) . First year students experiencing homesickness have found support in receiving AAI (Shellenbarger, 2015). University groups have come together through student organizations, like Campus Canines, to bring therapy dogs to campus and head off campus to walk shelter dogs.

Medical centers and hospitals are increasing including therapy dog and handler teams as volunteers. While visiting programs are the most common animal-assisted activity, AAIs have become an instrumental part of treatment planning for a variety of health needs. Studies of AAIs have reported positive outcomes of reduced anxiety pre- and post-medical treatment (Calcaterra et al., 2015; Coakley & Mahoney, 2009; Urbanski & Lazenby, 2012) along with post-surgery rehabilitative gains. The presence of an animal in these settings provides a positive distraction (Uglow, 2019). As an example, one study involving youth with autism spectrum disorder with long-term hospital stay(s) found that playing with the dogs in two 10-minute sessions supported a positive increase in emotions, receptiveness to social cues, and positive facial expressions (Germone et al., 2019).

In addition to, or in place of visiting therapy teams, medical centers may choose to have a resident facility animal. A UK university teaching children's hospital found that over a 12-month period, daily interactions with the facility dog decreased anxiety regarding procedures, from blood draws to radiographs. Staff also reported a positive view of the dog's presence and exhibited a decrease in work-related stress when engaging in daily interactions with the therapy dog (Uglow, 2019).

Case Study 9

Bonnie S. and Kimber, Therapy Dog visiting team, came together with the goal of training Kimber to be a service dog. When Kimber was not able to fulfill the requirements of the program, Bonnie thought of opportunities for putting Kimber's training and experience to good use. Kimber tested and easily certified with Pet Partners and the local hospital's program. Although certified with Pet Partners, working in a hospital setting required a retest and observation of Kimber's reaction to beeping machines, looming metallic IV poles, and unexpected patient and hospital noise. Once a month, Kimber visits pediatric patients at the hospital as one of a team of three dogs making rounds. With her very own hospital photo ID attached to her collar, she also visits adult hospital patients upon request. Kimber visits weekly at a neighborhood senior living facility that includes assisted living, memory care, and nursing care residents. Although groups vary in age and mental/physical ability, they each share common needs: comfort, compassion, joy, and hope—and for some, a renewed sense of purpose. The presence of a non-judgmental furry canine breaks down barriers, relieves stress, and increases happiness. That alone creates an environment of healing.

Dental clinics have recognized the impact of therapy dog teams and have opened their doors to volunteers and facility dogs. Dental fear is experienced across the life span; dental treatment for those with dental fear and anxiety typically includes the use of mild sedation (i.e., nitrous oxide), physical restraint, distraction, and/or dividing appointments into additional visits (Anthonappa et al., 2017; Casamassimo et al., 2009). Since dental care inherently positions the person in a vulnerable position—physically separated from other support persons (caregiver), reclined in a chair, mouth open—feeling safe may be associated with successful treatment. AAI can be provided in the waiting room before treatment, or even during treatment (Vincent et al., 2019). Studies have demonstrated that it is feasible to include AAI while maintaining high medical standards of care and successful dental treatment (Havener et al., 2001; Schwartz & Patronek, 2002; Vincent et al., 2019, 2020a).

The use of AAIs in nursing homes has historically been well received (Gammonley & Yates, 1991; Machova et al., Machová et al., 2020). The underlying thought is that "animals frequently elicit positive memories in older people, for example of previous pets. Animals are able to bridge communication between humans; they serve as a reason for and a topic of communication, and they enhance interpersonal contact as so-called 'social catalysts'" (Wesenberg et al., 2019, p. 225). One of the first research studies about the impact of animals in nursing homes was of watching fish in aquariums (Riddick, 1985). AAI with senior residents has yielded positive outcomes including increased psychosocial function, specifically emotional and social, during and post-AAI sessions (Aarskog et al., 2019).

The general implementation of AAI typically consists of weekly sessions with the therapy animal where residents either exercise together (walking), pet, or groom and socialize with the therapy animal and handler (Machova et al., 2020). A more specialized intervention with nursing homes and assisted living facilities is working with residents with Alzheimer's disease and/or dementia.

Case Study 10

Toby Cross, MOT, OT/L, CTRI, CPAM, works at Central Kentucky Riding for Hope as the Program Coordinator where she brings together her professional training of Occupational Therapist and a Certified Therapeutic Riding Instructor. As an OT, her role and primary treatment tool/intervention in interacting with individuals with mental health concerns is related to function. The day-to-day routine of caring for horses provides a clear functional activity or job to do around the horses, but allowing the horse to react to and interact with a client/individual in the structure of that functional task is the greatest benefit to the individual. The sensitivities and nuances of equine behavior allow for real-time, immediate feedback in the situation that often comes from a much more tolerable source than another human being.

Prison systems utilize two common dog training programs: (1) the retraining of aggressive shelter dogs that have been returned to the shelter for behavioral challenges for placement as service dogs and (2) vocational training for inmates with the aim of job placement upon reentry into the community. Retraining of behaviorally challenged shelter dogs includes socializing the dogs and desensitizing the dog so that the risk of behavior challenges decreases. This intervention not only allows the dogs more time and access for socialization and training but also increases interpersonal, job skills in inmates, with an aim to decrease environmental stress and recidivism (Corleto, 2018; Fournier, Geller and Fortney, 2007).

An example of a service dog training program is Working Animals Giving Service for Kids (W.A.G.S. 4 Kids). Founded in 2004, WAGS is dedicated to providing mobility and autism service dogs for children throughout northeast and central Ohio. The inmate trainers are guided by the professional training staff to prepare for reentry to the community with prospective job placement and work skill attainment (WAGS4Kids, 2020).

Just as prisons partner with dogs for the rehabilitative process, horses are also partnered with inmates for rehabilitation (Arditti et al., 2020). An example is the program that was highlighted in the acclaimed documentary "The Mustang" in 2019. Programs such as these partner inmates with Bureau of Land Management (BLM) mustangs or other horses with trauma history with the idea that they learn to rehabilitate each other. The newly trained horses are sold to the general public. This program, though not without controversy, has been shown to reduce recidivism and increase empathy and self-esteem in prison inmates (Arditti et al., 2020).

Community services that offer co-sheltering (sheltering of humans and animals together) are increasing through strategic initiatives such as the Purple Leash Project and Red Rover. Pets often serve as a source of companionship, as a confidant, and a vital member of an individual's support system (American Pet Products Survey, 2020; Wood et al., 2015). To that end, the relationships between humans and animals in a household may mirror the status of the health and safety of the people in that family (Krienert et al., 2012; Hoffer et al., 2018). This service is particularly important for individuals who are in need of services due to family violence. (For a discussion of the Link between interpersonal violence and animal abuse, see the chapter authored by Susan Hatters Friedman and colleagues in this volume.)

One example of at-risk populations and their pets living together is the *PALS (People and Animals Living Safely)* program in New York. *PALS* provides co-living residences for domestic violence survivors, their family, and their pets of all kinds. Another organization, *My Dog is My Home*, helps shelters obtain funding so that more shelters can offer beds to humans and animals together. Similarly, *Pets of the Homeless* provides veterinary care and food to pets whose owners face homelessness.

Case Study 11

Christine Kim, MSW, Senior Community Liaison, NYC Mayor's Office of Animal Welfare, serves as the Senior Community Liaison at the New York City Mayor's Office of Animal Welfare, the first office of its kind in the USA.

> *I have always been passionate about animals, as I was also passionate about ending homelessness, hunger, income inequality, racism, homophobia, and sexism. There is one case I largely credit to the trajectory of my career. While working in a permanent supportive housing program on Skid Row in downtown Los Angeles, a new resident moved in after years of being on the street. Unbeknownst to staff, he brought his dog with him. Staff eventually found out about the furry stowaway and gave the resident ultimatum that did not include housing and his dog. With the right support and advocacy, he found the path forward to staying with his dog in his new apartment. Being able to recognize the role of animals is the starting point of the contribution social workers can make in animals and human wellness.*

Case Study 12

Rosie Cross, MSSW, VSW, is Director of Homeless Outreach Services, Volunteer Ministry Center (VMC) at The Foyer in Knoxville, TN. My internship was focused on planning to open a low-barrier, housing-focused homeless shelter that would be LGBTQ-affirming and aimed to accommodate pets. Throughout my work, Rosie strives to provide a safe, inclusive, and affirming space.

> *When we have an animal in the residence, the neighbors treat the animal as a member of the family. I see neighbors who put their pets' needs before their own. If the person is ill, they may go without medical care if they do not have someone to care for their pet. They learn to trust people along with their pets, and they make friends the same way. I recently asked a neighbor what it meant for her to be able to stay at The Foyer with her dog.*
>   *This was the insight she shared: It gave me stability and peace of mind. I felt like I was part of something, and that gave me a sense of wholeness. It gave me one-on-one time with my baby. It allowed her to be a dog: to run, play, and lie in bed with me. She made friends and bonded with everyone. It gave her life outside of a cage... life outside of a car.... It was close to being home. It gave us an opportunity to work hard for what we wanted and accomplish something together.*

As veterinary social workers, we must help our clients access available resources. We must also empathize when our clients are faced with hard decisions, even when they make choices that we may not agree with.

Veterans who suffer from posttraumatic stress disorder (PTSD) may find a service dog helpful. The language around partnership with a services dog is different from therapy dogs because in service, the dog becomes an appendage to the person, rather than a collaborator. While service dogs differ greatly from companion and therapy dogs, the clinical understanding of the dog's importance and the role of alleviating symptomology of a mental health challenge is similar. In addition to self-identified impacts, partnerships with animals have been found to aid in managing psychiatric symptoms including depression, hyper vigilance, and anxiety—attributes of posttraumatic stress disorder—and reduction in sleep disturbances (Beetz et al., 2019; Nelson, 2017).

Research indicates that veterans with posttraumatic stress (PTS) can benefit from equine interaction due to the biopsychosocial impact (McKissock, 2018). Equine-assisted work with veterans often draws on the practice of mindfulness-based stress reduction. Equine-facilitated psychotherapy, also known as equine-assisted therapy, is a collaborative practice between an equine specialist and a licensed mental health provider.

Working with horses can include work on the ground, riding, carriage driving, or other modalities of partnership. The focus is on the quality of the time spent between person and horse, not the horsemanship skill learned and developed. The horses' innate ability to assess their environment and communicate nonverbally provides veterans with an opportunity to pause, breathe, relate, and, ideally, heal. Interaction with the horse promotes the development of self-regulation for people with PTS. Because horses may experience human hyper-arousal as uncomfortable or predatory, they may respond to those with PTS-associated hyper-arousal by not engaging with them. When the veteran learns to self-regulate, the horse engages in relationship, providing positive reinforcement. Interaction with horses can provide a unique platform where the veteran can practice positive relationship skills which can then be transferred to human relationships (McKissock, 2018).

Chapter 8 in this volume, authored by Sandra Breckenridge, focuses specifically on veterinary social work in the context of veterinary hospitals. However, the authors of this chapter would be remiss to not mention and give voice to a community member in practice. For more about this topic, refer to Chap. 6.

Case Study 13

Mary Beth Spitznagel, PhD, is a Clinical Neuropsychologist and Associate Professor at Kent State University. Her interest in human animal interaction work started with a senior mutt that she inherited from a family friend who unexpectedly passed away.

> Allo came into my home with little background information and multiple medical problems. Food refusal, incontinence, and night-time agitation led to many trips and phone calls to the veterinarian, diagnostic tests, and medication prescriptions. I was able to give Allo a good quality of life but was subsidizing her quality of life with my own. Trained as a clinical neuropsychologist, I see family caregiver burden all too often in the loved ones of my patients with dementia. I realized that I was a burdened caregiver...for a dog.

Through conversations and research, it became clear that caregiver burden occurs in veterinary medicine as well and stretches far beyond compassion fatigue. There appears to be a "burden transfer" due to common issues including daily hassles and confrontations, which are relatively rare in human medicine. She realized there was a previously unidentified risk factor for occupational distress in veterinarians. To learn more about Dr. Spitznagel, check https://www.petcaregiverburden.com/single-post/02272017-allosstory.

Virtual programming for AAI became critical in 2019, when the world experienced the unprecedented COVID-19 pandemic, which extends at the time of this writing. The entire AAI community of practitioners needed to respond to the restrictions for social distancing and preventative safety. And yet, the demand for AAI was still ever present. The PATH International community responded very quickly by developing and launching socially responsive programming to meet the service requests of participants who could not attend in person. One of the first web-based resources was The Virtual Education Co-Op, led by Stefani Zabala of the Colorado Therapeutic Riding Center. This resource was sourced by therapeutic riding instructors around the world, who uploaded content to teach horsemanship and provide equine-assisted services. Leaders in the field began to host virtual meet-ups to generate ideas, share learning, and support this new avenue of service delivery. Instructors facilitated sessions for typical clients of therapeutic riding centers. Through the virtual mediums, instructors taught lessons about horse colors, breeds, giants, and so much more. Horses even joined the learning through cameo appearances. Simultaneously, mental health clinicians took to secure platforms to deliver EFP services as well. Virtual education and virtual mental health offer a new mechanism for the provision of therapeutic services.

Case Study 14
Stefani Zabala is Head Instructor at Colorado Therapeutic Riding Center: I was involved with online education at both PATH Intl. and AHA, Inc. and worked for both organizations to deliver online resources to their members.

When the concerns about COVID-19 grew toward becoming a global pandemic, I knew we needed to bring virtual services to our participants. Virtual learning would not replace the experiences of physically being with horses, but as instructors, we could continue to connect and work with our students to provide a sense of continuity and comfort. More important than the collected resource, we created a supportive online community. As riding instructors, or in-person facilitators, most have not received training for how to translate in-person content to online effectively. I spent much of my time focused on developing strategies to empower instructors to feel comfortable teaching online. This was the starting point for our sustainable community to provide high-quality virtual equine-assisted services for programs and students. Developing the online platform and community has offered an entirely new stream of revenue and program opportunity for Centers worldwide.

Training and Preparation for Veterinary Social Workers and Their Animal Partners

Training Veterinary Social Workers

Formal education can begin at the outset of social work or aligned mental health education. Table 5.1 below provides a summary of the various training levels and their associated levels of skills for which individuals are trained. Internationally,

Table 5.1 Levels of training for VSW professionals

Level of education/training	Agency/organizations
Bachelor's degree	Can utilize AAI— no clinical diagnosis, no clinical lens
	Can utilize animal-assisted activities (AAA) or animal-assisted education (AAE)
Master's degree	Can utilize AAI as a treatment modality if clinically licensed within the scope of practice for your state and profession
	A number of colleges have faculties that teach units on animal/human interventions. Programs such as a master's in social work can utilize AAI
Veterinary social work certificate	Available through the University of Tennessee College of Social Work and College of Veterinary Medicine
Handler and dog certification	Available through Pet Partners, Therapy Dogs International, Alliance of Therapy Dogs, Bright and Beautiful Inc.

schools of social work may offer a course. There are other universities that have faculty who teach core courses, faculty engaged in research, and Centers for practice and research. Educational institutions in the USA and Canada offer explicit education in over 2 dozen universities, typically within schools of social work at the bachelor's and master's degree levels. Just like any specialization, opportunities to learn, role play, and experience are necessary to develop professional skills. At this time, there are two primary educational programs.

- The University of Tennessee, Knoxville, offers the Veterinary Social Work Certificate Program, a joint program between the College of Veterinary Medicine and the College of Social Work. The program focuses on the four modules of animal-assisted interventions, animal-related grief and loss, the link between human violence and animal abuse, and compassion fatigue and conflict management. The University of Tennessee launched a second certificate program, the Veterinary Human Support Certificate Program.
- The University of Denver offers several specialized educational certifications through the Institute for Human and Animal Connection: Animal-Assisted Social Work, Animal and Human Health Certificate, Canine-assisted Intervention certificate, Equine-Assisted Mental Health Practitioner, and Humane Education Practitioner.

Beyond university education, professionals are strongly encouraged to pursue certification for animal-specific practice. For example, the best practice for individuals working with canines is to obtain certification for therapy dogs through Pet Partners or Therapy Dogs International. Similarly, individuals working with horses and certification for therapeutic riding, driving, and mental health should include certification through the Professional Association of Therapeutic Horsemanship (PATH) International, the Equine Assisted Growth and Learning Association (EAGALA), or a country-specific organization. However, other countries have aligned organizations that cover foundational knowledge and serve to support professional practice, such as the Canadian Therapeutic Riding Association (CANTRA) in Canada. Although there are more certification or training program options, few have received

Table 5.2 Certification programs for dogs and horses

Certification	Organizations
Dog certifications	Basic obedience training American Kennel Club (AKC) Good Citizen Certification Therapy Dog International
Horse certifications	Equine Assisted Growth and Learning Association (EAGALA) Professional Association of Therapeutic Horsemanship (PATH) International

accreditation. Individuals interested in becoming trained are encouraged to investigate the credibility of any training program before pursuing a credential.

Training and Preparing Animal Collaborators

Table 5.2 provides a listing of the certifications that are available for dogs and horses that will be engaged in providing AAIs. While there are a number of organizations that help train and certify a dog as a therapy dog, the three most common trainings are the Canine Good Citizen test and screening from Pet Partners and Therapy Dogs International.

The Canine Good Citizen (CGC) test is a 10-skill training program that tests dogs on good manners, basic obedience, and different settings/stimuli (American Kennel Club, 2021). This showcases that the team of handler and dog have worked together and bonded and have been responding well to each other.

Building off of the GCG skills, becoming a team may require another form of training or endorsement from outside organizations such as Pet Partners or Therapy Dogs International. Volunteering for Pet Partners and Therapy Dogs International requires that a team be evaluated by the agency to establish that they have the foundation of basic obedience, the dog responds well to the handler, and the handler is aware of the dog's needs during the therapy visit (Pet Partners, 2021; Therapy Dogs International, 2021).

Professionals providing services in collaboration with horses require specialized training and education to ensure safety, knowledge, and best practice standards. There is a variety of modalities for engagement between horses and humans within the scope of AAI. To date, there is minimal, yet emerging, consensus on terminology (Wood et al., 2020). The intersection of social work practice and horses is most commonly referred to as equine-facilitated psychotherapy (EFP). The focus is on the credential of the professional facilitating the equine activity; the horse assists in the therapeutic process. In contrast, equine-assisted learning places the focus on education, personal growth, and organizational development with the assistance of horses. Modalities including adaptive riding, driving, and vaulting are considered horsemanship as the focus is on the acquisition of equine-related skills for the client rather than a treatment goal (Wood et al., 2020).

In 1996, the North American Riding for the Handicapped Association, Inc. (NARHA) founded a subsection, Equine Facilitated Mental Health Association

(EFMHA), with the purpose of "advanc[ing] the field for individuals who partner with equines to promote human growth and development so that our members, clients and equines can succeed and flourish" (PATH International, 2017, slide 14). This was the first explicit movement toward professionalization for a mental health practice that includes horses. In 2008, EFMHA was renamed Equine Facilitated Psychotherapy (PATH International, 2020). In 2010, NARHA changed its name to Professional Association of Therapeutic Horsemanship International (PATH International) to recognize the diversification of therapeutic benefit. At that time, EFMHA was absorbed into PATH and ceased to be a separate organization. Currently, there are two internationally dominant accrediting organizations providing therapeutic engagement with horses, PATH International and the Equine Assisted Growth and Learning Association (EAGALA). Members and centers of both organizations strive to meet standards of safety, client progress, and equine welfare. Both organizations offer mental health-specific training. There are also worldwide opportunities for furthering education through aligned models to further training specific to mental health, such as The HERD Institute (HERD, 2021) and Stable Moments (Stable Moments, 2020). While additional education and learning are fully supported, the best practice is to hold at least one worldwide-recognized certification from PATH International and/or EAGALA as a foundation for professional expertise to facilitate equine-facilitated mental health. (For more information about models of practice and the role of social work and practitioners, see Ballard et al., 2020).

One recurring concern of engaging with animals is that of general sanitation (Machová et al., 2020; See National Center for Health Statistics, 2001; United States Department of Health and Human Services, 2000). The leaders in training, e.g., Pet Partners and Therapy Dogs International (TDI), handler teams, delineate specific protocol for cleanliness of animal and preparation protocol, prior to and during visitation (Pet Partners, 2021). Organizations are encouraged to require the best practice standard of maintaining therapy dog teams to hold TDI or Pet Partners certification. The handler is responsible for looking after the animal throughout the interaction and for initiating its removal from the AAI if necessary. Preparatory protocols provide details on how to best prepare an animal to reduce dander and other debris from being brought into a hospital or other facility with immune vulnerable clients (McKissock, 2013; Therapy Dogs International, 2020).

Case Study 15

Bonnie, therapy dog handler of Kimber shared:

Like people, therapy dogs are all unique with different gifts and preferences. Some dogs like to cuddle. Others would rather do tricks or have children read to them. In whatever situation, the dog handler needs to know their own dog and monitor the dog's stress level. Dogs don't talk, but they do tell you when they're done. Physical signs are panting, a slowed pace, or a lack of their normal enthusiasm. Some days, an hour in a stressful setting is enough work for one day. The handler's job is to keep a watchful eye on the dog and know when to end daily visits so the dog can rest and re-energize. It is common for therapy dogs to keep their own internal clock and calendar, they may whine at the door on the days when it's time for work. Kimber loves her outings!

As a clinician facilitating an AAI session, it is imperative to assess the needs of your client. There are many considerations before bringing an animal into a session/ organization. Organizationally, it is important to consider the needs of others in the building including janitors, landlord's preferences, and others who share space (e.g., waiting room, hallways). Once the space is approved and established, it is important to assess the individual(s) who will be receiving the AAI. Assessments can be formal, such as with the BOAT inventory or the Companion Animal Bond Scale, or informal, such as asking about animals in the client's lives, prior pet ownership, and goals of AAI. If an individual has a history of animal abuse, AAI should be discussed and considered, potentially with consultation before proceeding.

Once a client is assessed and engaged in the opportunity of AAI, it is important to review shared goals and objectives. If the clinician is working with a team approach, as recommended, the collaborators (e.g., therapy dog handler, equine specialist) will need to be given instruction for the session and may need to sign an informed consent.

Throughout sessions, challenges will arise. As with all social work practice, clinicians should build a network of support and consultation. Since the partnership is explicitly with humans, having a veterinary accessible for discussion is highly encouraged. Resources to connect with other social workers include the Veterinary Social Work listserv, connecting with clinicians who provide similar services, developing peer networks, and using online social media forums. As with all social work practice, if there is a concern—professional, moral, value-based, financial, or others—connect and ask. Social work is an interdisciplinary, profession that thrives on the connection with others; the practice of AAI is no difference.

As the knowledge and training of how to implement AAIs increase, the more the field is seeing an increase in co-current handler and therapist teams. An increasing number of therapists are using their personal dogs or other pets as their therapy animal for their clients' sessions.

The great advantage to using one's personal dog as a therapy dog is that the therapist knows the animal better than anyone else. However, this dynamic also can lead to paying more attention to the animal than to the human client and anthropomorphism: "Does Fluffy like this person?" or "She only acts like that when someone doesn't like her." Feelings about the client's relationship with one's own dog can lead to transference and countertransference, a slippery slope (Hoy & Wehman, 2017).

Alternatively, the therapist-dog owner may feel the need to push the dog a little more, knowing the pet's limits. The usage of a personal dog does not consider the human client's preferences, e.g., the client is not receptive to a large dog, preferring instead to work with a small lap dogs. This could lead to overgeneralization and a "one dog fits all" mentality if one uses their personal dog (Schlau, 2017).

A different consideration is whether to allow one's client to bring their pet or emotional support animal to one or more sessions. A client's participation in a session with their own pet provides an opportunity to build on the current bond the pair has; practice exercises that could be used outside of the session, e.g., mindfulness exercises with the pet; or to better understand their dynamic if they are requesting an emotional support animal letter. It can also lead to concerns about training; is this dog safe to be around others, is it up to date on vaccines, or does it have basic obedience skills? Each time an owner brings their personal pet to be used as an AAI, it raises concerns of safety and should be taken into account.

One may also consider inviting a therapy animal team into sessions for AAIs. The team allows for the client and therapist to focus on the interventions and treatment goals, while the handler focuses on the needs of the therapy dog. This allows for a neutral relationship for all parties. However, a concern is confidentiality and if your client is comfortable bringing in a third party; an informed consent should be used.

Throughout each type of engagement, humans and animals are encouraged to complete training (together and independently). For example, an AAA and AAI can be led by a professional or a volunteer who has received training from an organization, e.g., Pet Partners or Therapy Dogs International, to safely facilitate therapeutic activities between a specific animal(s) and person(s). Many organizations offer training for human-animal teams to participate in on-site volunteer work. Similarly, sites such as schools, hospitals, and nursing homes may require attendance at an orientation or training prior to volunteering to learn policies regarding handwashing and hygiene in alignment with standards of practice (AAII, 2021).

Where to Go from Here

AAI is a developed practice with standards and competencies. And yet, it is ever expanding. AAIs started in medical settings, which remain the most common venue for its use. However, animals have reached their paws into a vast array of community settings. Nearly all professional social work spaces are also accessed by furry and hairy collaborators, and, if they're not yet, they may soon be. It is widely presumed that the number of people practicing AAI exceeds the number with formal certification and training, suggesting the need for more widespread education (Risley-Curtiss, 2010). It is through adherence to standards of education and practice that veterinary social work and practices of AAI will reach a level of professionalization that is on par with other social work specializations (Sterman & Bussert, 2020).

Research continues to flourish with support from international, national, and community funders. Funding through the National Institutes of Health has aided in creating a foundation for long-term commitment to this body of research (United States Department of Health and Human Services, National Institutes of Health, 2016). Institutions such as the Human Animal Bond Research Institute and Horses and Humans Research Foundation, Maddie's Fund, and the Kenneth Scott Charitable Trust aid in creating a sustainable future for AAI research. Consistent funding sources allow for researchers to engage in meaningful rigorous research (Esposito et al., 2011).

In addition to those engaged in research, and those providing funding, are those in academic and community settings that open the doors for students to learn about AAI and engage as collaborators of research. Within the last 10 years, AAI moved from a "nice to know'" to a "need to know." Research Centers such as OHAIRE (Organization for Human Animal Interaction Research) lab at Purdue University and CHAIRE (Center for Hyman-Animal Interactions Research and Education) at Ohio State University have responded to the developing field and the growing student interest by creating opportunities to foster future growth and interest. Together, researchers, practitioners, educators, and funders are continuing to move the field of AAI forward.

Appendix

Further Reading

Chandler, C. K. (2017). *Animal-assisted therapy in counseling*. Taylor & Francis.

Cusack, O. (2014). *Pets and mental health*. Routledge.

Fine, A. H. (Ed.). (2019). *Handbook on animal-assisted therapy: Foundations and guidelines for animal-assisted interventions*. Academic Press.

Friedmann, E., Son, H., & Saleem, M. (2015). The animal–human bond: Health and wellness. In A. H. Fine (Ed.), *Handbook on animal-assisted therapy* (pp. 73–88). Academic Press.

Hallberg, L. (2008). *Walking the way of the horse: Exploring the power of the horse-human relationship*. IUniverse.

Howie, A. R. (2015). *Teaming with your therapy dog*. Purdue University Press.

Hoy, J., & Wehman, S. (2017). *The relevance of human-animal interaction for social work practice*. NASW Press.

Levinson, B. (1997). *Pet-oriented child psychotherapy*. Charles C Thomas Publisher Ltd..

National Association of Social Workers. (2018). *Practice perspectives*. https://www.socialworkers.org/LinkClick.aspx?fileticket=MzB8oKdNVlw%3D&portalid=0. Retrieved 21 May 2021.

Ryan, T. (Ed.). (2014). *Animals in social work: Why and how they matter*. Springer.

Weil, Z. (2004). *The power and promise of humane education*. New Society Publishers.

Web-Based Resources

Assistance Dogs International: https://assistancedogsinternational.org/ Animal Welfare Institute: https://awionline.org/

Co-Sheltering Collaborative: https://www.co-shelteringcollaborative.org/

PAWS Act: https://awionline.org/content/pet-and-women-safety-paws-act

Pets of the Homeless: https://www.petsofthehomeless.org/

Sheltering Animals and Families Together: https://alliephillips.com/saf-tprogram/saf-t-shelters/

References

AAII. (2021). *Animal Assisted Intervention International*. Retrieved from: https://aai-int.org/

Aarskog, N. K., Hunskår, I., & Bruvik, F. (2019). Animal-assisted interventions with dogs and robotic animals for residents with dementia in nursing homes: A systematic review. *Physical & Occupational Therapy in Geriatrics, 37*(2), 77–93.

Adams, T., Clark, C., Crowell, V., Duffy, K., & Green, M. (2017). The mental health benefits of having dogs on college campuses. *Modern Psychological Studies, 22*(2), 50–59.

ADI. (2020). *Assistance Dogs International*. Retrieved from: https://assistancedogsinternational.org/

Agape. (2001). *Agape Therapeutic Riding Center*. Retrieved from: https://agaperiding.org/

Agape Therapeutic Riding Center. (2020). *Unbridled hope*. https://agaperiding.org/. Retrieved May 21, 2021.

Alcivar, C., & Gonzalez, L. (2020, March 15). *New airport therapy dogs programs that launched in USA 2018*. https://www.vanemag.com/new-airport-therapy-dogs-programs-launched-usa-2018/. Accessed 09 Dec 2020.

Allen, K. M., Blascovich, J., Tomaka, J., & Kelsey, R. M. (1991). Presence of human friends and pet dogs as moderators of autonomic responses to stress in women. *Journal of Personality and Social Psychology, 61*(4), 582–589.

American Kennel Club. (2021). *American Kennel Club*. https://www.akc.org/

American Pet Products Survey. (2020). *2019–2020 APPA national pet owners survey*. https://www.americanpetproducts.org/pubs_survey.asp. Accessed 14 Dec 2020.

American Psychiatric Association (Ed.). (2013). *Diagnostic and statistical manual of mental disorders* (5th ed.). American Psychiatric Association.

American Society for the Protection of Animals. (n.d.). *Position Statement on Ownership/Guardianship*. https://www.aspca.org/about-us/aspca-policy-and-position-statements/position-statement-ownershipguardianship. Retrieved on May 21, 2021.

Anthonappa, R. P., Ashley, P. F., Bonetti, D. L., Lombardo, G., & Riley, P. (2017). Non-pharmacological interventions for managing dental anxiety in children. *The Cochrane Database of Systematic Reviews, 2017*(6).

Arditti, J., Morgan, A., Spiers, S., Buechner-Maxwell, V., & Shivy, V. (2020). Perceptions of rehabilitative change among incarcerated persons enrolled in a prison-equine program (PEP). *Journal of Qualitative Criminal Justice & Criminology*. https://doi.org/10.21428/88de04a1.f0206951

Ballard, I., Vincent, A., & Collins, C. (2020). Equine facilitated psychotherapy with young people: Why insurance coverage matters. *Child and Adolescent Social Work Journal, 37*(6), 1–7.

Beck, K. R. (2015). The impact of canine-assisted therapy and activities on children in an educational setting. *Education*. https://fisherpub.sjfc.edu/cgi/viewcontent.cgi?article=1313&context=education_ETD_masters. Accessed 21 May 2021.

Beetz, A., Uvnas-Moberg, K., Julius, H., & Kotrschal, K. (2012). Psychosocial and psychophysiological effects of human-animal interactions: The possible role of oxytocin. *Frontiers in Psychology, 3*(234), 1–15.

Beetz, A., Schöfmann, I., Girgensohn, R., Braas, R., & Ernst, C. (2019). Positive effects of a short-term dog-assisted intervention for soldiers with post-traumatic stress disorder—A pilot study. *Frontiers in Veterinary Science, 6*(170). https://www.frontiersin.org/articles/10.3389/fvets.2019.00170/full. Retrieved on May 21, 2021.

Bekoff, M. (2007). Encyclopedia of human--animal relationships: A global exploration of our connections with animals [four volumes]. *Anthrozoös, 20*(2), 196–198.

Berget, B., & Ihlebæk, C. (2011). Animal-assisted interventions; effects on human mental health-A theoretical framework. In T. Uehara, T. (Ed.). *Psychiatric disorders-worldwide advances*. https://www.intechopen.com/books/psychiatric-disorders-worldwide-advances. Retrieved May 21, 2021.

Bikales, G. (1975). The Dog As "Significant Other". *Social Work*, 150–152.

Borrell-Carrio, F., Suchman, A. L., & Epstein, R. M. (2004). The biopsychosocial model 25 years later: Principles, practice, and scientific inquiry. *Annals of Family Medicine, 2*(6), 576–582. https://doi.org/10.1370/afm.245

Bowlby, J. (1988). Attachment, communication, and the therapeutic process. In J. Bowlby (Ed.), *A secure base: Parent-child attachment and healthy human development* (pp. 137–157). Basic Books.

Brelsford, V. L., Meints, K., Gee, N. R., & Pfeffer, K. (2017). Animal-assisted interventions in the classroom—A systematic review. *International Journal of Environmental Research and Public Health, 14*(7) https://www.mdpi.com/1660-4601/14/7/669/htm. Retrieved May 21, 2021.

Brensing, K., Linke, K., & Todt, D. (2003). Can dolphins heal by ultrasound? *Journal of Theoretical Biology, 225*(1), 99–105.

Brown, S. E. (2019). *Individuals with disabilities and their assistance animals: A brief history and definitions*. ADA National Network|Information, Guidance and Training on the Americans with Disabilities Act. https://adata.org/legal_brief/individuals-disabilities-and-their-assistance-animals-brief-history-and-definitions. Retrieved May 21, 2021.

Burd, K. A., & McQuiston, D. E. (2019). Facility Dogs in the courtroom: Comfort without prejudice? *Criminal Justice Review, 44*(4), 515–536. https://doi.org/10.1177/0734016819844298

Calcaterra, V., Veggiotti, P., Palestrini, C., De Giorgis, V., Raschetti, R., Tumminelli, M., ... Ostuni, S. (2015). Post-operative benefits of animal-assisted therapy in pediatric surgery: A randomised study. *PLoS One, 10*(6), 1–13.

Casamassimo, P. S., Thikkurissy, S., Edelstein, B. L., & Maiorini, E. (2009). Beyond the DMFT: The human and economic cost of early childhood caries. *Journal of the American Dental Association, 140*(6), 650–657.

Center for Disease Control. (2020). *Children's oral health*. https://www.cdc.gov/oralhealth/basics/childrens-oral-health/index.html. Retrieved May 21, 2021.

Chandler, C. K. (2012). *Animal assisted therapy in counseling*. Routledge.

Cirulli, F., Borgi, M., Berry, A., Francia, N., & Alleva, E. (2011). Animal-assisted interventions as innovative tools for mental health. *Annali dell'Istituto superiore di sanità, 47*(4), 341–348.

Coakley, A. B., & Mahoney, E. K. (2009). Creating a therapeutic and healing environment with a pet therapy program. *Complementary Therapies in Clinical Practice, 15*(3), 141–146.

Corleto, D. (2018). Prison rehabilitation: The sociological, physiological, and psychological effects of animal-assisted interventions. *Themis: Research Journal of Justice Studies and Forensic Science, 6*(8), 112–131.

Crittenden, P. M. (1995). Peering into the black box: An exploratory treatise on the development of self in young children. In D. Cicchetti & S. Toth (Eds.), *Rochester symposium on developmental psychopathology* (Vol. 5, pp. 79–148). University of Rochester Press.

Engel, G. L. (1977). The need for a new medical model: A challenge for biomedicine. *Science, 196*(4286), 129–136.

Engel, G. (1980). The clinical application of the biopsychosocial model. *American Journal of Psychiatry, 137*, 535–544.

Esposito, L., McCune, S., Griffin, J. A., & Maholmes, V. (2011). Directions in human–animal interaction research: Child development, health, and therapeutic interventions. *Child Development Perspectives, 5*(3), 205–211.

Farhat-McHayleh, N., Harfouche, A., & Souaid, P. (2009). Techniques for managing behaviour in pediatric dentistry: Comparative study of live modelling and tell-show-do based on children's heart rates during treatment. *Journal of the Canadian Dental Association, 75*(4), 283–283f.

Fieldstone Farm Therapeutic Riding Center. (2020). *A horse can change a life*. https://www.fieldstonefarmtrc.com/. Retrieved May 21, 2021.

Fine, A. H. (2019). *Handbook on animal-assisted therapy: Theoretical foundations and guidelines for practice* (3rd ed.). Academic Press.

Fournier, A. K., Geller, E. S., & Fortney, E. V. (2007). Human-animal interaction in a prison setting: Impact on criminal behavior, treatment progress, and social skills. *Behavior and Social Issues, 16*(1), 89–105.

Friedman, E., & Tsai, C. (2006). The animal-human bond: Health and wellness. In A. Fine (Ed.), *Handbook on animal-assisted therapy: Theoretical foundations and guidelines for practice* (pp. 95–120). Elsevier.

Gammonley, J., & Yates, J. (1991). Pet projects: Animal assisted therapy in nursing homes. *Journal of Gerontological Nursing, 17*(1), 12–15.

Gehrke, E., Myers, M., Mendez, S., Mckissock, B., Lindsley, J., & Tontz, P. (2019). Multi site psychophysiological analysis of equine assisted healing in combat veterans and first responders. *International Journal of Health and Science, 7*(4), 1–8.

Geist, T. S. (2011). Conceptual framework for animal assisted therapy. *Child and Adolescent Social Work Journal, 28*(3), 243–256.

Germone, M. M., Gabriels, R. L., Guerin, N. A., Pan, Z., Banks, T., & O'Haire, M. E. (2019). Animal-assisted activity improves social behaviors in psychiatrically hospitalized youth with autism. *Austim*, 1–12. https://doi.org/10.1177/136236131982741

Goldberg, S., Muir, R., & Kerr, J. (1995). *Attachment theory: Social, developmental, and clinical perspectives*. The New Atlantic Press.

Gray, S. W., & Zide, M. R. (2012). *Brooks/Cole empowerment series: Psychopathology: A competency-based assessment model for social workers* (3rd ed.). Cengage Learning.

Handlin, L., Hydbring-Sandberg, E., Nilsson, A., Ejdebäck, M., Jansson, A., & Uvnäs-Moberg, K. (2011). Short-term interaction between dogs and their owners: Effects on oxytocin, cortisol, insulin and heart rate—An exploratory study. *Anthrozoös, 24*(3), 301–315.

Handlin, L., Nilsson, A., Ejdebäck, M., Hydbring-Sandberg, E., & Uvnäs-Moberg, K. (2012). Associations between the psychological characteristics of the human–dog relationship and oxytocin and cortisol levels. *Anthrozoös, 25*(2), 215–228.

Harlow, H. F. (1958). The nature of love. *American Psychologist, 13*(12), 673. https://doi.org/10.1037/h0047884

Havener, L., Gentes, L., Thaler, B., Megel, M., Baun, M., Driscoll, F., … Agrawal, N. (2001). The effects of a companion animal on distress in children undergoing dental procedures. *Issues in Comprehensive Pediatric Nursing, 24*(2), 137–152.

Herd Institute. (2021, February 17). *HERD Institute – Equine facilitated psychotherapy & learning certification*. The HERD Institute. https://herdinstitute.com/

Hofer, M. A. (1995). Attachment and psychopathology. In *Attachment theory: Social, developmental, and clinical perspectives* (pp. 367–406). Atlantic Press, Inc.

Hoffer, T., Hargreaves-Cormany, H., Muirhead, Y., & Meloy, J. R. (2018). *Violence in animal cruelty offenders*. Online EBook. Springer International Publishing.

Hosey, G., & Melfi, V. (2014). Human-animal interactions, relationships and bonds: A review and analysis of the literature. *International Journal of Comparative Psychology, 27*(1), 1–26. Permalink: https://escholarship.org/uc/item/6955n8kd

Howe, D. (2009). *A brief introduction to social work theory*. Palgrave Macmillan.

Howie, A. R. (2015). *Teaming with your therapy dog*. Purdue University Press.

Hoy, J., & Wehman, S. (2017). *The relevance of human-animal interaction for social work practice*. NASW Press.

Hoy-Gerlach, J., Vincent, A., & Lory, B. (2019). Emotional support animals in the United States: Emergent guidelines for mental health clinicians. *Journal of Psychosocial Rehabilitation and Mental Health, 6*(2), 199–208.

International Association of Human-Animal Interaction Organizations. (2014). IAHAIO white paper. In A. H. Fine (Ed.), *(2019). Handbook on animal-assisted therapy: Theoretical foundations and guidelines for practice* (pp. 415–418). Academic Press.

Jacobson, T. (2019). The History of Equine Therapy. *Of Horse*. https://www.ofhorse.com/view-post/The-History-of-Equine-Therapy

Jalongo, M. R. (2018). An attachment perspective on the child-dog bond: Interdisciplinary and international research findings. *Children, Dogs and Education*, 21–41.

Karen, R. (1998). *Becoming attached: First relationships and how they shape our capacity to love*. Oxford University Press.

Katcher, A. H., Friedmann, E., Beck, A. M., & Lynch, J. J. (1983). *New perspectives on our lives with companion animals* (pp. 351–359). University of Pennsylvania Press.

Krienert, J. L., Walsh, J. A., Matthews, K., & McConkey, K. (2012). Examining the nexus between domestic violence and animal abuse in a national sample of service providers. *Violence and Victims, 27*(2), 280–296.

Machová, K., Procházková, R., Konigová, P., Svobodová, I., Přibylová, L., & Vadroňová, M. (2020). Acceptability of AAI from the perspective of elderly clients, family members, and staff—A pilot study. *International Journal of Environmental Research and Public Health, 17*(16), 5978.

MacLean, B. (2011). Equine-assisted therapy. *Journal of Rehabilitation Research & Development, 48*(7), ix–ix.

Malinowski, K., Yee, C., Tevlin, J. M., Birks, E. K., Durando, M. M., Pournajafi-Nazarloo, H., ... & McKeever, K. H. (2018). The effects of equine assisted therapy on plasma cortisol and oxytocin concentrations and heart rate variability in horses and measures of symptoms of post-traumatic stress disorder in veterans. *Journal of Equine Veterinary Science, 64*, 17–26.

Matuszek, S. (2010). Animal-facilitated therapy in various patient populations: Systematic literature review. *Holistic Nursing Practice, 24*(4), 187–203.

McCardle, L., Webster, E. A., Haffey, A., & Hadwin, A. F. (2017). Examining students' self-set goals for self-regulated learning: Goal properties and patterns. *Studies in Higher Education, 42*(11), 2153–2169.

McConnell, P. (2009). *For the love of a dog: Understanding emotion in you and your best friend.* Ballantine Books.

McKissock, H. B. (2003). *A model for using interaction with horses to increase reading motivation of first grade urban students* [Unpublished master's thesis]. Purdue University.

McKissock. B. (2013). *Reading with Rosie: Equine Assisted Literacy Implementation Manual.* Indiana: IBJ.

McKissock, H. B. (2018). *Equine assisted learning as a model of applied ecopsychology: Phenomenological study of the benefits of connecting with horses for people with post traumatic stress disorder* [Unpublished doctoral dissertation]. Akamai University.

McKissock, H. B., Bowen, A., Dawson, S., Eldridge, L., McIntire, J., Stanojevic, C., Tamas, D., & McCormick, B. P. (2022). *Manualized equine-assisted therapy protocol for clients with autism spectrum disorder. Therapeutic Recreation Journal, 56*(1), 39–54. https://doi-org.proxy2. library.illinois.edu/10.18666/TRJ-2022-V56-I1-10862

Miles, E. (2014). Biopsychosocial model. In M. Gellman & J. R. Turner (Eds.), *Encyclopedia of behavioral medicine* (pp. 227–228). Springer.

Morgan, M. (1894). *Xenophon, The Art of Horsemanship*. London: J.A. Allen.

NASW (2021). *National Association of Social Workers*, Retrieved from http://www.NASW.org

National Center for Health Statistics. (2001). *Healthy people 2000 final review*. Hyattsville, MD: Public Health Services. https://www.cdc.gov/nchs/data/hp2000/hp2k01.pdf

Nelson, N. (2017). *Use of animal-assisted therapy on veterans with combat-related PTSD.* https://ir.stthomas.edu/cgi/viewcontent.cgi?article=1769&context=ssw_mstrp. Accessed 21 May 2021.

Nimer, J., & Lundahl, B. (2007). Animal-assisted therapy: A meta-analysis. *Anthrozoös, 20*(3), 225–238.

O'Hare, T., & Montminy-Danna, M. (2001). *Evaluation report: Effectiveness of the Potter League humane education program.* https://digitalcommons.salve.edu/cgi/viewcontent. cgi?referer=https://scholar.google.com/&httpsredir=1&article=1001&context=fac_staff_pub. Accessed 21 May 2021.

PATH International. (2017). *Equine specialist for mental health and learning*. Faculty Presentation. Equine Specialist in Mental Health and Training, Certification: Denver, Colorado. Retrieved May 21, 2021.

PATH International (2020). *Professional Association of Therapeutic Horsemanship International.* Retrieved from: https://pathintl.org/

Pet Partners. (2016). *Pet Partners handler guide.*

Pet Partners. (2018). *Annual Report*. Retrieved from: https://petpartners.org/wp-content/ uploads/2019/06/AnnualReport2018_Web-Ready-File.pdf

Pet Partners. (2021). *Therapy animal program.* Retrieved from: https://petpartners.org/

Riddick, C. C. (1985). Health, aquariums, and the non-institutionalized elderly. *Marriage & Family Review, 8*(3–4), 163–173.

Risley-Curtiss, C. (2010). Social work practitioners and the human-companion animal bond: A national study. *Journal of Social Work, 55*(1), 38–46. PMID: 20069939.

Risley-Curtiss, C., Rogge, M. E., & Kawam, E. (2013). Factors affecting social workers' inclusion of animals in practice. *Journal of Social Work, 58*(2), 153–161.

Salgado, B. (2017, May/June). *Airports get their wag on with therapy animal programs.* https://airportimprovement.com/article/airports-get-their-wag-therapy-animal-programs. Accessed 09 Dec 2020.

Schlau, E. (2017). *Bring your dog to work day: What animal assisted therapy is not. In Ideas and research you can use: VISTAS 2017.* https://www.counseling.org/ docs/defaultsource/vistas/article_465ccd2bf16116603abcacff0000bee5e7.pdf?sfvrsn=c2db4b2c_6. Accessed 21 May 2021.

Schore, J. R., & Schore, A. N. (2008). Modern attachment theory: The central role of affect regulation in development and treatment. *Clinical Social Work Journal, 36*(1), 9.

Schwartz, A., & Patronek, G. (2002). Methodological issues in studying the anxiety-reducing effects of animals: Reflections from a pediatric dental study. *Anthrozoös, 15*(4), 290–299.

Serpell, J. (2000). Animal companions and human well-being: A historical exploration of the value of human-animal relationship. In A. H. Fine (Ed.), *Handbook on animal-assisted therapy: Theoretical foundations and guidelines for practice* (pp. 3–19). Academic Press.

Shellenbarger, S. (2015). To call mom or not? New help for homesick. *Wall Street Journal,* October 21. https://www.arboretum.umn.edu/UserFiles/File/Education %202015/WallStreetJournalHomesickness.pdf

Song, R., Liu, J., & Kong, X. (2016). Autonomic dysfunction and autism: Subtypes and clinical perspectives. *North American Journal of Medicine & Science, 9.*

Stable Moments. (2020). *Developmental Trauma: Equine assisted learning.* Stable Moments. (n.d.). https://www.stablemoments.com/

Sterman, J., & Bussert, K. (2020). Human-animal interaction in social work: A call to action. *Journal of Social Work Values and Ethics, 17*(1), 47–54.

Tedeschi, P., Fitchett, J., & Molidor, C. E. (2005). The incorporation of animal-assisted interventions in social work education. *Journal of Family Social Work, 9*(4), 59–77.

Therapy Dogs International. (2020). *About us.* Retrieved from: https://www.tdi-dog.org

Therapy Dogs International. (2021). *Therapy Dogs International.* https://www.tdi-dog.org/default.aspx

UD Department for Health and Safety. (2000). *Healthy people 2000.* Retrieved from: https://www.cdc.gov/nchs/healthy_people/hp2000.htm

Uglow, L. S. (2019). The benefits of an animal-assisted intervention service to patients and staff at a children's hospital. *British Journal of Nursing, 28*(8), 509–516.

United States Department of Health and Human Services, National Institute of Health. (2016). *Animal assisted interventions for special populations.* https://grants.nih.gov/grants/guide/rfa-files/RFA-HD-17-014.html. Retrieved May 21, 2021.

United States Department of Justice, Civil Rights Division. (2020). *ADA requirements: Service animals.* https://www.ada.gov/service_animals_2010.htm. Accessed 29 May 2021.

Urbanski, B. L., & Lazenby, M. (2012). Distress among hospitalized pediatric cancer patients modified by pet-therapy intervention to improve quality of life. *Journal of Pediatric Oncology Nursing, 29*(5), 272–282.

Vincent, A., McDonald, S., Poe, B., & Deisner, V. (2019). Beyond species, pets are family: The link between interpersonal violence and animal abuse. *Society Register, 3*(3), 83–101.

Vincent, A., Easton, S., Sterman, J., Farkas, K., & Heima, M. (2020a). Acceptability and demand of therapy dog support among oral health care providers and caregivers of pediatric patients. *Pediatric Dentistry, 42*(1), 16–21.

Vincent, A., Heima, M., & Farkas, K. J. (2020b). Therapy dog support in pediatric dentistry: A social welfare intervention for reducing anticipatory anxiety and situational fear in children. *Child and Adolescent Social Work Journal, 37*(6), 1–15.

WAGS4Kids. (2020). *Working animals giving service 4 kids* (W.A.G.S.4 Kids). Retrieved from: https://www.wags4kids.org/

Walsh, D., Yamamoto, M., Willits, N. H., & Hart, L. A. (2018). Job-related stress in forensic interviewers of children with use of therapy dogs compared with facility dogs or no dogs. *Frontiers in Veterinary Science, 5*, 46. https://doi.org/10.3389/fvets.2018.00046

Wesenberg, S., Mueller, C., Nestmann, F., & Holthoff-Detto, V. (2019). Effects of an animal-assisted intervention on social behaviour, emotions, and behavioural and psychological symptoms in nursing home residents with dementia. *Psychogeriatrics, 19*(3), 219–227.

Wilson, E. O. (1984). *Biophilia*. Harvard University Press.

Winkle, M., Rogers, J., Gorbing, P., & Vancoppernolle, D. (2022). *Animal assisted intervention international public document: Standards of practice and competencies for animal assisted interventions.*

Wood, L., Martin, K., Christian, H., Nathan, A., Lauritsen, C., Houghton, S., … McCune, S. (2015). The pet factor-companion animals as a conduit for getting to know people, friendship formation and social support. *PLoS One, 10*(4), e0122085.

Wood, W., Alm, K., Benjamin, J., Thomas, L., Anderson, D., Pohl, L., & Kane, M. (2020). Optimal terminology for services in the United States that incorporate horses to benefit people: A consensus document. *The Journal of Alternative and Complementary Medicine.* https://doi.org/10.1089/acm.2020.0415

Zilcha-Mano, S., Mikulincer, M., & Shaver, P. R. (2011). Pet in the therapy room: An attachment perspective on animal-assisted therapy. *Attachment & Human Development, 13*(6), 541–561.

Chapter 6
Animal-Assisted Interventions and Psychotherapy

Ellen Kinney Winston

Introduction

In 2018, almost 20 percent of adults and 16 percent of children and teens experienced mental illness, though less than half received treatment (National Alliance on Mental Illness, 2020). For many individuals, traditional talk therapy is not an effective or appealing option for treatment. As a result, people have increasingly been looking for varied methods of treatment, especially those who have experienced trauma or who may be resistant to or discouraged by previous efforts with traditional treatment methods (Chandler, 2005; Tedeschi & Jenkins, 2019). Animal assisted psychotherapy is a counseling and psychotherapy specialty that can meet the needs of many individuals, couples, families, and groups who are looking for something beyond talk therapy.

This chapter explains what is meant by the term animal assisted psychotherapy (AAP), reasons for incorporating AAP into treatment, and the unique benefits that AAP can have for both clients and clinicians. Some of the specific legal and ethical issues that arise with AAP are explored. Then, as it can be difficult to understand the therapeutic benefits and life-changing impact that AAP can have simply by reading about it, numerous case examples are presented to illustrate the power and flexibility of AAP and its implementation at Animal Assisted Therapy Programs of Colorado's Barking CAAT (Center for Animal Assisted Therapy) Ranch. Though it is beyond the scope of this chapter to explore how to become proficient in AAP or the scope of AAP practice, hopefully, it provides a good introduction into the strength of AAP as a growing clinical specialty.

E. Winston (✉)
Animal Assisted Therapy Programs of Colorado, Arvada, CO, USA
e-mail: ewinston@aatpc.org

© The Author(s), under exclusive license to Springer Nature Switzerland AG 2022   141
S. Loue, P. Linden (eds.), *The Comprehensive Guide to Interdisciplinary Veterinary Social Work*, https://doi.org/10.1007/978-3-031-10330-8_6

Animal Assisted Psychotherapy

Animal assisted psychotherapy (AAP) is a unique and expanding field in which mental health professionals incorporate trained animals into counseling sessions. Clinicians are educated and certified in a counseling field, such as counseling, social work, psychology, or marriage and family therapy, and then receive additional training and certification in the inclusion of animals into their practice (Fine et al., 2015; Parish-Plass, 2013; Winston, 2015a, b). AAP diverges from the more commonly understood animal-assisted therapy (AAT) in several important ways. First, AAP occurs specifically in mental health/counseling/psychotherapy sessions, whereas AAT takes place in hospitals, physical therapy offices, or a variety of other settings. Second, AAP is conducted by a mental health clinician working within their[1] area of expertise, responsible for both the client and the animal. AAT is conducted by volunteer handlers and animals who have been taught how to safely interact with people but are not necessarily trained in the field in which they are volunteering; for instance, a lawyer may be volunteering with her dog in a hospice setting. These volunteer, visiting AAT programs are certainly powerful for both the participants and the volunteers, but AAP's focus on mental health, the depth and complexities of the therapy, and the training of clinicians make it a distinctive professionally led intervention (Fine et al., 2015; Winston, 2015a, b).

There is no specific theoretical or clinical focus that an AAP practitioner needs to have; rather, AAP is an additional clinical specialty that supplements therapeutic work and may enhance the practitioner's ability to work within a specific theoretical orientation. AAP can be incorporated into most styles of counseling (directive or non-directive, individual, couple, family, or group), as its interventions and techniques can be adapted to best fit the theory, counselor, and client (Chandler, 2005; Fine, 2015). AAP is not an adjunct to another therapy but is "a form of psychotherapy which is conducted with the same rationales and goals as mainstream psychotherapy" (Parish-Plass, 2013, p. xviiiit); this means that all clinicians who practice AAP should be specifically trained in the specialty and work with an animal that has been evaluated for safety in working with clients. The clinician must determine that the client and animal are safe to work together, that AAP aligns with and enhances the client's treatment needs and goals, and that the AAP relationship benefits both the client and the animal (Parish-Plass, 2013; Winston, 2015a, b). An AAP clinician also does not "use" or "utilize" their therapy animal; rather, the animal is the therapist's partner, and the therapist includes, incorporates, or works with the animal as appropriate and safe. Most AAP clinicians work primarily with their own trained therapy animal, but increasingly, therapists may also work with animals that reside at a mental health facility or therapeutic ranch setting such as Barking CAAT Ranch, AATPC's urban therapy farm. Barking CAAT Ranch has currently has about 25 resident animals, including four horses, two donkeys, two alpacas, three

---

[1] For the purposes of inclusion, this chapter will use the terms they/them/their rather than individual gendered pronouns even when referring to one individual.

goats, six cats, two rabbits, two three guinea pigs, and two rats; many staff clinicians also have their own certified therapy dogs.

AATPC counselors decide which animal they are going to work with, and it may change multiple times a day, depending on various factors including the needs and comforts of the client, stage of treatment, treatment goals, safety considerations, the animal's work/rest balance, presence of other counselors and clients, weather, and animal health. Sessions may take place either inside or outside and are generally a mix of free, non-directive interactions and directive, structured interventions. Clinicians can also choose to work with animal representations, such as puppets, stuffed animals, figurines, or pictures, particularly if a client is not ready for a live animal or the animal is not present or able to participate. The specifics of the session, including the interventions and the interactions, depend on all the previously mentioned factors and will be discussed later in the chapter and throughout the case examples.

Legal and Ethical Issues

Though AAP has innumerable benefits, it also comes with added legal and ethical risks that are not present in more traditional therapeutic settings. As of this writing, there is little in the way of national or international standards or laws for practicing animal assisted therapy/psychotherapy. Several different organizations have created their own standards or guidelines for practice, including the American Counseling Association (Stewart et al., 2016), the International Association of Human-Animal Interactions Organizations (IAHAIO) (Jegatheesan et al., 2018), and the Israeli Association of Animal-Assisted Psychotherapy (Hazut et al., 2006). Each paper proposes guidelines for animal-assisted issues including knowledge and skills the therapist should possess, professional training and education, animal training and skills, animal selection criteria, and animal welfare issues. However, the guidelines/ suggestions vary and do not always align. As there is no formal requirement to follow these recommendations, there is often misinformation, confusion, and a lack of guidance for individuals looking to start practicing AAP.

An AAP clinician is responsible for managing both the client and the animal during sessions. Therefore, it is essential that the clinician monitors the safety, welfare, behavioral changes, and emotional well-being of both parties (Parish-Plass, 2013; Winston, 2015a, b). A clinician needs to understand how to combine the strengths, challenges, needs, and desires of their client and their animal in a way that is safe, ethical, and beneficial to all participants in the therapeutic session (Winston, 2015a, b). The health and safety of all parties involved are a top priority. The following section outlines some basic guidelines for legally, ethically, and safely practicing AAP and includes some steps and precautions that AATPC takes to create the safest and most enriching environment for all parties involved, human and animal alike.

Animal Selection and Welfare

One of the first steps in deciding to begin AAP is to ensure that the animal is a good fit for therapy work and "wants" to be a therapy animal. AAP should not be conducted unless the animal enjoys and benefits from interacting with clients on a regular basis: "Those who involve animals in their work to help improve the lives of others have a strict, moral, and enduring responsibility to the animal participants" (O'Haire et al., 2019, p. 34). When therapists choose to partner with animals in therapy, it is essential to treat them as sentient beings who have emotional responses to events and interactions. Just as clinicians respect clients, it is also our responsibility to show our animal partners the respect they deserve.

There is no one way to select a therapy animal, but general guidelines state that the animal should be healthy, predictable, reliable, behaviorally and medically evaluated, and temperament tested and enjoy human interaction (Ng, 2019). The therapy animal also needs to be a good fit for the environment. For instance, there are unique and varied demands asked of a therapy animal working in a private practice office, school or mental health center, or a therapeutic ranch. A dog who enjoys and thrives at working in a quiet private office may be unhappy and stressed when introduced to a busy, loud school environment and thus may be a good AAP companion at a quiet setting, but a poor choice for a more chaotic setting. As there are many intricacies and steps to choosing a therapy animal, it is important to seek advice from a skilled AAP practitioner, animal trainer/behaviorist, and veterinarian.

Some basics of animal welfare in AAP include allowing the animal access to food/water, having regular bathroom and rest breaks, freedom to express normal behavior, and freedom from discomfort, fear, or distress (Chandler, 2005; Ng, 2019; Stewart et al., 2016). This work can be emotionally challenging and stressful for animals and "arguably, only when an animal is properly cared for will there actually be a therapeutic transfer" (O'Haire et al., 2019, p. 38). AAP clinicians need to ensure that their animals are healthy, rested, happy, and enjoying their work in order to be practicing AAP in safe and ethical manner.

Identifying the primary population with whom the therapy animal will be working is another consideration in selection. Mid-sized, sturdier animals such as larger dogs are fairly well tolerated by most clients, but small animals such as rats may be too fragile or fast-moving for younger or older clients, or for individuals with motor control or impulse issues. Large animals such as horses can be a good choice because they are not easily injured by clumsy handling; however, horses can also more easily injure a person by accident, and so may not be appropriate for clients who struggle to follow directions or have impulse-control issues. Medium-sized animals such as guinea pigs and rabbits may be a good choice for a smaller office setting but tend to be more timid and can easily be hurt if not picked up correctly. Therefore, these animals may be a good fit for calmer clients with good self-control, but not a good option for impulsive or young clients.

Once a clinician has selected a therapy animal, it is essential to have a strong relationship with and understanding of that animal, including species-specific behavior, and the individual animal's unique behavioral cues and nuances. In addition, it is important that the clinician is able to competently and appropriately respond to these cues (Ng, 2019; Stewart et al., 2016). For example, prior to working with any of AATPC's facility animals, clinicians are trained on each animal species and each individual animal at the facility. AATPC clinicians must spend time with each animal prior to including it in sessions, to ensure they are knowledgeable about each animal's likes, dislikes, preferences, fears, health issues, stress signs, and behavioral cues, both typical and stress related.

Animals communicate nonverbally, and with subtle behavioral cues, that can be easy to miss. In order to ensure the safety of the client and the animal, the therapist must learn the animal's communication style and "language" as much as possible. All animals demonstrate signs and signals of stress and fear, as well as pleasure. Behaviors that are often seen as problematic, such as biting or kicking, usually occur when an animal is increasingly stressed or fearful but has not had its needs for safety met. Therefore, knowing the signs for each species and each individual animal is part of the clinician's training. One strategy with clients to address animal communication is to talk about animals "whispering, talking, and yelling" when they are stressed, explaining that each animal does this differently but generally through behavior rather than vocalizations. Ideally, the clinician will identify that the animal is stressed because it is whispering. The clinician should then redirect the activity or give the animal a break, to avoid escalation to a yell, often expressed often by an animal biting or kicking. Animals should always have the ability to choose if they want to participate in a session and should have a quiet place to retreat or rest if necessary. At AAPTC, animals are generally in a session off leash or without a harness unless it is part of a direct intervention such as a walk. Thus, the animal can walk away if they are feeling unsafe, unwell, or simply not interested in being social. Smaller animals can choose if they come out of their enclosures. It can often take weeks for a client to win an animal's trust and be able to interact freely.

Clinicians are expected to respond appropriately when they notice that an animal is stressed, but also to integrate the animal's negative and positive responses smoothly into a therapy intervention. For instance, if a cat moves to the door and begins to meow, a clinician may ask the client to interpret this behavior. While the cat will always be allowed to leave the room, a therapeutic response may also include processing with the client their feelings and beliefs about the cat leaving the session. The client's interpretation and projection onto the cat's behavior can reveal powerful information to the therapist and lead to impactful therapeutic discussions and future goals.

A common misconception is that therapy animals must be perfect or have no misbehaviors. Though therapy animals certainly need to be safe with clients, they do not need to be perfect. Allowing for imperfection in animals is powerful for numerous reasons: it allows clients to feel connected to an animal's unique challenges or issues; clients are able to help solve an animal's issues, which often relates to the clients' own challenges; clients see their therapists being gentle and patient with an imperfect animal; and clients witness that it is acceptable to make mistakes.

Though these legal and ethical issues are critical in AAP, it is also beyond the scope of this chapter to explore every possible issue that could arise when a clinician introduces one or more animals into their therapy practice. Prior to implementing any AAP interventions, those interested in this field should research the literature, enroll in training programs, find a skilled and experienced mentor/supervisor, and seek the advice of an animal behaviorist or trainer if necessary.

Benefits of Animal-Assisted Psychotherapy

The impact of the human-animal bond (HAB) and human-animal interactions (HAIs) is receiving recognition in not only the United States but across the world. Some of this impact may be rooted in the biophilia hypothesis, which states that humans have an innate attraction to nature and other forms of life, including animals (Wilson, 1984; O'Haire et al., 2019) (For additional discussion, see the chapter by Vincent et al., in this volume.). Humans may be drawn to and feel a deep sense of connection to animals. In fact, research has found that humans have many positive physiological benefits from engaging with animals. Being with or petting an animal can reduce heart rate and blood pressure and self-reports of fear and anxiety. These benefits may contribute to an increased sense of well-being while in therapy (VanFleet, 2008; Winston, 2015a). Interacting with animals may also increase oxytocin, the hormone that contributes to social bonding and attachment relationships (O'Haire et al., 2019; VanFleet, 2008; Olmert, 2009). In addition, cortisol, a hormone that increases during periods of stress, has been shown to decrease during and after interactions with animals (O'Haire et al., 2019; Olmert, 2009). These physiological changes may help clients feel better physically and allow clients to experience therapy as less threatening, thus enabling them to engage in therapy.

Animals offer many individuals a sense of support and comfort, especially during initial therapy sessions. Animals can enhance feelings of emotional safety, trust, and social support (VanFleet, 2008; Winston, 2015a). Having an animal present can make a therapy setting seem more welcoming and less threatening, as well as helping the therapist appear more empathic and trustworthy, therefore facilitating rapport with the therapist and increasing the client's willingness to disclose (Chandler, 2005; Fine, 2015; Parish-Plass, 2013; Schneider & Harley, 2006; VanFleet, 2008). The therapeutic environment can often feel strange or uncomfortable to a new therapy client, especially one who finds it difficult to interact with others or who has struggled in therapy in the past. Working with animals can enhance the therapeutic alliance for these clients in the early phases of therapy (Chandler et al., 2010, O'Haire et al., 2019; Parish-Plass, 2013). Animals may encourage social interactions, as the client and therapist can discuss the animals and build a relationship while talking about neutral topics. The therapist and client are not focusing on the "problem" but instead are connecting over a mutual interest in the animal. This ability to have a simple conversation can lower defenses and lead to increased comfort with the therapist, encouraging more willingness to disclose more personal or therapeutic issues (Winston, 2015a).

Furthermore, animals demonstrate unconditional acceptance and nonjudgmental interaction. They are ready and willing to interact with clients regardless of the client's presenting issue, diagnoses, appearance, etc. Interactions with the animals are often seen as more genuine by the client (Chandler, 2005; Fine, 2015; Tedeschi & Jenkins, 2019; Parish-Plass, 2013; VanFleet, 2008; Winston, 2015a, b). Moreover, animals can provide a physical connection that therapists often cannot: petting the animal can release tension and soothe anxiety, playing with the animal can reduce the serious nature of a session, and the animal can provide physical touch and affection in a safe and appropriate way (Chandler, 2005; Tedeschi & Jenkins, 2019). Animals also offer companionship, help reduce loneliness, create connections, and often act as a social lubricant, making social interactions start and develop more smoothly and at a higher comfort level for the parties involved (O'Haire et al., 2019; VanFleet, 2008). The combination of the physiological and social impacts of having an animal in the session enhances the potential effectiveness of therapy, by enhancing the critically important therapeutic relationship.

Building empathy is an important therapeutic goal for many clients, but one that can be hard to address in traditional therapy. Through building relationships with the animals, AAP has an inherent ability to teach empathy (VanFleet, 2008; Winston, 2015b). Since all of AATPC's animals were rescued or adopted, they come from complicated backgrounds that often include trauma, abuse, neglect, or physical ailments. The animals' stories can be shared, and often clients feel a connection to a certain aspect of the animal's history. Since animals are less complicated than people, clients are often able to feel empathy with an animal, which can help them develop and practice their empathic skills. For this reason, AATPC prefers to work with rescued animals and encourages others to do so as well, when possible.

Working with animals has been found to increase positive social behavior and decrease behavior problems (Chandler et al., 2010). Therapy animals can help clients learn and practice verbal and nonverbal social and communication skills through many relationship-based activities. Talking to the animal, about the animal, or giving the animal training commands helps clients share difficult feelings, feel understood, and practice clear and assertive communication (Chandler, 2005; VanFleet, 2008). Clients can practice necessary social skills such as learning to read nonverbal social cues and body language and practicing reciprocal engagement. Interacting with a therapy animal helps clients practice and develop these social skills with less at stake, because animals are not worried about social norms and do not judge. Interventions with animals also encourage problem-solving, patience, frustration tolerance, and emotional awareness and regulation (VanFleet, 2008; Winston, 2015a, b). While paying attention to the animals' body language, clients learn how to decipher and process the animals' communications. Clients then have to modify their behavior to respond to the animals' behavior. During this process, clients practice patience and frustration tolerance, as they work to understand and successfully engage with the animal. In addition, clients develop emotional awareness and regulation skills in order to maintain successful interactions with the animal. Over time, clients will reap the benefits of these interactions through the animals' increasing trust and reciprocal interest in the clients. (Please see the case examples at the end of this chapter for examples.)

Working with animals in session can also be empowering and esteem building for clients (Chandler et al., 2010; Parish-Plass, 2013; VanFleet, 2008). Teaching an animal a new trick, learning to harness and walk a horse or a goat, or simply discovering a special connection with a rabbit can allow clients to feel a sense of pride, mastery, and belief in their abilities. Moreover, in order to train a dog or harness a horse, clients must be assertive and have a sense of control over themselves and assert confidence to the animal. Clients learn a gentle and authoritative sense of control, rather than a physically or emotionally domineering sense. Clients therefore learn how to assert themselves and manage situations around them in a healthy, positive way. When clients successfully work with animals, they also feel accomplishment and pride, helping to build their sense of esteem, a positive sense of self, and trust in their own abilities. Being with the animals may also help clients recognize skills or unique traits that help them create a positive sense of identity.

Working with an animal encourages acceptance and allows for a sense of freedom to be oneself (Fine, 2015; Parish-Plass, 2013; VanFleet, 2008). As many of AATPC's animals struggle with challenging behaviors, clients can see that perfection is not expected of animals or humans. Though animals are not allowed to harm clients, they also have the freedom to be imperfect while still being accepted, valued, and loved. Working with the animals allows for a sense of self-acceptance while also learning to embrace one's best self.

An important element of AAP is that it is experiential; rather than talking "about" issues and discussing what clients could or should do in the future, the client is actively doing the work and practicing the necessary skills in the moment within each session. In their interactions with the animals, clients are showing their behavior, their thought processes, and their emotional experiences. Thus, clinicians are able to witness and work on all of these elements together. Clients can try new behaviors with the animals, modify their interactions, practice new skill sets, and then process and discuss their thoughts and feelings in the moment. Counselors encourage the clients to take these skills and practice them with their own pets at home and/or to generalize them to other activities in their life.

In addition, clients are often outside during AAP, experiencing the many benefits of nature (which are numerous but beyond the scope of this chapter). Moreover, as clients do this work, it feels fun! Working with animals allows for lightness and laughter in session, which is often lacking in traditional mental health treatment. Clients can experience levity and happiness while also experiencing fun in a safe setting, demonstrating that therapy can be both fun and effective. Whether walking a horse, cuddling with a rat, or playing fetch with a dog, the focus moves from the negative and internal to the positive, external experience of a loving, playful animal.

Animal assisted psychotherapy is not just for individual therapy. Rather, many benefits can be extended to work with families, couples, and groups. The discussed benefits of AAP apply, but the inclusion of animals in family and group counseling adds another way to discuss relationships, social skills, and group/family dynamics.

It allows a clinician to see how clients engage with others, not just with the therapist. For example, the clinician can ask a family to do an obstacle course with a dog and see directly how the members work together, communicate, problem solve, disagree, tolerate frustration, and celebrate successes. Clients are not just reporting to a therapist how they interact with others but are showing the therapist, who is then able to process and address challenges in the moment. Additionally, group members can bond over activities and shared experiences with the animal, and the animal can normalize some of their issues. For instance, clients can discover that animals may also experience social anxiety or have dealt with trauma and feel more willing to share their own experiences in a group setting. Case examples presented at the end of the chapter describe how AAP can be successfully integrated in family and group work.

Benefits to Clinicians

A unique benefit to AAP is the support it offers to clinicians. Being a mental health professional is hard work and can lead to burnout and stress. A 2012 Health and Human Services (HHS) review of the literature found that up to 67% of mental health professions may be experiencing some level of burnout and "mental exhaustion" (Morse et al., 2012). Working with animals can offer clinicians a more relaxed environment and provide incentive to spend time outside. Therapists are also able to be more genuine and share their own love of animals, an element of their life and personality that may not otherwise be shared. Adding an animal to therapy also allows clinicians to be more creative in their work with clients and the interventions they do, which can keep clinicians invigorated. Therapy animals can create more motivation for clients, which can lead to increased progress, which in turn feels rewarding and motivating to clinicians. In addition, the animals can aid clinicians in the same ways they help clients, offering emotional support and affection. Clinicians can pet and engage with the animals during sessions, but also before and after sessions, seeking a comfort after a hard session or a reset before their next client. The case example with Cody and Avery is a powerful depiction of an AATPC clinician benefitting from the support and love of the therapy horse, Cody.

Case Examples

Case studies demonstrate the power of AAP. The following AAP case examples come from this author's professional experience and that of the AAPTC clinical team. All clients' names and identifying details have been changed, and some client stories were combined in order to preserve privacy and present a cohesive example of AAP. The following case examples are categorized by animal type: dogs (many

AAP practitioners work only with canines), large farm animals (horses, alpacas, donkeys, goats), and small indoor animals (rats, rabbits, guinea pigs, cats).

In these examples, there are instances in which animals experience and display signs of minor stress, such as moving away from a client or other behavioral cues. The clinicians in these situations were carefully monitoring and noting the animals' cues and stress levels. In all examples, the stress signs were minor; the animals were still "whispering" and were not stressed above a tolerable level, akin to daily stressors they would encounter with other animals or out in pasture. The animals were able to leave the situation and/or self-regulate in all cases. If the situations had become more stressful for the animals, the clinicians would have intervened and in order to keep the animals safe and happy. At the end of every session, clinicians check in with animals to ensure they are doing well. Animals also get a break after each session, and staff will spend time with them going for walks, petting or playing with them, and generally ensuring that the animals are calm and happy.

Dogs

Dogs are one of the most common and popular animals for inclusion in therapy work for a variety of reasons: dogs are familiar and acceptable to most people; dogs are often active, playful, and friendly and enjoy physical contact; dogs are trainable and adaptable; dogs seem accepting and nonjudgmental during interactions; and dogs are social animals with a focus on attachment that appears to demonstrate empathy (VanFleet, 2008). Therapy dogs should be eager to engage in sessions, excited to meet new clients, respond appropriately to clients' energy level by playing actively or snuggling quietly, and demonstrate affection and acceptance. Below are a few examples of dogs as powerful therapy partners.

Rupert and Joe While playing fetch with therapy dog Rupert, 10-year-old Joe became very frustrated because Rupert was no longer dropping the ball as quickly as earlier. Joe, a self-proclaimed "tough kid," quickly became frustrated and began yelling "drop it" at Rupert. The therapist observed to Joe that he seemed frustrated and asked him what Rupert might be trying to say when he kept the ball in his mouth. They talked about how Rupert was tired and how holding the ball was his way of telling Joe, "I need a rest!" Joe was able to choose another activity to do for 10 minutes while Rupert took a rest, and Joe talked with the therapist about how angry and frustrated he had felt when Rupert ignored the "drop it" command. Joe also suggested that Rupert might need some water to help him cool down while he rested. The simple activity of playing fetch with a dog allowed Joe to demonstrate empathy, notice another's body language and communication, pay attention to and control his own emotional reactions, and take a break when he got angry.

Sasha, Kim, and Mike Kim and Mike initially contacted AATPC for therapy during their divorce as a support for their children, but soon the therapist realized the parents would need some guidance to manage the stress and feelings surrounding the familial shift. Mike and Kim initially stated that it was an amicable divorce and that their children had no idea about the reason behind the divorce (infidelity) or the anger that both parents felt toward each other. However, it became clear that the children were picking up on and absorbing the animosity at home, so the therapist asked the parents to come in for some sessions. Sasha, an older and calmer therapy dog, was present for the sessions and provided much needed feedback to the parents about their affect and behavior. For instance, during the first session, Sasha was asleep on the couch, and the parents sat on either side of her. They stated that they were able to have tough conversations with each other at home while staying calm; they were certain that their children were unaware of how angry and stressed they were. Yet, almost as soon as they began sharing their stories with the therapist, Sasha woke up and started licking her paws and yawning, subtle signs of stress for her. Within several minutes, Sasha got up from the couch, shook off several times, and went to stand by the therapy room door, all clear signs of escalating stress or discomfort. The therapist asked the couple what they noticed about Sasha's behavior and what they thought that Sasha may be communicating. Though both clients noticed that Sasha had gotten up, neither commented on her specific behaviors or what they might mean. The therapist shared that Sasha had waken up; demonstrated several subtle signs of stress, then several larger signs of stress; and was asking to leave the therapy room, a sure sign that she was uncomfortable with the shift that had happened during the discussion. This observation led to conversation about how the parents may not be as calm as they had hoped during communications at home and that their children may actually be picking up on their emotion and anger and then acting out, just as Sasha had responded with several stress related behaviors. It was easier for the parents to see, understand, and appreciate Sasha's behaviors, because she was a neutral presence and they were not impacted by any emotional investment toward her. It then became a goal of the session to keep Sasha asleep on the couch between them as they had discussions about the divorce, their children's behaviors, and the custodial agreement. Mike and Kim were able to practice emotional awareness and regulation and subsequent behavioral change and then implement these strategies at home with their children. Dogs (and other animals) can help individuals see how they come across to others and how they may be impacting those around them.

Small Animals

Small animals, such as cats, rabbits, guinea pigs, and rats, are less traditionally included in therapy animal discussions. However, there are benefits to working with these animals, assuming the individual animal enjoys human interaction and that the client population is safe to engage with small, delicate animals. Working with small, often shyer animals such as cats and rabbits can be an excellent way for clients to practice being gentle, calm, and regulating their own emotions and behaviors. A rabbit will not come play with a loud, unregulated client but will come out for a calm client who is sitting quietly. This experience may give clients the motivation needed for self-regulation in sessions, and in other settings, as well as an opportunity for more therapeutic discussion.

Clients are often surprised to find out how clever and trainable the small animals are. The opportunity to set up obstacle courses or mazes or teach skills to the animals allows clients to be creative, problem-solve, tolerate frustration, build empathy, and celebrate successes. Some small animals species may be novel to clients, providing them excitement and motivation to engage in and return to therapy sessions. In addition, small animals can provide powerful metaphors for the clients, for example, a client who feels like a rat because people judge her based on her appearance or a client who feels like a quiet rabbit that gets overlooked in a family of exuberant dogs.

Rosie and Lena Rosie is one of AATPC's most unique therapy animals; she is a hairless guinea pig with numerous health issues and as a result had to have one of her eyes removed. Rosie has also struggled to get along with other guinea pigs, as they often targeted and injured her, so she was in an enclosure on her own for several months to heal from injuries, which is a lonely situation for a social creature such as a guinea pig. Regardless of her past, Rosie is sweet, friendly, and always eager to interact with and be petted by clients. Though some clients hesitate to interact with her initially, due to her unusual appearance, many are also drawn to her, because she is like no other animal they have ever met. Some clients feel connected with her specifically because of her appearance, feeling a kinship with her in being different or having others judge them based on their appearance.

One such client, Lena, had several physical disabilities and was diagnosed with high functioning autism and anxiety. Lena had recently moved to a new area and struggled with feeling different from and connecting with her new peers. Her physical differences and autism caused her to feel isolated, and her anxiety contributed to struggles with social interactions. Immediately upon meeting Rosie, Lena lit up and began asking questions about Rosie's history, how she lost her eye, how Rosie felt about being different, and how she got along with the other guinea pigs. She asked whether Rosie got enough love and attention, and when her therapist asked her to say more, Lena noted, "Well, some people probably ignore her or don't want to play with her because she looks different. But I really like her." She then gave Rosie a kiss on the head and several gentle pats. Lena said, "Just because Rosie looks or acts different doesn't mean she's not sweet and really fun." These comments were projections of the client's own struggles in feeling different, being judged by her peers, and not connecting meaningfully to those around her.

As Lena's anxiety about moving to a new home and school were a big issue in therapy, the therapist described how Rosie's move into her own enclosure caused her to show signs of "guinea pig anxiety" and the staff needed to find ways to make her feel safe. Since Lena enjoyed doing art, she and the therapist created a book about "Rosie's Big Move," in which the client wrote and illustrated Rosie's story before, during, and after the move. She told how Rosie would scratch herself too hard when she felt nervous, which paralleled the client's own experience with scratching herself until she bled when upset. Lena described the issues that caused Rosie anxiety, such as looking different from other guinea pigs, having other guinea pigs be mean to her, moving to a new enclosure, being alone, and not knowing how to make friends with "regular" guinea pigs. Lena then listed several ways that Rosie could feel better, such as taking deep breaths, snuggling with a person, and remembering how strong she was to survive losing her eye. The book ended with Lena's picture of Rosie as a superhero and with a list of all her positive qualities. In essence, Lena had created a book about her own struggles, negative thoughts, and anxieties and had then created a list of ways to overcome those issues but in a way that felt safer and less personal. It is often easier for clients to solve an "animal's issue" which relates to their own struggles, rather than problem-solving for themselves. Therapists can then choose to make this connection for the client, with comments such as, "Wow, you and Rosie have some things in common! I wonder if you could try those strategies too and let Rosie know how it goes!" Some clients respond well to making these overt connections, while for other clients, it is better to let the underlying message stay as a metaphor.

Lena loved to see Rosie play, run, and jump, despite her vision loss. Lena would set up increasingly harder mazes and obstacle courses for Rosie, encouraging Rosie and celebrating excitedly when Rosie completed each one. She made comments such as "Rosie doesn't let anything stop her!" and "Rosie can do it, even though she is different from the other pigs!" These comments demonstrated how Rosie was acting as a metaphor for the client's own physical differences and struggles and how she saw that it was possible to overcome them and succeed. During one session, the client observed that Rosie climbed onto an elevated platform a different way than the other guinea pigs had and noted, "It is so cool that she did it her very own way!" The client saw that Rosie was able to find a different solution to a challenge, but one that ultimately led to success. Again, Rosie was a metaphor for the client's own issues and the client was able to see that there were ways to solve problems that were different than how others may do it. Often, children can resist hearing comments such as "You can do it too!" or "Don't let your struggles stop you" from adults. But because this therapeutic lesson took place in the context of a fun game and a strong bond with an animal, the client was able to absorb and internalize the message.

Maggie and Greg   Because rabbits tend to be more shy and reserved, clients have to work hard to gain their trust and engage with them. Often, this process can take weeks of sitting in the rabbit room, keeping one's body calm, and regulating emotions until the rabbits feel the client is a safe presence. As with all animals, AATPC never forces rabbits to interact with clients. Therefore, it is entirely up to the client to find a way to help the rabbits feel safe and happy during interactions. Though it can be a long process, it is also very rewarding for the clients once they earn the rabbits' trust and are able to sit quietly with them, gently stroking the rabbits' soft fur.

Greg was a teenage client who was referred to therapy due to angry outbursts stemming from his parents' contentious divorce. Though reportedly physical and aggressive when angry at home, Greg was always calm and polite during therapy sessions. This is a common dynamic at AATPC: clients are often able to regulate emotions and follow limits when at the Ranch, in part due to the motivating factor of interacting with the animals and the sense of safety they have at the Ranch. Greg's favorite activity during session was to sit in the rabbit room and pet Maggie as he talked about his struggles and his anger at his parents. Though he was clearly hurting and feeling intense emotions, he was able to share his experiences and feelings with some level of control over his emotions. He would comment that it felt really good to "just sit still and breathe," which was much different than his daily life of school, sports, dealing with three younger siblings, and switching houses every 4 days. Greg shared that his dad would get frustrated and angry with him very quickly and start to yell, which made Greg scared and angry, so he yelled back. Greg and his therapist worked on mindfulness activities while he petted Maggie and focused on the physical sensations inside and outside of his body.

Greg and his father then planned on doing a session together, to discuss some of his struggles and feelings about the divorce. In the session prior to their joint session, Greg began to get agitated, raising his voice, standing up, and starting to pace the room. Maggie woke up from her traditional spot and began to slowly and loudly thump her foot on the floor, a rabbit behavior when they sense danger. Maggie had never done this in session before, particularly with Greg, who was usually her safe, gentle friend. The therapist immediately pointed out this behavior to Greg and asked, "What do you notice about Maggie?" and then followed with, "What do you think made her respond like that?" Greg was able to observe that his tone and volume of voice were elevated and that he was pacing, likely making Maggie feel unsafe and unhappy. He then said "Huh... I wonder if my parents get mad when I act like that too." He was able to use some of the mindfulness techniques that they had practiced in previous sessions to calm himself down, and Maggie resumed her calm behavior. Greg's therapist noted that he was able to observe and ultimately change his behavior, successfully deescalating himself and controlling his own response to a situation. Greg nodded as they discussed this and also reflected that it might "be helpful to remember that next week when my dad is yelling at me." This brief observation and interaction with a small rabbit was deeply powerful for Greg. He was able to witness how his behavior affected those around him and to take stock of his own emotions, manage them successfully, and repair the brief rift in his relationship with Maggie. This ability to self-reflect, deescalate, and fix a negative interaction were skills that until now had been missing in Greg's life.

The following week, Greg and his father came in for their joint session. Greg had requested to have the session in the rabbit room, since it was a safe space for him, and the therapist agreed, but reminded both of them that if they became too escalated and the animals felt unsafe, the session would be moved to a new space. Almost immediately, Greg's father became frustrated and angry while discussing Greg's behavior at home. Maggie took two big jumps and began thumping her leg loudly. Greg said, "Dad, do you see the bunny? She's really upset." The therapist supported Greg's assertion and briefly educated the father about rabbit stress signs, noting that even though the father was not yelling or acting out physically, his tone of voice, volume, and aggressive posturing felt scary and threatening to Maggie. Rather than having to tell the father that he was scary and intimidating to his son, the therapist was able to use the interaction with Maggie as a gentle teaching point in how the father's actions came across to others. Greg's father nodded slowly and said, "Yeah I guess I can be a lot sometimes." This comment led to a powerful discussion about Greg's father's approach to conflict, particularly with Greg, and how it can intensify quickly, causing Greg to escalate and react with anger as well. Greg then shared some of the activities he had done with Maggie to calm himself and her down, showing his dad where to sit in the room and how to breathe calmly until Maggie felt safe. Though it took a while, Greg and his father were able to get Maggie to come sit between them and took turns patting her gently. The therapist asked if they could continue their discussion while keeping Maggie between them, thus giving both of them an incentive to regulate their emotions while talking to each other, something they clearly struggled with at home. In this session, Maggie provided feedback about and was a gauge for behavior and emotions. She was a motivator to practice self-soothing and emotional regulation techniques but also a way to facilitate a special father-son moment and connection.

GusGus, Oscar, and Rachel AATPC's rats are some of the most popular animals, particularly with children. Though some adults have beliefs about rats being dirty, mean, or stupid, these are common misconceptions. The gentle, friendly, sweet, and clean rats at AATPC can usually change the minds of those who are willing to give them a chance. Having unique animals such as rats is powerful because it allows clients to connect in a different way than with traditional therapy animals and it allows those clients who feel different or misunderstood to feel a connection to animals with a similar story.

Rachel was a 12-year-old who struggled with identity issues, perfectionist tendencies, and a fear of failure, to the point where she refused to try anything new. Rachel was born a female but was beginning to think that she may identify more as a male, though she was too afraid to tell her parents. In her first session, Rachel and her therapist discussed how people were sometimes wary of the rats because they were not used to being around them but that the rats showed people how wonderful they were, regardless of what people thought of them initially. Rachel was then introduced to two female rats named GusGus and Oscar. She delighted in learning that they had traditionally male names despite being female, because AATPC had initially believed them to be males. These discussions about people having preconceived notions and then holding certain beliefs based on gender resonated with Rachel and helped her feel safe and comfortable with her therapist. She was also able to witness how gentle and kind her therapist was to the rats, regardless of what anyone else thought about them, what their names were, or what gender they were. This helped Rachel feel a connection and affinity with her therapist and feel safe disclosing her own struggles about gender identity.

Rachel and her therapist then worked on helping the four new rats become trained therapy rats, because they were young and new to the Ranch. They discussed what a therapy rat "should" be like and then explored whether each rat fit that description. Not surprisingly, the rats were not perfect and did not meet all the expectations to be the "right" kind of therapy rat! Rachel and her therapist talked about how each rat was different and how their individual personalities and quirks actually made them more helpful and wonderful therapy animals. For example, some of the rats were more apt to snuggle and be calm, while others liked to run obstacle courses and mazes. Some liked to be put on harnesses and go on walks outside, while others preferred to stay in their rat room. Rachel was able to see that there is not one "right" way to be good at something and that various qualities are valuable for different reasons. Sometimes, however, the rats did engage in undesirable behaviors, such as nipping a finger or taking another rat's food. Rachel commented, "Wow, GusGus isn't being nice and that's not a good therapy rat behavior, but I still love her anyway! She is still a great therapy rat!" She and her therapist were then able to process that it is acceptable to act differently from those around you, and to make mistakes, and that did not impact how lovable or worthy one was.

Rachel created obstacle courses for GusGus and Oscar, noticing that Oscar often fell short of her expectations. She observed that Oscar did not seem bothered when she did not complete the obstacle course and did not berate herself, as Rachel was apt to do. Watching both rats struggle and sometimes fail also helped normalize failure for Rachel and recognize that everyone fails at something, sometimes. As they tried to complete various obstacles, Rachel would encourage the rats and then say, "That's ok, you tried so hard!", or "You did your best and I love that!" Over time, Rachel was able to apply these lessons of encouragement and acceptance to her own life. She would come to sessions and unhesitatingly report times when she was different than those around her or times she failed. Through her interactions with the rats, Rachel was able to see and experience that difference and failure were acceptable and even valuable parts of herself.

Siggy and Jenny   Jenny was a 14-year-old client who felt very connected to Siggy the cat. During one session, when Jenny was holding Siggy and did not let him go when he gave her subtle nonverbal cues, he tried to bite her. (She was not harmed.) Jenny and her therapist discussed what had happened with Siggy, and she reflected that he was "just like me" because when people did not listen to her right away, she became quickly angered and would lash out verbally and physically. They processed how Siggy's attempt to bite did get Jenny to put Siggy down, but it also made her mad at him and nervous to play with him again. They talked about how Siggy had tried to communicate nonverbally, and if she had noticed and responded to those signals, perhaps he would not have resorted to more severe actions. Jenny was able to connect this to her own experience and noted that she tried to communicate her frustration to friends or her parents, but when they kept "bothering" her, she would feel forced to yell, kick, or hit. These behaviors often got Jenny what she wanted initially, but it also made her parents angry or her peers reluctant to play with her. Jenny and her therapist then observed how Siggy could make his needs more evident, by wiggling away, meowing, or standing up. They discussed how Jenny could make her needs or desires more clear. Jenny came up with several solutions, including stating what she wanted, asking her parents for a few more minutes, and compromising with friends about activities. Thus, Jenny began by identifying emotions and problem-solving for Siggy but ended the session focusing on her own emotional awareness and creating solutions for her bullying triggers.

Large Animals

Horses are the most common large animal incorporated in therapy, though they are certainly not the only large animal that can be included in AAP work. AATPC works with full-size horses, miniature horses, alpacas, donkeys, and goats. There are many benefits to working with large animals: it is often a new experience for a client to interact with a horse, goat, or alpaca, helping the client to become excited, engaged, and eager to return to sessions. Clients may need to pay close attention to learn communication for these animals and therefore to practice observation, social skills, and awareness of others. New and large animals can also be intimidating or anxiety provoking, so clients may be able to work on self-awareness, signs of stress, mindfulness, and self-soothing before they interact with the large animals. Clients may be able to learn and practice new skills, such as harnessing a horse or grooming an alpaca, which can build confidence and self-esteem. These larger animals are also prey animals used to living in a herd, which can lead to powerful discussions and parallels about intuition, relying on others, vigilance and hyper-vigilance, trauma responses, and intuition. Because they are so adapted to respond to those around them, herd animals can be very sensitive to clients and often mirror their emotions or struggles. Goats, donkeys, alpacas, and even horses can also be very playful and silly, lending a lightness and joy to therapy that many clients need and benefit from.

Krunk, Kuzco, and Sam Krunk and Kuzco are AATPC's resident alpacas, adopted from an Alpaca rescue. Alpacas are wonderful therapy animals for a variety of reasons, in part because they are unique but also because they are silly and have funny mannerisms. Clients are eager to see them, and therapy feels fun with them. Moreover, alpacas are independent and curious but also quite cautious and need those around them to prove that their trustworthiness before they are comfortable interacting with them. Thus, clients need to demonstrate that they are safe, using calm mannerisms and staying regulated, which are good therapeutic practices for many of clients.

Kuzco is more shy and anxious than his brother and often looks to Krunk for cues. Though he was becoming much more confident after spending time with staff and clients, Kuzco reverted to some of his shy ways after the COVID pandemic reduced the number of interactions he had daily. In order to help both alpacas (but particularly Kuzco) reduce his anxiety and gain more confidence around people, staff and clients have begun to use a clicker to train Kuzco, encouraging him to engage with people and getting a reward for it.

Sam began in-person therapy several months into the pandemic due to severe anxiety and fear of interacting with people because of concerns about illness. His therapist asked him to help the alpacas gain their confidence back because they had also gotten more nervous during the pandemic and really needed Sam's help. This seemingly small comment helped Sam feel valuable, special, and needed simply by being present at the therapy session. It also gave him motivation to come to session each week, something he had struggled with during past attempts at therapy. When they entered the alpaca enclosure for the first time, the alpacas made anxious vocalizations, and the therapist and Sam stood still and discussed what the alpacas might be feeling and why the pandemic increased their anxiety. Sam was able to share that he had felt more anxious and "nervous about people and new things" since the pandemic began.

During the next several sessions, Sam and his therapist did clicker training work with the alpacas. Sam was in charge of the process, deciding what to teach the alpacas and how to teach them. Sam needed to be confident in deciding what he wanted to do, problem-solve how to do it, and then being assertive but gentle in his work with the alpacas. Though initially both the alpacas and Sam were nervous, after several sessions, Sam had trained the alpacas to turn in a circle with the command "turn" after which they were rewarded by a click, treat, and gentle pats. Additionally, the alpacas began to run over to Sam when he arrived in their enclosure, giving him positive reinforcement for being at therapy and making him feel valued. He would often smile shyly and even noted, "Wow, I guess they are so glad to see me." The alpacas gained confidence being around Sam and he gained confidence during his interactions with them and during his interactions with the therapist. His mother also noted that he was showing less anxiety at home and was willing to try activities that he had previously been fearful about doing. His mother was also able to see that Sam had the capacity to stay calm, be patient, and be a leader, which impacted how she approached and engaged with him, thus benefitting their relationship as well.

Millie and Sue Millie and Daisy, AATPC's therapy donkeys, are popular because of their sweet nature, exuberant voices, and connection to people. However, they can also be quite stubborn and can hold their boundaries very well with clients. Sue was an adult client who had tried therapy many times in the past but had never felt a positive connection to a therapist. She decided to give therapy one more try and sought out AATPC because of the therapy animals and her preference for animals over people. Sue's therapist noted that Sue showed resistance to deeper level work and resisted any discomfort in sessions. During one session, the therapist asked Sue to halter and walk Millie to a nearby field where there were several natural formations, such as logs and boulders, that served as an obstacle course. Though Sue was able to halter Millie, once Sue tried to walk her, Millie completely refused. Sue tried pulling Millie gently, going first, and going behind Millie, even using treats, but Millie refused to budge. This situation provided an interesting parallel to Sue's resistance in sessions to move beyond surface level work and delve deeper into her psyche.

After 20 minutes of trying various strategies, Sue finally conceded and asked her therapist for help. Although AATPC encourages clients to problem-solve on their own, it is always an option for clients to ask their therapists for help. Sue seemed defeated, and her therapist reflected her frustration and noted that it seemed she and Millie were well matched in their stubbornness and strong wills. Sue's therapist shared that sometimes a lack of success is not for a lack of trying but may mean we need to ask for help, slow down, use our senses, and pay attention to the moment, rather than focus on the goal, because sometimes an exclusive focus on a goal makes us miss the power of the moment. Sue absorbed this information for a moment and then walked back to Millie, standing next to her quietly. Millie turned and rested her head on the client's shoulder, sharing the quiet moment with Sue, who started crying and acknowledged that she had been pushing down her emotions for years in order to meet her definition of success and that she was so tired of doing that. Sue took a deep breath and said she was finally ready to do some of the hard work of therapy, and in that moment, Millie picked up her head and walked through the gate. Though it is impossible to say what was going on for Millie during this session, it seems that her behaviors were a reflection of what the client was experiencing and that her response to each aspect of the session was meaningful and paralleled Sue's internal emotional state.

Goats and Group Example The goats are some of our most popular animals; they are sweet, affectionate, and funny, but also stubborn, willful, and troublemakers! When doing group work, AATPC often incorporates the goats because they so love to be part of the pack but are also very clear about their own desires and intention. A fun and effective intervention is the goat obstacle course. A clinician can either set up a series of obstacles for the client and the goat to complete or the clients can choose the obstacles that they would like to complete with the goat. As they work to complete the challenge, clients often find that the goats have a mind of their own and do not always comply. This situation can bring out frustration, impatience, and even anger, as clients have to work through their emotional reactions, uncover the thought processes behind these feelings, and then find new ways to interact and behave with the goats. During group or family work, we see how individuals interact not only with the goats but with each other and what social skills, challenges, and dynamics are coming into play.

A residential substance abuse group visits AATPC's facility weekly. There are often group dynamics that impact the activities, especially because the participants live together and deal with many issues arising from a shared living space. One week, the group split into two teams, and each team worked with a goat to complete similar obstacle courses. One team worked with the Nubian goat Wally and though he was defiant at first; he quickly adapted to their requests and finished the course. The team was able to notice where Wally got stuck or confused and make small adjustments in their behavior, including how and where they stood, where they held treats, who gave the commands, and how they celebrated the successes. They observed that Wally got overwhelmed when they all stood close to the obstacles or stood behind him; he shut down if more than one person gave a command; and the treats got him too distracted to focus if they were held out. One group member noted that Wally was like an addict in that way and they could understand how hard it was to focus and stay on track when your substance of choice was dangled in front of your face!

In contrast, the group working with the pygmy goat, Dahlia, felt overwhelmed from the start and was unable to get her to complete a single obstacle. Group members kept trying different tactics but often several would speak to Dahlia at once. As some members gave her commands, others wandered around the yard, distracting Dahlia, who would then wander over to explore what they were doing. During the session debrief, group members shared that it was hard to work together as a team, and so they each decided to do their own thing, which was ultimately overstimulating and confusing for Dahlia. Members shared that having so many mixed messages and demands from various people around you was often how it felt to be in recovery.

This activity led to a powerful discussion about what aspects of life clients are able to control, such as where to stand and who gives treats and what aspects we cannot, such as who we have around us and what we have to accomplish. The group related this to how it felt to seek sobriety and that there are certain aspects of life they can control, such as their social circle and the small goals they set for themselves on their way to their bigger goal of sobriety. The Dahlia group was also able to process that it felt really hard to see the other group succeed and that this paralleled their feelings when they saw others "succeed" in sobriety. The Wally group noted that while they felt really proud of themselves, they also kept wondering when they were going to mess up, and this was how they felt every day.

Cody and Avery AATPC is open seven days a week, and sometimes, clinicians are at the Ranch on their own, which can be difficult after a tough session. One therapist, Avery, had a difficult client on Sundays and would often struggle to regroup afterward. While she was in the horse paddock after a session, the therapy horse, Cody, joined her and stayed by her side as she cleaned up. Avery felt a sense of calm and companionship, which helped her feel more grounded, present, and ready to see the rest of her clients. After that week, Avery would go sit in the paddock every week after tough sessions, and Cody would always come to see her. Sometimes, he would lay on the ground next to her, while other times, he would stand next to her as she leaned on him and talked or cried. She shared that it truly felt as though Cody was listening to her and that she felt more ready and able to work with clients after her moments with Cody.

Conclusion

Animal assisted psychotherapy is a growing and powerful field that can greatly benefit clients facing mental health challenges and the clinicians who work with them. This chapter explored some of the benefits of AAP and the ways it can be integrated into counseling sessions to create impactful and lasting change. With the proper education and training, clinicians with varied backgrounds and expertise can safely and ethically integrate animals into their profession.

Acknowledgments Thank you to the amazing team at Animal Assisted Therapy Programs of Colorado for supporting me in the writing of this chapter, sharing their experiences and clients' stories, and being a wonderful group of people to work with! Special thanks to Linda Chassman for her advice, insight, and support; to Alyssa Weidman for sharing her perspective as a clinician and client examples; and to Lindsey Chadwick, Mike Lathrop, Julie Maerz, Anna Miller, Kailey Mulvihill, and Elizabeth Worth for sharing case examples.

References

Chandler, C. (2005). *Animal assisted therapy in counseling*. Routledge.

Chandler, C., Portrie-Bethke, T., Minton, M., Fernando, D., & O'Callaghan, D. (2010). Matching animal-assisted therapy techniques and intentions with counseling guiding theories. *Journal of Mental Health Counseling, 32*(4), 354–374.

Fine, A. H. (2015). Incorporating animal-assisted therapy into psychotherapy: Guidelines and suggestions for therapists. In A. Fine (Ed.), *Handbook on animal-assisted therapy: Theoretical foundations and guidelines for practice* (4th ed., pp. 141–155). Academic Press.

Fine, A. H., Tedeschi, P., & Elvove, E. (2015). Forward thinking: The evolving field of human-animal interactions. In A. Fine (Ed.), *Handbook on animal-assisted therapy: Theoretical foundations and guidelines for practice* (4th ed., pp. 21–35). Academic Press.

Hazut, T., Tzur, D., Maayan, E. Barel, I., Tirosh, O., Brill, I., Besser, M., Gal, A., Hadari-Karkum, L., Yulius, H., & Parish-Plass, N. (2006). *Code of ethics*. Retrieved from https://e4198ad0-b1fd-4d28-b188-236f086d3fc9.filesusr.com/ugd/aa2bac_fc496572f1394a1e-ab78b10f2adef1f3.pdf

Jegatheesan, B., Beetz, A., Choi, G., Dudzik, C., Fine, A., Garcia, R. M., Johnson, R., Ormerod, E., Winkle, M., & Yamazaki, K. (2018). *White paper: The IAHAIO definitions for animal assisted intervention and guidelines for wellness of animals involved*. Unpublished report. Retrieved from https://iahaio.org/wp/wp-content/uploads/2020/07/iahaio_wp_updated-2020-aai-adjust-1.pdf

Morse, G., Salyers, M. P., Rollins, A. L., Monroe-DeVita, M., & Pfahler, C. (2012). *Burnout in mental health services: A review of the problem and its remediation*. https://www.ncbi.nlm.nih.gov/pmc/articles/PMC3156844/pdf/nihms290021.pdf

National Alliance on Mental Illness. (2020). *Mental health by the numbers*. https://www.nami.org/mhstats

Ng, Z. (2019). Advocacy and rethinking our relationships with animals: Ethical responsibilities and competencies in animal-assisted interventions. In P. Tedeschi & M. A. Jenkins (Eds.), *Transforming trauma: Resilience and healing through our connections with animals* (pp. 55–90). Purdue University Press.

O'Haire, M. E., Tedeschi, P., Jenkins, M., Braden, S. R., & Rodriguez, K. E. (2019). The impact of human-animal interaction in trauma recovery. In P. Tedeschi & M. A. Jenkins (Eds.), *Transforming trauma: Resilience and healing through our connections with animals* (pp. 15–53). Purdue University Press.

Olmert, M. D. (2009). *Made for each other*. Da Capo Press.

Tedeschi, P., & Jenkins, M. A. (2019). Human trauma and animals: Research developments, models, and practice methods for trauma-informed animal-assisted interventions. In P. Tedeschi & M. A. Jenkins (Eds.), *Transforming trauma: Resilience and healing through our connections with animals* (pp. 1–13). Purdue University Press.

Parish-Plass, N. (2013). *Animal-assisted psychotherapy: Theory, issues, and practice*. Purdue University Press.

Schneider, M. S., & Harley, L. P. (2006). How dogs influence the evaluation of psychotherapists. *Anthrozoös, 19*(2), 128–142.

Stewart, L. A., Chang, C. Y., Parker, L. K., & Grubbs, N. (2016). *Animal-assisted therapy in counseling competencies*. Developed in collaboration with the Animal-Assisted Therapy in Mental Health Interest Network of the American Counseling Assocation. https://www.counseling.org/docs/default-source/competencies/animal-assisted-therapy-competencies-june-2016.pdf?sfvrsn=c469472c_14

VanFleet, R. (2008). *Play therapy with kids & canines: Benefits for children's developmental and psychosocial health*. Professional Resource Press/Professional Resource Exchange.

Wilson, E. O. (1984). *Biophilia*. Harvard University Press.

Winston, E. K. (2015a). Animal assisted psychotherapy for grief and loss with children and adolescents. In S. L. Brooke & D. A. Miraglia (Eds.), *Using the creative therapies to cope with grief and loss* (pp. 373–391). Charles C. Thomas.

Winston, E. K. (2015b). Animal assisted psychotherapy in the healing of childhood depression. In S. L. Brooke & C. E. Myers (Eds.), *The use of creative therapies in treating depression* (pp. 291–309). Charles C. Thomas.

Chapter 7
Veterinary Social Work and the Ethics of Interprofessional Practice

Jeannine Moga

Introduction

A clinical social worker, employed by a veterinary specialty referral hospital to assist with case management, is called to the Emergency Room to consult on a "hit by car." The patient, a 6-month-old mixed breed puppy, is dropped off by a bystander who saw the puppy run into traffic. The medical team evaluates the puppy before contacting the puppy's family; the puppy has a compound fracture of the femur and a dislocated hip and will require surgery to address his many injuries. The veterinary team is also concerned about the puppy's overall condition, as the puppy is covered in parasites and appears unkempt. The puppy's owners are unable to afford surgery and insist that the puppy be discharged to home care. One of the owners describes the puppy as her emotional support dog, saying she got the puppy from a neighbor after the owner's psychiatrist suggested that a pet might help with her depression. The owner also remarks, though, that she "didn't know the dog had gotten away," noting that she "just puts the dog outside when it makes a mess in the house." The veterinary team asks the social worker for guidance, as doctors and nurses were concerned about the patient's acute injuries, as well as his long-term well-being with a family that may not be equipped to care for him. The social worker, on the other hand, felt pulled between two parties in conflict, a distressed veterinary team and a distressed client, with an injured patient hanging in the balance.

This case is a potent example of how ethical dilemmas manifest in interprofessional veterinary care. It is not the only way ethical dilemmas arise when human and animal needs intersect, however. Veterinary social workers, who may be found in a wide range of practice settings including, but not limited to, veterinary medical

J. Moga (✉)
Banfield Pet Hospital, Vancouver, WA, USA
e-mail: Jeannine.Moga@banfield.com

facilities are likely to confront conflicting principles, values, and goals throughout their careers. As argued by Goldberg (2019), mental health professionals who intersect with human-animal interactions and relationships should have familiarity with the ethical terrain of veterinary medicine – and not just when they are working in veterinary settings:

> Veterinarians are the only health-care professionals simultaneously trained to preserve and end life. Human-animal relationships… are complicated. The intersection of these realities creates a myriad of ethical issues which feature prominently, not only in the role of mental health professionals within veterinary settings but also wherever mental health professionals encounter animal-related grief, loss and bereavement (p 396).

Indeed, the capacity to recognize, respect, and engage the ethical terrain of human-animal relationships and interactions is key for any social worker who is tasked with addressing those relationships in practice. This chapter will explore how ethical thinking and ethical dilemmas present for veterinary social workers, particularly those who collaborate with professionals and paraprofessionals of other disciplines. Practice ethics, conceived of as the *ought factor*, will be explored through an interprofessional lens alongside models of ethical decision-making and recommendations for creating both ethical practice and ethical culture.

Interprofessional Practice and Boundary Spanning

Social workers are the most prevalent mental health professionals in the United States, uniquely trained to attend to systems issues, intervene with a person-in-environment lens, and operate in host settings. Host settings are agencies in which social workers are "resident guests," working in organization where social work is neither the primary language nor the core professional community (Dane & Simon, 1991). The work conducted in host settings often brings with it the challenges that erupt when professionals are working from diverse (and potentially contrary) assumptions, ways of knowing, and methods. While host settings such as human hospitals, correctional institutions, and schools have enabled social workers to serve individuals and families for many decades, the organizations in which veterinary social workers are found are still relatively novel by comparison. The novelty of veterinary social work, despite its growth as a subspecialty in the past 20 years, increases the likelihood that social workers will find themselves on teams that do not understand what social workers do, thus amplifying the possibility of value discrepancies, role dilemmas, and identity confusion – both for the social worker and the interprofessional team.

Understanding the concept of interprofessional practice is key to understanding the interprofessional nature of veterinary social work. Interprofessional practice aims to improve healthcare quality, accessibility, and outcomes while reducing associated costs by leveraging the coordination, collaboration, and cooperation of professionals from multiple backgrounds (Interprofessional Education Collaborative,

2016). Also known as IPC, interprofessional practice has become commonplace in human healthcare, employing social workers to support patient care and recovery, to promote quality of life, and to address both the risks and disadvantages that influence overall well-being. Engel and Prentice's (2013) paper on the ethics of interprofessional practice explains the difference between interprofessional work and inter−/multi-disciplinary work: "What moves interprofessional beyond multidisciplinary is a much greater intent to have professionals engage in interaction with one another and for decision-making to be shared, rather than to be an autonomous activity…" (p. 432). And as noted by Bronstein (2003), this type of active interaction and collaboration "… facilitates the achievement of goals that cannot be reached when individual professionals act on their own" (p. 299).

According to the Interprofessional Education Collaborative (IPEC) (2016, p. 10), there are four competencies of interprofessional practice:

1. Working with other professionals to maintain mutual respect and values
2. Using the knowledge of one's own role and those of other professions to appropriately assess and address the healthcare needs of patients and to promote and enhance the health of populations
3. Communicating with patients, families, communities, and professionals in health and other fields in a responsive and responsible manner that supports a team approach to the promotion and maintenance of health and the prevention and treatment of disease
4. Applying relationship-building values and the principles of team dynamics to perform effectively in different team roles to plan, deliver, and evaluate patient/population-centered care and population health programs and policies that are safe, timely, efficient, effective, and equitable.

While each of these competencies, applied expansively, *may* be seen in any setting of which a veterinary social worker is part, the first competency is most important for the purposes of this discussion. This competency includes sub-competencies such as valuing diversity, respecting dignity and confidentiality, acting with integrity, and managing ethical dilemmas in a manner that is patient-centered (IPEC, 2016, p. 11). We will return to some of these topics later in the chapter.

Interprofessional care in veterinary health is less widespread than in human medicine – particularly in general medicine – and this likely reflects the fact that "…veterinary, and allied, professions continue to be taught almost exclusively in isolation" (Kinnison et al., 2016). Kinnison and colleagues' study of interprofessional veterinary practice, which involved social network analysis, clinic observation, and staff interviews, revealed that interprofessional work often involves blurring of roles and the existence of "boundary spanners" that serve as key links between different members of the interprofessional team (2016, p. 54). Veterinary social workers, whose skills and training prepare them to communicate and collaborate across people and systems, may find themselves fulfilling the role of boundary spanners as they strive to meet the needs of families, organizations, and communities when troubling human-animal issues arise (Moga, 2020).

Boundary spanning in social work, as both an interprofessional skill set and an identity, is skillfully reviewed by Oliver (2013), who notes that many social workers begin careers on interprofessional teams that require that we locate ourselves at the intersections of systems, negotiate and leverage relationships in those systems, and take practical risks that enable perspective-taking and problem-solving across culture and profession. She argues that social workers, particularly those employed at the intersections of health and social care, are uniquely prepared to address complex problems as change agents with diverse partners and across contexts. Doing so, though, requires social workers to immerse themselves in the culture, language, and norms of other disciplines in order to productively interact with other professionals, manage interprofessional relationships effectively, and advocate for clients/patients (Craig et al., 2020). Regardless of the language that is used to describe the work, the requirement to conduct the work ethically is paramount to its success. In the case of veterinary social work practice, the difference between social work roles, values, and ethics, and those not only of other human service professions but of animal health and welfare fields, provides much grist for the mill.

McAuliffe's text on interprofessional ethics (2014) serves as a useful bridge between the "what" and the "how" of ethical practice for boundary spanners and their colleagues alike. McAuliffe provides a thorough exploration of not only moral philosophy and ethical theory but also how these ideas influence how different professions regulate the professional behavior of their people and how those professionals negotiate interprofessional work. Interprofessional work, by its very nature, requires professionals to understand similarities and differences in the principles, structures, and processes for behavior across disciplines as those influence moral obligations, roles, and hierarchies, as well as the duties that propel both conflict and problem-solving. It is in understanding these differences while pursuing common ground – and a unifying purpose – that interprofessional practice shines: "An interdisciplinary or interprofessional approach to ethics provides an opportunity to search out those relationships and connections that will provide a more holistic outcome for our clients and service users" (McAuliffe, 2014, pp. 15–16).

The Challenge of Anthropocentrism for Veterinary Social Work

The requirements of *ethical* boundary spanning may look very different for the veterinary social worker than for social workers in human medical settings, if only because patients in veterinary settings – as well as the key stakeholders in animal-related service organizations – are not fully represented in social work's code of ethics. As the number of social workers trained in human-animal relationships and interactions grows, so, too, will their placement in settings both within and outside veterinary clinics. As noted by Arkow (2020), veterinary social workers may be employed in child (or adult) welfare, domestic violence programs, courthouse services, and homeless shelters (anywhere a human-animal crisis or opportunity may arise). Additionally, clinical social workers in private practice – and macro social workers in positions of policy and program development – may apply their knowledge and skills with human-animal interactions in myriad ways. Regardless of setting, veterinary social workers regularly confront challenges that come from having to bridge concerns about both human and animal well-being while addressing organizational or social policies that make doing so difficult. Counterbalancing competing needs and demands – from their interprofessional colleagues, their clients, and the animals who companion and/or serve both colleagues and clients – requires guidance, agility, and an acknowledgement that animal well-being directly impacts the well-being of humans.

Despite the proliferation of animals in human spaces, whether wild or domesticated, chattel, or companion, social work – and, indeed, veterinary social work – prioritizes human well-being. This focus is historical, and there will be many who argue that this split is necessary and appropriate. The "humans come first" edict does, in fact, reflect social work's emphasis on social justice, the centralization of underserved and marginalized populations, and the necessity of attending to the needs of humans who otherwise do not have the power or resources to affect their own well-being. However, the field's person-in-environment perspective, which *could* uniquely position social workers to leverage the relationships between humans, animals, and their shared environments (MacNamara & Moga, 2014), marginalizes animals and the ecosystem in its approach to understanding, if not influencing, individual, family, and community health (Coates, 2003).

It is therefore no surprise that an acknowledgement of animals is absent in social work codes of ethics in the context of both clinical care and research. (See the chapter authored by Loue in this volume for a discussion of ethical issues pertaining to social work research with humans and animals.) This is true for all Anglo-American societies, despite the fact that animals work *alongside* social workers in practice with increasing frequency and as central players in the context of veterinary social work (Taylor et al., 2016). Professional silence about the ethics of animal relationships, animal care, and animal use is particularly problematic because it leaves practitioners with little guidance about how to pre-empt, prevent, and resolve dilemmas involving increasingly complex human-animal interactions and relationships, other than to put the needs of humans first and refer concerns about animals to other professionals. This false, "human or animal" bifurcation is both anthropocentric and monocultural; it also places veterinary social workers in the difficult position of both making space for the diverse human-animal relationships and simultaneously ignoring potentially impactful animal issues and needs, particularly when situations get sticky.

A familiar refrain that "veterinary social workers should leave the animal issues to animal professionals" to handle is problematic for multiple reasons – particularly in interprofessional practice. Not all veterinary social workers – particularly those in rural or under-resourced areas – will have easy access to the consultation and cooperation of other professionals who can skillfully evaluate and problem-solve the animal side of complicated human-animal dynamics. Cross-training, collaboration, and cross-reporting are simply inadequate at this time, making it critical that boundary-spanning social workers learn to include non-human animals in the process of ethical problem-solving, if only to do a better job of meeting the health and well-being needs of humans. Further, animal care/control and welfare laws differ significantly by jurisdiction and by species, and these policies do not provide equal care, guidance, or protection for all animals with whom veterinary social workers may interact or work. For instance, most laws protecting the health and welfare of companion animals, including those employed by animal-assisted therapy programs, do not equally extend to the livestock (such as horses) or wild animals (such as dolphins) often utilized in such programs (Ianuzzi & Rowan, 1991). While some might advise that this is beyond the scope of social work's concern, it goes without saying that how the therapist approaches and relates to the animals, both within and outside the "therapy hour," may influence how consumers of these services interpret the presence/behavior of the animals and their relationships with them. The condition of such animals has much to do with the strength – or weakness – of the therapeutic milieu.

The false bifurcation of human and animal well-being – and absence of animals in social work ethical codes – is also contrary to the One Health paradigm. "One Health" is "…a worldwide strategy for expanding interdisciplinary collaborations and communications in all aspects of health care for humans, animals and the environment" (One Health Initiative, 2021). One Health explicitly connects the well-being of humans, animals, and the environment in order to improve problem-solving around increasingly complex and interconnected health problems. As observed by Hanrahan in her evaluation of this paradigm, social work has been largely absent from One Health research, training, and education (2014). While One Health provides a provocative and powerful inspiration for interprofessional collaboration, the omission of animals from social work theory and ethics – and the absence of social work in One Health discussions – belies the ecology shared by humans and animals, as well as the very existence of veterinary social work practice.

The absence of animals in social work ethical thought, theory, and training is perhaps best illustrated by examining some of the more common ethical dilemmas in veterinary social work practice. Learning how to identify ethical problems unique to animal relationships and interactions and what those mean for the humans in the interprofessional space is the first step toward untangling the "oughts," the "musts," and the "ought nots" that make up a social work-informed ethical decision-making process.

Red Flags and Ethical Dilemmas in Veterinary Social Work

Veterinary social workers will find themselves in positions to provide leadership in situations involving both situations of acute ethical distress on the interprofessional team and requests for ethics consultation that addresses both potential and actual risk/harm. These situations trigger what can be called the *ought factor*: a marked feeling of tension between what one wants to do, what one ought to do, and what is possible to do. The ought factor is challenging enough to manage on teams (and in situations) when there is consistency of values, roles, and goals; it is exponentially more difficult in interprofessional settings, in which professionals with diverse values, operating principles, practice standards, and ideas are engaging the same dilemma from different angles. Veterinary social workers, though, are uniquely positioned to provide leadership in such situations because their graduate training and post-graduate practice licensure require extensive education in ethics generally and ethical decision-making specifically. This training puts veterinary social workers at the apex of interprofessional processes related to solving ethical dilemmas. As such, veterinary social workers will be called upon to model ethical deliberation and decision-making from an integrative, systems-informed perspective. Listed below are some of the more common ethical dilemmas in veterinary social work practice, along with a discussion of the core issues they represent.

Conflicts of Interest

A certified therapy dog bites another dog while in the lobby of local veterinary clinic while the dog/owner dyad is waiting to be seen for routine care. Thankfully, there was no visible injury to the bite recipient. The veterinary practice, in accordance with local regulations, requires that all dog bites be reported to Animal Control, regardless of context or severity. The therapy dog's owner, a veterinary social worker who works both with local veterinary teams around issues of compassion fatigue and burnout and with her dog in a local visiting animal program implores the veterinarian not to report the bite out of concern that her dog may lose therapy dog certification. The veterinary social worker is well-known and well respected in her community and hopes that her good reputation will support the unusual request of avoiding a formal bite report.

Reamer's (2012) comprehensive evaluation of boundary issues in human services settings notes that conflicts of interest can take many forms, including when a practitioner leverages a personal or professional relationship with a colleague, client, or other party to produce a personal benefit for themselves. These "self-serving motives," which involve disregarding one duty in favor of another (Reamer, 2012, p 148), are problematic because they may put others at risk. In this case, the practitioner is likely concerned about what it will mean (both personally and professionally) if her therapy dog loses certification status due to a bite incident. However, asking another professional to ignore reporting requirements carries with it potentially significant impact on their liability and compliance status.

Boundaries and Dual Relationships

Veterinary social workers often have their own companion animals, and having animals means having to navigate those animals' social lives and physical needs. Regardless of the size of the community, being an animal caregiver is likely to require consulting or working with the people with whom veterinary social workers are otherwise engaging with socially/personally. Communities of animal people tend to be small and densely interconnected, so engaging in animal health interactions involving personal animals and friends/colleagues can quickly go from boundary crossings to boundary violations. As discussed by McAuliffe (2014), *boundary crossings* are departures from standard practice that may benefit a client (like providing a professional discount to a client who is also a peer or giving the same person extra attention or time that might not be afforded to someone without the same status); *boundary violations*, on the other hand, represent breaches of acceptable behavior and/or policy/law that result in potential (or actual) harm to others (p. 132).

Both boundary crossings and boundary violations are more likely when dual relationships are in play. In veterinary social work, this might occur when the veterinary social worker is both a client *and* a consultant with the veterinary practice in question. This dynamic is also present, though, when veterinary social workers employ personal animals in professional programs, which puts them in the position of simultaneously serving as the clinician, the animal handler/trainer, and the animal's voice/best friend. When social workers are emotionally tied to their [working] animals, it can be difficult to see – let alone address – problems arising out of blurry boundaries. This challenge is illustrated in the following case:

> An equine-assisted therapy program for youth employs three horses who rotate through service (both mounted and ground work); all of the program horses are privately owned by the clinicians on staff with the program. One of the horses has proven to be highly reactive and unpredictable when in the presence of youth with impulse control issues. This horse was adopted from a hooved animal rescue organization 2 years ago with a known history of abuse and neglect. The horse, however, is a compelling presence on the farm, not only for his physical attributes but because some youth find that the horse's history reminds them of their own stories. The clinician/owner insists that pairing the horse with impulsive clients may "help both the horse and the clients learn self-control." The horse's owner is reluctant to remove the horse from programming despite the horse's increasingly unpredictable behavior, as neither she nor the program is financially able to procure another working horse. The owner/clinician loves her horse and is committed to his rehabilitation, insisting that working is, in itself, a form of trauma treatment and that metaphor makes for powerful bonding between her horse and clients.

While not directly examining the role of dual relationships in animal-assisted therapy, Evans and Gray (2012) argue that practitioners of AAT ought to consider those interventions as reciprocal transactions that directly impact the health and well-being of all participants – animals included. Further, they note that the safety, well-being, and learning capacity of both clients and animals are the result of an ecological process that is constantly negotiated – and should involve keen attention to the effects of interactions on humans and animals alike. It is notable, though, that their assessment of practice ethics does not account for how practitioners' personal relationships with animal colleagues may influence this process – particularly when difficult decisions must be made about withdrawing personal pets from the work the social worker and pet perform *together*. At its best, this work is likely engaging and meaningful for pets and their people; at its worst, the work may put animals and/or clients at risk when a social worker's relationship with her/his animal clouds clinical – and ethical – judgment.

Confidentiality

A veterinary social worker on contract with a small group of regional veterinary clinics receives a referral for family support services, all of which services are provided at the social worker's private office. The veterinary social worker requires all clients to sign consent paperwork that includes the option to approve or deny the release of information to referring partners. This particular referral involves an older female who recently presented the family dog for veterinary care with concerns about urinary incontinence and submissive urination; at the time of that veterinary consult, she admitted to feeling overwhelmed with child and dog care. The client, who has a long relationship with her veterinary practice, is the legal guardian for her 9-year-old granddaughter, who has a number of behavioral challenges.

During the first counseling appointment, the client confided that her granddaughter has a history of sexual and physical abuse; the dog has been seen urinating on the floor after playing with the child. The social worker continues with the interview, focusing on the details of these situations, the client's efforts to manage them, the veterinary teams' treatment recommendations (antibiotics for a UTI), and the other support/treatment available to the family. As the conversation unfolds, the social worker becomes increasingly concerned that the child is re-enacting sexual abuse with the dog. Because re-enactment is problematic for both the child and the dog, the social worker would like to share this information with providers serving the family – including the veterinarian. The client refuses to give consent to release any of this information to associated providers, though, preferring to "keep family matters private" and expressing concern over how that information might be used. The social worker is unable to persuade the client to share her concerns about the grandchild and dog with the veterinarian, or her granddaughter's case worker, directly.

This case brings up multiple ethical concerns, the most glaring being how to manage client confidentiality. Reamer (2018) acknowledges the difficulty of managing private health information in integrated healthcare, noting that not all partners in integrated health settings, where professionals from diverse professions are coordinating care (sometimes under one roof), will share the same level of training and expectations about the handling of confidential and privileged information. This challenge is also true in interprofessional veterinary social work practice, particularly because veterinary medicine is not included in the Health Insurance Portability and Accountability Act of 1996 (HIPAA) (USDHS, 2017), which established national standards for the privacy of health information. It is also essential to recognize that each state's laws and standards related to veterinary confidentiality are different. As such, veterinary social workers are wise to remember how these discrepancies in policies and standards influence concerns about confidentiality across providers and how to root themselves in social work's edict to preserve clients' confidential information:

> Clients' confidentiality rights arise when they entrust others with private information. Thus, when social workers' clients in integrated health care settings choose to share private information with them, social workers have a moral duty to respect clients' confidentiality rights in accord with the profession's ethical standards and relevant federal and state laws and regulations. (Reamer, 2018, p. 120–121)

In this and similar cases, veterinary social workers will need to be nimble and creative problem-solvers to work in a manner that upholds confidentiality while still pursuing necessary collaboration and cooperation across providers. Privacy concerns may be easier to address, and less vexing, when they do not overlap with mandated reporting issues. The next case is an example of how confidentiality and mandated reporting issues dovetail in veterinary social work practice.

Mandated Reporting

> An elderly woman, whose primary relationship is a small dog belonging to her recently deceased spouse, is referred to a local veterinary specialty practice for a behavioral evaluation. The dog has a documented history of bites, primarily toward the owner (most recently on the face and requiring emergency treatment). The client is vision-impaired and socially isolated; she relies on home visits for psychosocial support by those in her church, as well as the delivery of meals and other provisions. The client is informed that she will have to implement multiple changes to household management in order to reduce the likelihood of bites to herself and others; she is then referred to a veterinary social worker in the local community for additional support. The veterinary social worker talks with the client multiple times, learning that not only does the dog continue to bite her but that the client is unwilling to implement management changes because she thinks her deceased spouse – who engaged in a lengthy pattern of physical abuse toward the client –"left the dog in charge" upon his death. The veterinary social worker is unable to secure a release to share this information with the veterinary team and grows increasingly concerned about the client's lack of understanding about her dog's behavior. The social worker is unclear how to proceed, knowing that the dog may ultimately be removed from the home if another serious bite occurs. He contacts Adult Protective Services in an effort to explore his concerns about the risks this dog poses to the client; the APS worker listens with interest before responding, "The perpetrator is a DOG?"

Having cross-reporting requirements and protocols in place well before they are needed can help clinicians manage these issues of what to share with whom and when. As social services/behavioral health providers, animal care providers, and human healthcare providers learn to recognize signs of abuse, neglect, and risk across species (as well as what those signs mean for the health of systems), there are increased calls to require cross-reporting and to develop cross training in how to identify, and work with, complex concerns about risk and welfare (Long et al., 2007). These protocols are still relatively rare, however, making it both difficult and incredibly important to consider the limits of confidentiality when veterinary social workers confront injury, neglect, and abuse in practice – or are otherwise the recipients of confidential client disclosures that may be important for health and safety outcomes.

It is also crucial to acknowledge the implications of mandated reporting on collegial relationships in interprofessional practice, particularly when there is disagreement about what – or whether – a reportable concern is present. McAuliffe (2014) states: "The implications for practitioners working together are that some members of the team may be required to notify by law, while others may not. Again, it is important to not only be aware of the requirements of our own discipline but also of the potential implications for others when we engage in discussions around suspicions of possible abuse" (p. 125). Openly and honestly discussing concerns about reporting can go a long way toward managing the outcomes of those processes.

Competence

> A graduate student in social work pursues a clinical internship with a local animal-assisted therapy organization, with the goal of running her own therapeutic riding center after graduation. The organization serves youth with emotional and behavioral disorders as well as veterans with co-occurring disorders. The organization also serves as a hooved animal rescue, with a key part of its mission being "pairing survivors, together for healing." The program does not employ any social workers, so the graduate student receives supervision from an off-site clinical social worker whose animal-assisted therapy experience involves visiting a local nursing home with her own dog once per week. The student's task supervisor is the Program Director, a retired veteran in recovery, who has an Associate's Degree Small Animal Care and a professional background in marketing. Most programming is delivered by a small group of graduate student interns who receive help from two volunteers, both of whom are retired psychologists with experience in early childhood development and developmental disorders. The social work student's most recent supervision session included a disclosure by the student that she feels uncomfortable facilitating group work with clients, particularly the adults, because she isn't clear how grooming and handling the program's farm animals is contributing to symptom management and reduction – a concern other program staff have not been able to answer for her.

This example begs multiple questions, not the least of which is why trainees are providing client services without the guidance and tutelage of licensed practitioners who have demonstrated experience with the program's target populations *and* a deep knowledge of how to apply the theory and methods of animal-assisted therapy to their work with clients. This criticism applies not only to task instruction but also to the field instruction in this case, which was being delivered by a practitioner without critical experience in equine-facilitated therapy methodologies. The NASW Code of Ethics covers these issues in its discussion of competence as a core standard that reflects social workers' responsibility to protect and serve clients (NASW, 2017). Unfortunately, animal-assisted intervention programs that are delivered without the oversight and direction of clinicians who are trained in both animal behavior/handling and the application of human-animal interactions to mental and behavioral health issues proliferate because facilitated animal contact engenders positive feelings, fueled by the ardent faith of supporters, practitioners, and sponsors who are "animal people" (MacNamara & Moga, 2014).

Competence in veterinary social work does not arise from a history of animal-keeping or a passionate interest in human-animal relationships. Instead, competence is a core social work value reflecting the importance of practicing within the scope of our training and expertise, allowing ourselves to be inspired – but *not* clinically informed – by personal experiences. Further, the capacity to skillfully administer interventions – whether those interventions are widely accepted or innovative in nature – is key to serving clients effectively and, quite frankly, protecting the public (Reamer, 2013). The situations in which most veterinary social workers operate likely involve widely accepted interventions, such as medical case management or cognitive behavioral therapy, applied in practice settings that make human-animal relationships central. However, there are circumstances (like the above example) in which the greatest risk to clients involves the *negligent* application of an otherwise accepted intervention – often reflecting a dearth of training and/or skill, despite the best of intentions. Otherwise framed as misfeasance, or the commission of proper act in a manner that is improper or injurious (Reamer, 2006), this occurs in veterinary social work when practitioners and paraprofessionals proceed with work in which they are not properly schooled, skilled, and/or supervised.

Competence is not a destination, but an ongoing process involving critical self-evaluation, training, and consultation to ensure that necessary understanding and skills are applied to the professional situations in which human services professional find themselves (Corey et al., 2018). An example of competence building in veterinary social work is described by Moga (2020), as this author fielded a professional request to provide forensic social work services for a legal team litigating the case of multiple equine fatalities at a large show barn. While my professional training and experience includes working with traumatic grief, disaster response, and assessing/addressing human-equine relationships, this request for service still fell outside the scope of my expertise. Forensic social work is a specialty with its own set of unique competencies, and it took many hours of research and study, as well as ongoing consultation with an expert forensic practitioner, before I felt prepared to pursue this project with intention and ethics aligned.

Working with the "Ought Factor" in Practice

It is one thing to evaluate an ethical dilemma – *any situation in which there are competing obligations, values, or principles* – from the outside and entirely another to problem-solve it as a key stakeholder in the process and/or outcome. Models for working through ethical dilemmas in practice abound, with roots in various ethical theories and varying amounts of prescription. It is beyond the scope of this chapter to review ethical theory in any detail; however, Featherstone's notion of an ethic of care (Featherstone, 2010) provides a sound foundation from which to understand the importance of relationships in creating mutually beneficial outcomes when complex ethical dilemmas erupt. This perspective, which is less abstract than many others, acknowledges the influence of identities, interdependence, and power on how problems arise and are solved, with the ultimate goal of creating caring responses to tough situations. The strength of this theory, and its applicability to the unique dynamics found in veterinary social work practice, rests in its ability to address veterinary social work dilemmas from a more biocentric perspective.

As for particular models of ethical decision-making, all are intended to integrate principles, values, and obligations in a structure that enables critical thinking to produce a path out of vexing "sticky wickets." Problem-solving systematically, instead of intuitively, inoculates practitioners from the impulse to follow an internalized ethical code that could lead to biased and subjective solutions (Boland, 2006). Furthermore, the skill of *ethical bracketing* (Kocet & Herlihy, 2014), or identifying and intentionally separating the practitioner's personal and professional values, provides clarity about where conflicts truly arise, as well as how to move beyond sometimes deeply personal ideas about how ethical dilemmas ought to be solved. Ultimately, bracketing is a skill that enables us to work with – and serve – others whose values, beliefs, and decisions diverge from our own.

With that in mind, a succinct review of contemporary models of ethical decision-making reveals multiple methods of working through ethical dilemmas. The first of these, courtesy of Frederic Reamer (2013, p 78), proposes seven stepwise components:

1. Identify the core ethical issues, including any values, obligations, and duties in conflict.
2. Identify all parties likely to be affected by the ethical problem.
3. Begin to identify possible courses of action and their potential risks and benefits for the various parties involved.
4. Consider the pros and cons of each potential course of action, with an eye toward ethical codes and guidelines, practice theory/principles, legal principles, and personal values.
5. Consult with experts and colleagues.
6. Make your decision, with full documentation about the process by which it was reached.
7. Monitor, evaluate, and document your process.

Reamer's (2006) discussion of working through ethical concerns in nontraditional and unorthodox practice also points to the importance of following the procedural standard of care when making practice decisions. This suggestion, which is particularly important when practitioners are implementing innovative/novel approaches that do not yet have a solid empirical base (such as some animal-assisted therapies), involves asking oneself what an "ordinary, reasonable, and prudent social worker would do" (Reamer, 2006, p 194). More completely, this standard of care includes securing peer consultation and appropriate supervision; obtaining full informed consent (with disclosure of any practice methods that are not yet evidence-based); the full review of all relevant laws, regulations, and ethical standards; obtaining legal consultation; and engaging in evaluation/documentation. The consequences of not following the standard of care are potentially grave for clients, practitioners, and organizations – particularly when new areas of practice (and new practice methods) are being developed and pursued.

Another popular model is found in the *ethical principles screen* (Dolgoff et al., 2009), which proposes a hierarchical set of principles that can guide decision-making in difficult situations when alternative options for proceeding need to be weighed against one another. This model, also constructed for a social work audience, revolves around principles that are widely applicable in interprofessional conversations:

1. Protection of life
2. Equality and inequality
3. Autonomy and freedom
4. Least harm + quality of life
5. Privacy and confidentiality
6. Truthfulness/full disclosure

These models function as assistive devices, providing the scaffolding for ethical solution-building. However, they are also challenging to remember – let alone model – in the time-pressed and complex interprofessional conversations in which veterinary social workers take part. Bruce Hartsell's (2006) *life-choice-relationship model* provides a concise and flexible alternative that represents three values, thereby reducing the possibility of conflicts *among* the elements of the model itself. Noting that all decisions are based in the values of life (supporting life processes), choice (allowing the opportunity to select among multiple options for resolution), and relationship (the voluntary interaction between individuals, including spoken and unspoken rules of engagement and communication), Hartsell emphasizes that all ethical decision-making ought to maximize these values in the deliberative process. Further, he notes that by keeping to just three essential elements, practitioners' thinking will be streamlined, and the inability to resolve ethical dilemma will be marked by any situation that requires the practitioner to sacrifice one element for another. This model, as simple and straightforward as it seems, provides a spacious and inclusive framework to address ethical dilemmas with a biocentric lens, acknowledging that all human-animal interactions involve life, choice, and relationships that may be maximized for the benefit of all.

Last, the *inclusive model of ethical decision-making* (Chenowith and McAuliffe, in McAuliffe, 2014) reflects four basic dimensions and five stages, each of which allow for ethical problem-solving in interprofessional contexts. Succinctly stated, these dimensions (accountability, consultation, cultural sensitivity, and critical reflection) reflect the value base of social work, as well as other affiliated disciplines, and account for a sense of shared responsibility for both ethical thinking and ethical solution-building. Next, the five stages of this model reflect a nimble and inclusive process: defining/redefining the dilemma, mapping/remapping legitimacy, gathering/regathering information, identifying alternative approaches/re-approaches and actions, and critical analysis and (re)evaluation. Each of these allows interprofessional teams to deepen reflexive conversations in a way that honors diversity of experience and perspective, permits robust and respectful debate, encourages open reflection, and engages transparent evaluation. Interestingly, this model also reflects some of the processes found among ethics consultation teams, which are commonly located in human healthcare settings.

Bridging Principles and Process: Ethics Consultation

A critically ill cat is presented to a team of veterinary specialists at a large hospital by a distressed and devoted family that is looking for any possible way to prolong their cat's life. While there is no cure for the cat's complicated medical issues, the team presents a number of options to the family, including an expensive experimental treatment that might either improve the cat's condition or cause marked decompensation and death. This treatment, if chosen, would be a landmark event for the team and the hospital, requiring significant resources to plan, execute, and support through its conclusion.

The voices among the team were many and markedly divergent, both for and against the experimental treatment. Some on the team were excited to forge new ground and contribute to scientific discovery, holding onto hope that their hard work might result in the remission of this cat's symptoms. Others, however, expressed strong concerns about the impact of the experimental treatment on the patient, on the family, and on the functioning of the team. There were realistic concerns about patient suffering, the diversion of valuable resources to a single patient (not just for the procedure but also for the prolonged hospitalization and recovery), and the high potential for burnout among team members involved in this patient's intensive care. One nurse summed up the situation succinctly as she remarked, "what will we do if we pour everything we have into this patient, and the patient suffers and dies? How is that ethical?" Meanwhile, the family rallied around their cat, managing to pull together the financial resources to underwrite treatment. They were committed to pressing forward, recognizing that their cat might not survive the attempt to help him.

Cases like this are not unusual in medicine, veterinary, or otherwise. Concerns about how treatment decisions are made – particularly by surrogates who are trying to intuit what a loved one would want – are complicated by nature and fraught with pressure. Recent research reveals that veterinary practitioners confront ethical conflicts frequently – often weekly – and also experience high levels of emotional distress as a result (Batchelor & McKeegan, 2015; Moses et al., 2018). When professionals feel caught between professional obligations to provide treatment and limitations on what they are actually able to do, or when those obligations conflict with their values and moral standards, or when two or more principles apply in a situation but point to different courses of action, the result is often *moral distress* (Fourie, 2015). Whether triggered by situations of overtreatment and undertreatment, complicated by the unique financial dynamics of veterinary care, reflecting the tension between almost unfettered property rights and humane treatment (Rosoff et al., 2018), or arising out of euthanasia, moral distress is commonplace in interprofessional veterinary practice. Providing practitioners with the tools to identify and resolve conflicting ideas, values, and principles is the key to neutralizing that distress.

This author was serving as the primary veterinary social worker on the hospital team at the time the case described above arrived in hospital, and the experience of navigating these conversations (both between and among team members) made it clear that the open communication, collaboration, and negotiation required for resolving ethical dilemmas don't naturally occur, particularly in emotionally charged situations. The similarities between my experience and those of pediatric medical social workers are striking, as ethical dilemmas arising out of caring for patients who cannot advocate for themselves and over whom guardians have both great responsibility and great power are significant. Delaney et al. (2017) note that ethical dilemmas in pediatric medical settings bring with them communication challenges both between team members and between teams and the patient's family; the tall bar of upholding/balancing rights and responsibilities and confidentiality issues; and, for social workers in particular, the added hurdle of managing the hierarchy of medical settings with diplomacy and skill. Regardless, it was necessary for both organizational learning and organizational culture to find an approach to resolve the complex ethical dilemmas inherent in this case, as concerns about case management and resolution were erupting throughout the organization. It was also evident that any approach to problem-solving needed to be attentive to both human and animal needs; sensitive to client, clinician, team, and organizational values; and conducive to problem-solving in a time- and resource-pressed environment.

The process of problem-solving and program generation began with targeted outreach to a local University that housed both a renowned human hospital and expert consultants in bioethics and ethics consultation. Forging a collaborative relationship with the Chair of this university's Ethics Program led to a multiyear process of creating a functioning ethics consultation team in the host veterinary hospital. This process, described in Adin et al. (2019) and Rosoff et al. (2018), embodied a spirit of shared learning in which clear communication became an ethical endeavor in and of itself. All structures and processes, meticulously crafted, needed to ensure that collaborative problem-solving could occur in the face of sometimes disparate ideas, principles, and values. At the recommendation of our expert consultants and collaborators, an "ethics committee" was recruited to represent doctors and nurses from both small animal and large animal practice; this team, including the veterinary social worker, received extensive training in bioethics consultation based on the core competencies set forth by the American Society for Bioethics and Humanities (2011). The Committee adopted an ethics facilitation approach, which focuses on providing consultation and communication to help medical practitioners identify core ethical conflicts (as well as the values, obligations, and principles that undergird them), analyze the nature of uncertainty, and use skilled communication to facilitate principled ethical resolution (ASBH, 2011, p 7). Further, it chose to utilize a concise and systematic model of case facilitation called *CASES*. Created by the National Center for Ethics in Healthcare, the CASES model was designed to help ethics consultants guide medical professionals through a systematic and deliberative process of identifying and problem-solving ethical problems (Berkowitz et al., 2015). The similarities to other stepwise models are evident, with discussion in each phase being facilitated by one or two consultants affiliated with the ethics committee:

C: Clarify the request and formulate the ethics question.

A: Assemble all relevant information from stakeholders, focusing on objective medical information, client/patient preferences, ethical and legal guidelines, and institutional policies.

S: Synthesize the information, analyze it, and facilitate moral deliberation between ethically justifiable options.

E: Explain the synthesis and proposed resolution to key stakeholders, provide additional resources for those who need additional information and support, and document the process.

S: Support the consultation process and its participants through follow-up, process evaluation, and the identification and discussion of any relevant systems issues.

The role of veterinary social work here was to provide leadership through education, particularly with hospital administration and the within the ranks of hospital staff, many of whom were concerned that ethics consultation equated with "the ethics police"; advocacy, particularly in crafting a process that made space for inclusion and transparency for all members of the team and eventually the client; facilitating ethics team processes, including formal and informal consultations and record keeping/data collection; and brokering resources and services as the Ethics Committee launched.

Admittedly, not every veterinary social worker will find themselves in a medical setting, per se. However, it is critical to note that all veterinary social workers engaging with interprofessional teams in some form or fashion are likely to confront the need to lead deliberative conversations about shared ethical dilemmas. The good news is that social work has long been part of these conversations. As more veterinary social workers are diffused into interprofessional teams, I expect the opportunities to develop and lead ethics consultation/conversation processes will expand considerably.

Moving Forward: Ethical Literacy and Ethical Courage

While discussions about ethics in practice are often reactive in nature and focused on individual ethical decisions, shifting to a more proactive and interprofessional stance is congruent with all functions of veterinary social work practice: increasing attention to the diversity and depth of human-animal relationships; improving our collective capacity to support those relationships in individuals, families, and communities; advancing awareness and support of the health and well-being of animal care professionals; and creating interprofessional interventions and programs that support the health and well-being of humans, animals, *and* the environments in which they live. As a community, veterinary social workers will only accomplish these goals if we place the ethics of our work in the forefront of our thinking, our partnerships, and our processes.

Doing so effectively requires creating and seeking opportunities for interprofessional education that makes space at the table for professionals in human healthcare, social services, veterinary and animal science, public health, and environmental science to learn about, and alongside, one another. Ideally, this type of learning should be case based in nature because ethics learned in silos and devoid of real-world context do not generalize well and can lead to misunderstandings (about professional values, methods, and goals) when difficult issues arise. In fact, creative solutions to our most challenging (and complex) problems require that we be willing to have detailed conversations about the philosophies, epistemologies, values, and methods informing our work, particularly if we wish to successfully navigate shared practice space (McAuliffe, 2014).

Donna McAuliffe makes a compelling case for interprofessional education, noting that having interprofessional conversations early and often provides a framework and expectation for respectful dialogue based in a solid understanding of how diverse professionals understand their work and navigate their roles (McAuliffe, 2014). Building familiarity with team-based ethics consultation, such as the model discussed in this chapter, also increases the possibility that ethical dilemmas will be swiftly identified, discussed, and debriefed before significant moral injury erupts among interprofessional teams.

Interprofessional ethics training is also a valuable mechanism for producing *ethical literacy*. When professionals across disciplines enter shared practice spaces with a solid understanding of professional integrity, clearly defined practice boundaries, a sound knowledge of ethical theory and ethical decision-making models, and a willingness to maintain transparency and accountability, the quality of their independent and collaborative work dramatically improves (McAuliffe, 2014). Unfortunately, not all allied professionals in the veterinary social work space receive focused training on practice ethics and ethical decision-making strategies; in fact, a recent survey of North American veterinarians revealed that about 70% of respondents reported having no education in how to resolve ethical conflicts in care (Moses et al., 2018). These discrepancies in training practically beg for social work's attention and advocacy.

Veterinary social workers who serve as "lone rangers" in host agencies, where they are the only voice for social work values and ethics, should also be prepared to discuss and manage ethical dilemmas up front, recognizing that they will likely be called to lead problem-solving efforts when cases trigger significant ethical concerns among the interprofessional team. Social workers with a solid foundation of ethics training are better prepared to operate from a place of social courage, which is necessary when tasked with helping to identify, and negotiate resolution for, ethical issues impacting both clients and colleagues. Applying that courage to difficult situations in practice often looks – and sounds – like advocacy, which is both a key social work role and a skill based in sound ethical reasoning.

Last, and perhaps most provocatively, social work as a profession would do well to address the anthropomorphism in its ranks. When our codes of ethics do not reflect increasingly diverse attitudes toward, and relationships with, animals for individuals, families, and communities, practitioners are left with little guidance in how to attend to these relationships – particularly when divergent values, goals, and ideals about animals emerge in practice. The placement of service animals and emotional support animals in households with increasingly diverse needs, as well as the application of animals in wide-ranging physical, social, emotional, and behavioral health interventions, begs the question of why social workers can work alongside (and, indeed, prescribe) animals on the one hand while simultaneously marginalizing their needs on the other. This is particularly true because animals, unlike art supplies, sand trays, or genograms – some of the tools employed by social workers – are living beings with physical, emotional, and social needs of their own. What message are we sending to our clients, particularly those who are disenfranchised and whose voices are marginalized, by supplanting animals' needs in service to humans?

Parting Thoughts

Much, if not all, veterinary social work is interprofessional in nature. Even if veterinary social workers find themselves in private practice or solo work, they are likely to encounter client situations that challenge their sense of what is ethically appropriate. We must think expansively about how veterinary social work is defined, beyond work with veterinary practices and issues, in order to fully understand what interprofessional dynamics influence the presence and resolution of ethical concerns that arise for professionals in these areas. Social workers are often in the position to serve multiple stakeholders simultaneously, and those stakeholders often have competing interests and demands.

Donna McAuliffe, whose text on interprofessional ethics has been referenced throughout this chapter, provides a rich history of, and ample guidance for, ethical theory and ethical practice. While speaking the language of ethics, knowing one's own ethical boundaries, and committing to open and respectful dialogue are key to McAuliffe's argument, her ability to differentiate between a wise and brave practitioner is perhaps most powerful:

> A wise practitioner will always engage with critical reflection so that they take nothing for granted; so that they remain aware that no two situations will automatically demand the same response; and so that they explore every situation for evidence of structural disadvantage or potential injustice. A brave practitioner will not remain silent when there is a need to speak out, or take a stand, on a principle that upholds professional ethical responsibilities. (2014, p 181)

The challenge of veterinary social work is to be both wise and brave in practice such that we activate values in our work with clients and interprofessional teams. Foregrounding human-animal relationships in our work – and attending to the ethics of these relationships – is the vehicle through which we demonstrate the very best of social work theory, thinking, and practice. This is not an easy endeavor, mind you, if for no other reason than our own profession struggles with the place and consequence of animals – and the natural environment – in human life. But if we want to do more than encourage and model healthy relationships for clients, colleagues, and communities, we must lean into the ethics of human-animal relationships, interactions, and interventions – particularly when they go awry (Moga, 2019).

Nevertheless, it is in working the margins that social workers shine. Our history, our values, and our unique perspective on the world prepare and demand that we stand for justice, fairness, diversity, and equity in our public and private spaces. This is the ethic of social work, and it should not be absent from veterinary social work practice. Forging relationships, inspiring conversations, and advocating for humane interactions between and among all species should serve as the guiding principles we all share.

References

Adin, C., Moga, J., Keene, B., Fogle, C., Hopkinson, H., Weyhrauch, C., Marks, S., Ruderman, R., & Rosoff, P. (2019). Clinical ethics consultation in a tertiary care veterinary teaching hospital. *Journal of the American Veterinary Medical Association, 254*(1), 52–60.

American Society for Bioethics and Humanities. (2011). *Core competencies for healthcare ethics consultation* (2nd ed.). American Society for Bioethics and Humanities.

Arkow, P. (2020). Human-animal relationships and social work: Opportunities beyond the veterinary environment. *Child and Adolescent Social Work, 37*(6), 573–588.

Batchelor, C., & McKeegan, D. (2015). A preliminary investigation into the moral reasoning abilities of UK veterinarians. *Veterinary Record, 177*(5), 124.

Berkowitz, K. A., Chanko, B. L., Foglia, M. B., Fox, E., & Powell, T. (2015). *Ethics consultation: Responding to ethics questions in healthcare* (2nd ed.). National Center for Ethics in Healthcare. https://www.ethics.va.gov/docs/integratedethics/ec_primer_2nd_ed.pdf

Boland, K. (2006). Ethical decision-making among hospital social workers. *Journal of Social Work Values and Ethics, 3*(1). https://jswve.org/download/2006-1/JSWVE-Spring-2006-Complete.pdf

Bronstein, L. (2003). A model for interdisciplinary collaboration. *Social Work, 48*(3), 297–306.

Coates, J. (2003). *Ecology and social work: Toward a new paradigm.* Fernwood Publishing.

Corey, G., Corey, M., & Callanan, P. (2018). *Issues and ethics in the helping professions* (10th ed.). Brookes/Cole.

Craig, S., Eaton, A., Belitsky, M., Kates, L., Dimitropoulos, G., & Tobin, J. (2020). Empowering the team: A social work model of interprofessional collaboration. *Journal of Interprofessional Education & Practice, 19*, 100327. https://doi.org/10.1016/j.xjep.2020.100327

Dane, B., & Simon, B. (1991). Resident guests: Social workers in host settings. *Social Work, 36*(3), 208–213. https://doi.org/10.1093/sw/36.3.208

Delaney, C., Richards, A., Stewart, H., & Kosta, L. (2017). Five challenges to ethical communication for interprofessional paediatric practice: A social work perspective. *Journal of Interpersonal Care, 31*(4), 505–511.

Dolgoff, R., Loewenberg, F., & Harrington, D. (2009). *Ethical decisions for social work practice* (8th ed.). Thomson Brooks/Cole.

Engel, J., & Prentice, D. (2013). The ethics of interprofessional collaboration. *Nursing Ethics, 20*(4), 426–435.

Evans, N., & Gray, C. (2012). The practice and ethics of animal-assisted therapy with children and young people: Is it enough that we don't eat our co-workers? *British Journal of Social Work, 42*, 600–617.

Featherstone, B. (2010). Ethic of care. In M. Gray & D. Webb (Eds.), *Ethics and value perspectives in social work* (pp. 73–84). Palgrave Macmillan.

Fourie, C. (2015). Moral distress and moral conflict in clinical ethics. *Bioethics, 29*(2), 91–97.

Goldberg, K. (2019). Issues in serious veterinary illness and end-of-life care. In L. Kogan & C. Blazina (Eds.), *Clinician's guide to treating companion animal issues: Addressing human-animal interaction* (pp. 395–419). Academic Press.

Hanrahan, C. (2014). Integrative health thinking and the One Health concept: Is social work all for 'one' or 'one' for all? In T. Ryan (Ed.), *Animals in social work: Why and how they matter* (pp. 32–47). Palgrave Macmillan.

Hartsell, B. (2006). A model for ethical decision-making: The context of ethics. *Journal of Social Work Values & Ethics, 3*(1). https://jswve.org/download/2006-1/JSWVE-Spring-2006-Complete.pdf

Ianuzzi, D., & Rowan, A. (1991). Ethical issues in animal-assisted therapy programs. *Anthrozoös, 4*(3), 154–163.

Interprofessional Education Collaborative. (2016). *Core competencies for interprofessional collaborative practice: 2016 update*. Interprofessional Education Collaborative.

Kinnison, T., Guile, D., & May, S. (2016). The case of veterinary interprofessional practice: From one health to a world of its own. *Journal of Interprofessional Education & Practice, 4*, 51–57.

Kocet, M., & Herlihy, B. (2014). Addressing value-based conflicts within the counseling relationship: A decision-making model. *Journal of Counseling & Development, 92*(2), 180–186. https://doi.org/10.1002/j.1556-6676.2014.00146.x

Long, D., Long, J., & Kulkarni, S. (2007). Interpersonal violence and animals: Mandated cross-sector reporting. *Journal of Sociology & Social Welfare, 34*(3), 147–164.

MacNamara, M., & Moga, J. (2014). The place and consequence of animals in contemporary social work practice. In T. Ryan (Ed.), *Animals in social work: Why and how they matter* (pp. 151–155). Palgrave Macmillan.

McAuliffe, D. (2014). *Interprofessional ethics: Collaboration in the social, health, and human services*. Cambridge University Press.

Moga, J. (2019). Integrating clients' animals in clinical practice: Insights from an animal-informed therapist. In L. Kogan & C. Blazina (Eds.), *Clinicians' guide to treating companion animal issues* (pp. 253–266). Academic Press.

Moga, J. (2020). Animal loss and interprofessional practice: A primer in "boundary spanning" for mental health professionals. In L. Kogan & P. Erdman (Eds.), *Pet loss, grief, and therapeutic interventions: Practitioners navigating the human-animal bond* (pp. 323–337). Routledge.

Moses, L., Malowney, M., & Boyd, J. (2018). *Ethical conflict and moral distress in veterinary practice: A survey of North American veterinarians* (pp. 2115–2122). Journal of Veterinary Internal Medicine.

National Association of Social Workers. (2017). *Code of Ethics of the National Association of Social Workers*. NASW Press.

Oliver, C. (2013). Social workers as boundary spanners: Reframing our professional identity for interprofessional practice. *Social Work Education, 32*(6), 773–784.

One Health Initiative. (2021). *About one health*. Retrieved from https://onehealthinitiative.com/

Reamer, F. (2006). Nontraditional and unorthodox interventions in social work: Ethical and legal implications. *Families in Society, 87*(2), 191–197.

Reamer, F. (2012). *Boundary issues and dual relationships in the human services* (2nd ed.). Columbia University Press.

Reamer, F. (2013). *Social work values and ethics* (4th ed.). Columbia University Press.

Reamer, F. (2018). Ethical issues in integrated health care: Implications for social workers. *Health & Social Work, 43*(2), 118–124.

Rosoff, P., Moga, J., Keene, B., Adin, C., Fogle, C., Ruderman, R., Hopkinson, H., & Weyhrauch, C. (2018). Resolving ethical dilemmas in a tertiary care veterinary specialty hospital: Adaptation of the human clinical consultation committee model. *The American Journal of Bioethics, 18*(2), 41–53.

Taylor, N., Fraser, H., Signal, T., & Prentice, K. (2016). Social work, animal-assisted therapies and ethical considerations: A programme example from Central Queensland, Australia. *The British Journal of Social Work, 46*(1), 135–152. https://doi.org/10.1093/bjsw/bcu115

United States Department of Health and Human Services. (2017). *HIPAA for professionals.* Retrieved from https://www.hhs.gov/hipaa/for-professionals/index.html

Part III
Veterinary Social Work and the Veterinary Setting

Chapter 8
Veterinary Social Work in Veterinary Hospital Settings

Sandra Brackenridge, Lisa Hacker, and Alyssa Pepe

Introduction

Literature is sparse with regard to social work programs within veterinary hospitals. Most articles describe particular programs and the veterinary social workers who created the programs (Cima, 2020; Cohen, 1985; Crocken, 1981; Holcombe et al., 2016; Larkin, 2016). Therefore, most of the knowledge shared in this chapter has been learned through the professional experiences of the authors. The authors are well-acquainted with the needs of an entire veterinary hospital, the hospital clients, and various staff, and how to navigate through initiation of a program evolving into obvious success. There are strikingly no data yet compiled in the published literature which address the efficacy of these programs, although some data have been presented at veterinary conferences. We provide some statistics at the end of this chapter which will demonstrate the utilization of the programs by hospital staff and the clients of the hospitals served by the authors.

Sandra Brackenridge created an early comprehensive program at Louisiana State University School of Veterinary Medicine in 1990. The program there included pet loss counseling and quality of life counseling to clients, counseling for staff and students, teaching about communication with clients and about grief due to pet loss in rounds and in the curriculum, and an animal-assisted therapy program. It also incorporated social work students who were doing their required internships for the Master's degree in social work. This program at LSU is still in operation today

S. Brackenridge (✉)
Counseling and Consultation for Veterinarians and Hospitals, Corinth, TX, USA
e-mail: sandra@sbrackenridgelcsw.com

L. Hacker
1st Pet Vet Centers, Madison, WI, USA

A. Pepe
Orchard Park Veterinary Medical Center, Orchard Park, NY, USA

under the direction of one of the original interns in the program. Through trial and error, the program at LSU flourished, and Brackenridge learned about the pitfalls and the effective efforts in development of a veterinary social work (VSW) program. Brackenridge left LSU to become a professor of social work, retiring from teaching in 2017. She built on her experience at LSU in 2013 when she was asked by an undergraduate social work student to create an internship in a veterinary hospital so that the student could complete her Master's degree in social work and the Veterinary Social Work certificate with the University of Tennessee School of Social Work online. A specialty and emergency veterinary hospital agreed to give the VSW internship a try. Brackenridge continued to provide field instruction for students at the hospital for years, eventually becoming an employee of the hospital. As an employee, she was able to build a more robust program to serve needs of staff as well as to continue client care. As she began to receive requests from other hospitals for assistance in developing a VSW program, Brackenridge began to consult, develop, and ensure the success of other programs. Today, Brackenridge consults and provides counseling services to veterinary professionals full-time while practicing privately.

Two of those successful programs are now directed by the other authors of this chapter. Lisa Hacker became the VSW for a specialty and emergency veterinary hospital in the upper Midwest in 2018. This hospital had a strong culture of compassion for clients and staff, and it had multiple locations of various sizes. Hacker had already had extensive previous experience in pediatric medical social work and program development. In consultation, Hacker was able to shadow a program as part of her training in veterinary social work. Hacker built a comprehensive VSW program, serving clients and serving staff. The hospital quickly recognized the value of a VSW program, and Hacker eventually became the Program Manager with two other social workers serving the hospital's locations. Hacker incorporated social work interns into the program and served as field instructor as well.

Alyssa Pepe developed a VSW program in the northeast United States beginning in 2019. Pepe had extensive experience in psychotherapy and mental health, as well as a wealth of experience as a volunteer in wildlife rehabilitation. Pepe also traveled to learn about development of a program. The program that Pepe built and enhanced received accolades from staff and social media alike, and due to her work, she was awarded the New York State's National Association of Social Work award for Exceptional Service in 2020. Pepe also incorporated VSW interns into the hospital program.

The authors argue that social work services should be provided within any large veterinary hospital, daily and with regularity. We define a large hospital as one that has 100 or more employees. The veterinary profession, veterinarians and their technicians, nurses, and support staff are struggling with their mental health, and the rate of suicide within the profession is well-documented as a concern (Skipper & Williams, 2012; Tomasi et al., 2019; Volk et al., 2018, 2020). Some hospitals have implemented programs which provide mental health and client services as per need and by request from the hospital or individual staff members, but the mental health provider or VSW is not on-site with regularity. For example, a mental health professional may visit the hospital 1 or 2 days each month. Within those types of programs, debriefing, crisis counseling, and support is offered without much acquaintance and without a working trust between the VSW and the person needing assistance.

More importantly, this type of program does not address the needs of clients for emotional support which was demonstrated by Spitznagel et al. (2019) to be perhaps the greatest indicator of stress and burnout for veterinary professionals. The researchers studied the effect of burden transfer from clients to the veterinary professionals: "The frequency that veterinarians reported encountering BTI [Burden Transfer Inventory] items was positively correlated with measures of stress and burnout, which suggested burden transfer from owners to veterinarians. The extent to which veterinarians reported being bothered by BTI items was a more robust predictor of stress and burnout than the frequency with which those items occurred" (Spitznagel et al., 2019). In fact, the literature provides irrefutable evidence that a mental health practitioner who works with clients within the hospital may reduce the stress and risk of compassion fatigue for staff and increase well-being among staff in general (Spitznagel et al., 2017, 2018, 2019, 2020).

We describe a day in the life of a veterinary social work program in order to explain the reasoning underlying in-hospital social work. It is our argument as authors that hiring a VSW to direct a social work program in a veterinary hospital is a minor and justifiable expense in a hospital's budget which results in valuable benefits in terms of client satisfaction, staff recruitment and retention, and overall employee wellness.

A Day in the Life of an In-Hospital VSW Program

It may be helpful to describe what an in-hospital VSW program looks like, in a broad sense, even before we detail the development of a program. We can attest to the unpredictability of any particular day within a large veterinary hospital, especially when emergency services are offered as well as specialty services. Specialties generally have appointments scheduled throughout the week, but emergency can vary from moment to moment. For our example, we are describing a VSW program with one program lead who is an employee of the hospital. Our program example includes social work interns who are completing their hours toward the Master's in Social Work (MSW). The interns are unpaid and complete their hours while in school. They may complete anywhere from 16 to 32 hours a week, depending upon how they are enrolled in the school curriculum. We are describing a weekday rather than a weekend.

7 am: VSW intern (VSW-I) arrives and prints the current list of hospitalized patients, names of owners, department providing service, and location of the patient in the hospital. If time allows, the VSW-I will read the history of the patients in the

hospital documentation program, and then they will check the separate documentation system for VSW-view-only for notes made by any other social worker.

7:30 am–8:30 am: VSW intern attends rounds at shift change with doctors. As doctors update one another on the cases, referrals of owners needing support or quality of life counseling are made to the VSW-I. Doctors may also share with VSW-I that certain patients with poor prognosis may lead to the family considering euthanasia. Cases which were difficult, and owners who presented with intense emotion during the night, may also be discussed during rounds, and VSW-I may debrief with doctors at this time or inquire as to whether other staff need a debriefing. They will inquire as to whether it is recommended that a VSW follow up with the client.

8:30 am–9:30 am: VSW-I finds patients mentioned to familiarize themselves with the animals. They then return to the computer to read the histories thoroughly.

9:30 am–10:30 am: Employed VSW (lead and field instructor) arrives. Information from rounds is shared. Cases are discussed, and possible approaches to the clients or staff for support are taught to the VSW-I. It is determined as to who should reach out to the clients or the staff members. The supervision time is interrupted by a client services representative informing the VSW and VSW-I that a family is coming in to euthanize patient X and that they are on their way. This patient was discussed in rounds as a possible euthanasia. During this supervision hour, a doctor comes to the VSW office to get some candy and debriefs with the VSW and VSW-I about a difficult case and angry client from the day before.

11:15 am–noon: Family of patient to be euthanized has arrived. VSW lead obtains the folder of grief materials and goes to talk with the family. The VSW facilitates introductions and provides pre-euthanasia counseling, describes the euthanasia process, shares and describes the materials available in the folder, and provides information about counseling through the VSW program including the pet loss support group. The VSW provides tools for a hair clipping if the family desires and makes a bed so the family can lay with the pet. If the pet is still eating, the VSW may also provide treats and water for both the pet and the clients. When the clients indicate that they are ready (by ringing a button), the VSW confirms that they are ready, goes to determine if the doctor is aware, and accompanies the doctor to the room. (In times of the pandemic, the VSW may also assist the doctor with PPE). If the family expresses a need, the VSW may remain with them during the euthanasia. The VSW may provide further counseling post-euthanasia and make certain the clients are safe to drive.

While the VSW lead is working with the family, the VSW-I may be working with another euthanasia case, or perhaps a patient has coded and they are working with that family. They may be supporting a client family whose pet has just been brought in and rushed to ICU. They may be introducing VSW services to clients waiting in exam rooms, or during the pandemic, to clients waiting in their cars. They may be visiting with an owner of a chronically or terminally ill patient whose doctor requested that a VSW provide the tools in the quality of life (QoL) folder.

Noon–1 pm: VSW and VSW-I process and debrief regarding the cases worked during the previous hour. Each social worker records their activities in two documentation systems. In the hospital's system, brief factual notes about activities are recorded so that staff can see that the VSW has been involved. Notes in this system will include any information relevant to enhance the treatment of the patient, but client disclosure irrelevant to treatment is recorded in a documentation system available only to the VSW and VSW-Is. In the VSW documentation, a more in-depth description of the interaction with clients is recorded so that any other VSW or VSW-I can continue to work well with the client. Supervision and teaching for refining social work skills are offered during this hour as well.

1 pm–2 pm: VSW-I finishes documentation and ends their day at the hospital. VSW lead attends a staff meeting for the internal medicine department. During the first portion, a structured debriefing is conducted.

2 pm–2:45 pm: VSW lead consults with a manager who is concerned about an employee. VSW sends an email to the employee asking for a check-in.

3 pm–5 pm: VSW lead welcomes the second intern who will continue until 9 pm. VSW lead updates VSW-I2 on all cases. VSW-I2 walks through the hospital familiarizing themselves with patients and speaking to doctors about their cases. VSW-I2 calls clients to inform them that their pet's cremains have returned to the hospital and provides follow-up and pet loss counseling. VSW-I2 or VSW will also provide counseling to clients when they arrive to retrieve remains. Clients and VSW or VSW-I meet in exam rooms (or during pandemic, at their cars).

4 pm–5 pm: VSW lead provides a presentation to all staff able to be present about communicating with clients. Presentations to occur in the upcoming weeks include those about burnout and compassion fatigue, stress and anxiety techniques which can be practiced at work and, for doctors only, a presentation on *The Serious Veterinary Illness Conversation Guide* (Goldberg, 2019). Other duties which may happen during this hour may be facilitation of stress-reduction activity.

5:30 pm: VSW lead ends their day.

5:30 pm–9 pm: VSW-I intervenes with two additional families whose pets are euthanized and provides pet loss counseling to two more clients who arrive to retrieve remains in exam rooms (or curbside during the pandemic).

Development of a VSW Program

Every large veterinary hospital, defined by the authors as a hospital employing 100 or more people, could benefit from a veterinary social work program. Each hospital is unique in terms of size, location, clientele, work environment, number of employees, and culture. Some of the differences are due to geographic location, but hospitals are also differentiated by the history and character of ownership, mission and values, diversity among employees, as well as financial solvency or constraints. Types of veterinary services offered vary from hospital to hospital; some offer emergency only, some offer both emergency and specialty services, and some offer general practice in addition to emergency/specialty. Within the specialties offered, some hospitals have only one or two specialists, whereas others may have a complete list of specialists that include those trained specifically in internal medicine, critical care, surgery, oncology, cardiology, neurology, physical rehabilitation, dental, reproduction, radiology, pathology, nutrition, holistics, and more. There are even sub-specialties within many of the specialties. So a plethora of variables can determine the personality of each hospital, and therefore the need within each hospital for a social work program.

A thorough examination of the hospital as an organization, community, and workplace is warranted before concluding that an in-hospital veterinary social worker is a correct prescription for clients and staff. A program can and should be designed to fit each hospital. Doctors, nurses, and staff can help define what would be useful for their unique community. Some VSW responsibilities are necessary and welcome in one hospital and not valuable in another. Many veterinary hospitals have hired a social worker or a mental health professional without a clear understanding of all the variables we have discussed. These programs either failed or took years to become successful largely because the hospital had not been studied thoroughly, the program may not have been tailored to the unique hospital, and/or the doctors and staff may not have had an opportunity to express their needs and questions about how a program would work. Doctors and staff may have lacked adequate information about what a veterinary social work program could actually do to assist them in their daily work and personal life. Unfortunately, a person may have been hired for the hospital who was not a good fit for that particular community. In addition, veterinary professionals have a limited understanding of social work qualifications and licensure, and they may have hired someone who could not perform the responsibilities of the position.

Needs Assessment

The authors believe that a thorough understanding of the personality, structure, culture, and working environment of the hospital is essential in developing a successful veterinary social work program. This can be accomplished by conducting a comprehensive needs assessment. "The assessment of needs is perhaps the most important part of planning or evaluating any new program. Informal discussions or opinion polls are simply inadequate" (Scriven & Roth, 1978). The type of needs assessment suggested when developing and planning a new program for a community is called a strategic needs assessment. "Needs assessment involves carefully analyzing a situation and building support for action" (Sleezer et al., 2014). The needs assessment process begins with the planning and organizing phase, data collection, summarizing and disseminating the needs assessment, and sharing the results to facilitate action planning (Sharma et al., 2000). We recommend several steps in the data collection process to gain a thorough understanding of each hospital's clientele, staff, structure, culture, and working environment as well as the unique stressors experienced by staff for which a VSW program will be beneficial.

Planning and Organizing   The first step in this process is an in-depth discussion with personnel who will be directly involved with a VSW program and potentially gain approval for implementation. The personnel might be the hospital manager, administrator, chief executive officer (CEO), or medical director. The discussion should be designed, first, to educate the influential personnel about VSW programs in general, the potential roles and responsibilities of the VSW, associated costs, and licensure requirements for social workers. Veterinary professionals are generally unaware of how social workers are educated and trained. This discussion will help them learn about the uniform curricula within schools of social work and which degree or licensure level is possible. These discussions often reveal a concern from the stakeholders about how the VSW themselves will handle the responsibility of such a position; the discussion provides an opportunity to explain that social workers are trained to recognize and implement self-care. Since internships for veterinarians are mostly paid positions and completed after the award of the Doctor of Veterinary Medicine, it is useful to educate them about social work internships. They should learn that social work interns are usually unpaid, how many hours are required for completion, and what depth and duration of experience their potential VSW must have attained in order to supervise interns. Ethical considerations for services rendered by a VSW are an additional topic for discussion, in that confidentiality and documentation mandated of a social worker will be something that the hospital will need to consider.

Data Gathering Step 1   The second goal of this initial discussion is data gathering. It is useful to learn about the demographics of the hospital, number of employees, number and type of specialties, etc. Examination of the organizational chart and knowledge about how human resources functions within the organization is helpful. A veterinary social work program will interface with other opportunities for wellness which may already exist through benefits offered employees, so it is helpful to know about resources which are already in place. In addition, the personality of the hospital helps shape the type and intensity of stressors which are faced by employees. Exactly why a hospital may have a need for a veterinary social work program and what led the hospital to recognize the need for social work services should be understood before proceeding with the creation of the position. The personnel in charge may in fact be looking for solutions that a VSW program cannot address. For example, Brackenridge has talked with hospitals who are in need of a business consultant rather than assistance in development of a VSW program.

Data Gathering Step 2   After this discussion, if the hospital chooses to go forward, we recommend that a thorough interactive tour of the hospital be conducted for the person helping to develop a program. One goal for the person receiving the tour is to learn about the environmental stressors experienced by clients and by staff that the VSW may help to ameliorate. Another goal is to learn how the VSW will most effectively establish a presence and where. There are many questions to be asked and answered as the tour is conducted, beginning with outside of the hospital and within each area of the hospital.

The tour should include a discussion of the size and function of the reception and client services team, which is often the face of the hospital. Each hospital structures this department differently. Some hospitals require that they answer the phones only, while in others they also handle euthanasias, remains, payment, and issues with estimates. They may also witness client emotion and family distress and mediate with unhappy clients.

It is helpful to know whether the hospital already provides materials for pet loss, bereavement, or quality of life tools. If it does, the person receiving the tour should review the services provided to learn how efficient the current system is for locating doctors/nurses, alerting a doctor that someone is ready to euthanize, or alerting personnel about the need to take a body to the back. These are elements which a VSW can enhance. Analysis of the waiting area is important in terms of learning about chaos versus calm for clients, and the division of waiting areas per specialty.

During the tour, a good look at exam rooms should be included; it is especially important to note whether or not there is a room dedicated to euthanasia and whether it is designed according to the standard for best practice (Hart et al., 1990; Lagoni, 2011; Lagoni et al., 1994; Leary and Johnson 2020; Morris, 2009, 2012). If not, the VSW who will be hired will need to upgrade and enhance this feature of the practice. In addition, all elements surrounding death of patients should be observed during the tour, including how bodies are handled after death, where they are kept, and whether clients are protected from visually observing these activities. The authors of this chapter have found through experience that the euthanasia process as well as the handling of deceased bodies can profoundly affect staff wellness in terms of compassion fatigue and burnout.

The tour should also include observation and analysis of ICU and treatment areas in regard to stressors for staff. There may be space concerns, traffic flow stressors, ability/inability of nurses/techs to have eyes on patients, etc. An important factor for the VSW's responsibility for staff mental health might involve where and how controlled drugs are kept. Further concern for staff may involve learning during the tour where doctors make phone calls and do documentation. Contributing stressors to staff well-being are noted. In terms of client concern, the VSW may or may not need to supervise and/or develop rapport with clients who are visiting patients, so it is important to note whether clients have free access or are supervised for visitation.

Because the tour is interactive, many more notes and observations may occur. The tour should also include a discussion about how the VSW program will function. The person receiving the tour may be able to speculate about the ideal location for the VSW, where they will visit with clients, and where they will meet with staff confidentially. Perhaps the hospital has designated an area already. The VSW will want to inquire whether the hospital has designated an area, such as a conference or meeting room, in which the VSW can perform other responsibilities, e.g., debriefings in groups and presentations. Again, in terms of analyzing how the VSW might assist in ameliorating staff stressors, a view and analysis of the staff breakroom/

lounge should be included. It will be important to have some space for stress reducing activities to be held. The VSW's job description will reflect some needs exposed during the tour.

Data Gathering Step 3 We recommend a third step in an accurate assessment of need for a VSW program within a veterinary hospital. Conducting several focus groups with employees can yield much information. In the literature, there are many sources which prescribe procedures for focus groups (Morgan, 1997; Morgan and Lobe, 2011; Sharma et al., 2000; Toseland & Rivas, 1995). "Focus groups are well suited for gathering in-depth data about the attitudes and cognitions of participants" (Toseland & Rivas, 1995). Through her many years in academia, Brackenridge became familiar with the many benefits of focus groups when introducing a new concept, product, or program, or when studying a problem in order to select a solution. Focus groups are utilized in academia for research projects, and to understand the needs of students as well as faculty. Focus groups are utilized in business before rolling out a new product, and they are utilized in entertainment when determining how an audience may respond to the concept of a movie or a television show. Effective focus groups should be led by a trained leader who can keep participants on topic, structure the discussion, eliminate monopolization of time by any one participant, and ensure tolerance and non-judgment when participants express their opinion. There should ideally be 6–12 voluntary participants in a focus group. Depending upon the amount of time allotted to the group, the leader should be prepared with 8–12 questions. Focus groups should be recorded and transcribed as they are data-gathering tools for the needs assessment. (Morgan, 1997: Morgan and Lobe, 2011; Sharma et al., 2000; Toseland & Rivas, 1995)

Participants in the focus groups in veterinary hospitals should be voluntary. When it is announced that the groups will be discussing development of a VSW program, participants are often curious and receptive. Groups can ideally be divided with similar roles in mind; for example, there may be one group of client service representatives, another group of technicians/nurses/assistants, a group of administrative personnel, and a group of veterinarians. There may also be a group of managers or a group of owners, depending upon the ownership or administrative structure of the particular hospital. When leading focus groups with the goal of obtaining data for the needs assessment, the groups begin with an introduction of the facilitator's background and experience in the veterinary arena. The facilitator continues with statements about the purpose of the group, setting boundaries, and explaining how confidentiality will be maintained, especially with respect to staff disclosures to the VSW. In a round-robin fashion, the participants then are instructed to say their first name, their position in the hospital, what veterinary school they attended (for doctors only), if they have ever had experience or interaction with a social worker, and if the experience was positive or negative.

Next, the participants are asked to describe two of the stressors that they experience at work, again in a round-robin fashion. The facilitator has the opportunity as each participant speaks to probe a little deeper to gain information about the workplace, management, morale, etc. Many times, the participants become emotional during the discussion of stressors. When leading focus groups in a veterinary hospital, a facilitator should be prepared and experienced to effectively moderate and follow up with the emotionality. Participants may never have had the opportunity to say, particularly in a group setting, what the difficulties of their job are or to have group support when management has been a stressor. Indeed, the validation, agreement, support, and shared experiences may be therapeutic in and of themselves.

Next, an exhaustive list of sample job responsibilities for a VSW is given to each participant, and the participants are asked to review the list and state what they feel would apply or be valuable in their hospital, and also what and why they think some of the duties would be unnecessary. During this discussion, the facilitator has many opportunities to provide information about veterinary social work programs, what social workers are trained to do, how the program may look in the hospital, and the training of social workers for their own self-care. Moreover, gathering even more information about the workings of the hospital and what is important to the participants is helpful. Some participants may fear the VSW would usurp their relationship with other staff or with clients, and these concerns are aired and either ameliorated, noted, or validated. Finally, the facilitator asks participants to describe a person that they feel would fit with their hospital in terms of personality characteristics, background, experience, etc.

The importance of successful focus groups to the success of a VSW program cannot be understated. Participants, called stakeholders in literature, become educated about the possibilities of the program and how it could make their work lives better. They leave the groups feeling as though they have had a voice in not only the new program but also who might be their VSW. The participants "buy in" and promote enthusiasm among all other employees of the hospital.

Summarizing and Disseminating Now that all data have been gathered, the information can be summarized and disseminated. The focus group recordings should be transcribed. It is important to protect the confidentiality of participants. Although there may be one or two people in the hospital who know which individuals were in each group, the transcription should be written so that the identity of the person making each statement is unrecognizable. Utilizing all data collected from the tour, from earlier discussions, and from the focus groups, a summary with recommendations can now be written. The summary should detail strengths already present in the hospital such as wellness initiatives, receptiveness of human resources for wellness, environmental/workplace strengths which help in wellness, and attention to detail with regard to policies and work environment influences about euthanasia, quality of life counseling, and so forth.

The summary should also address barriers to wellness which were learned from the data gathering. These barriers may be due to environmental or financial constraints of the hospital as a facility, but more often information from the needs assessment has led to identification of management or organizational problems. Recommendations following the summary should address possible solutions to these issues and indicate how the addition of a VSW program may be one solution. Often, when transcriptions, summary, and recommendations are rendered, hospital owners or administrators learn for the first time what is seriously ailing their employees' morale. There may be some recommendations which can be implemented even before a VSW comes on board.

Lastly, the summary should include the creation of the job description for the VSW position. A large amount of data was collected in steps 2 and 3 that is relevant to the job description, including the previous experience and characteristics that would be required, tailored to the particular hospital.

Potential VSW Duties

The delineation of VSW duties should be refined and entered into the job description. Our previous section describing a day in the VSW program included many of the usual job responsibilities. However, there are many administrative tasks that may occupy the VSW's time which were not mentioned previously. Materials for bereavement and quality of life tools should always be ready for distribution. There should be a brochure about safety planning for pets in domestic violence situations. Information should be readily available for staff regarding the recognition and reporting of suspected animal abuse. We recommend a poster for each bathroom that provides information about how to recognize suicidal ideation, risk factors for suicide, and how best to respond. These posters should include hotline numbers and other referral sources. For financially compromised clients, we recommend the development of a trove of resources not only for funding but also for rescue groups that may be of help with finances. Although there may be many more responsibilities allotted to the VSW program, we will include the most common here (Tables 8.1 and 8.2).

On-Boarding the VSW

When beginning a program, as a very different profession from social work, hospitals enjoy guidance from an experienced VSW in screening applicants and in interviewing social workers for the position. The experienced VSW may screen applications for the position of VSW for qualifications, perform preliminary interviews remotely, and record the audio/visual of each interview for the hospital to view. The experienced VSW may interview and rate candidates based upon all of the data gathered during the needs assessment, using a numerical ranking of candidates to the hospital with a summary of the strengths and weaknesses of each candidate. The interview may also provide an opportunity to inform applicants who are new to veterinary social work about the program and about veterinary medicine, and the career and its associated challenges.Interview questions should be designed to target the applicant's potential ability to handle constant death and euthanasia, their knowledge of or interest in the challenges faced in particular by this profession, and

Table 8.1 Sample duties of veterinary social worker for clients

Grief Folders given to every client family in bereavement. Folders regularly updated and maintained by interns
Maintenance of resources for clients and staff (includes the following and more which is given to clients as per need):
Complete list of funding organizations for medical needs of pets
Exhaustive materials on dealing with the euthanasia decision and grief due to pet loss
Exhaustive list of articles and books on veterinary stress and compassion fatigue
Quality of Life folder which includes several tools and reading materials
List of At Home Euthanasia service and Palliative & Hospice Care Services in the area
Intervention with individuals/families sitting alone in exam room, waiting for long periods
Intervention with individuals/families by referral from any department
Help CSR (client service reps) place in rooms when CSR is very busy
Accompany individuals/families to ICU for visitation and/or facilitate Facetime visits
Facilitate communication leading to euthanasia and accompaniment during euthanasia when requested by clients
Documentation in hospital system and Smartsheet
VSW assessment of clients for hospital digital documents
Facilitate pet loss group 2x month
Assess animal abuse/child abuse/domestic violence and properly report (for animal abuse report in conjunction with veterinarian)
Follow up with clients:
Meet with clients when they arrive to get remains, assess grief, and inform of pet loss group
Follow up phone calls:
Clients who euthanized
Clients considering quality of life issues
Clients who, by social work assessment, need support
When requested by any department or attending

© Sandra Brackenridge, LCSW, BCD (2019)

how the applicant may deal with the ethical dilemmas and moral distress inherent in the veterinary specialty/emergency hospital.

The hospital will view the recordings and consider what is submitted; hospital personnel should be encouraged to interview top candidates in person; during these interviews, the candidates will visit with as many staff members and departments as possible. It is also strongly recommended that the candidates provide a presentation on a relevant topic to all staff and that all staff be surveyed as to their opinion of each candidate. This process helps to ensure "buy-in" by the majority of staff and gives the new VSW a head start in developing the trust of staff members.

After hiring a VSW, consultation with an experienced VSW may still be very helpful. To avoid reinventing the wheel, the new VSW can utilize relevant existing materials, allowing the program to commence more quickly. Additionally, to facilitate the program start-up, the new VSW should also:

- Be advised about the software and other communication equipment needed to begin the program

Table 8.2 Sample duties of veterinary social worker for staff

Debriefing
Crisis intervention
Suicide assessment and prevention
Provide support for staff:
Short-term supportive counseling and appropriate referrals for mental health care
On-the-spot interventions as per need
Trainings for staff (possible examples):
Grief and how to help yourself and clients
Communication skills
Wellness/self-care
Stress management
Redefining success and failure: shedding inner dialogues
Animal abuse recognition and tools
Recognizing co-workers in need
Tools for suicide prevention
Training on the serious illness conversation guide
Stressbuster activities frequently throughout the year
Collaborate with administration and team leads on staff distress and help to analyze organizational contribution to distress with recommendations (note: social workers are uniquely trained in "macro" social work which is about community and organization)
Speak and publicize program at veterinary meetings, local and national
Meet with candidates for positions at hospital to explain the services offered to them through this program as recruitment tool
Meet with new hires to explain services
Measure compassion fatigue, burnout at least once per year

© Sandra Brackenridge, LCSW, BCD (2019)

- Be provided with the transcripts of the focus groups
- Work with an experienced VSW to develop a protocol about how to work with a VSW and disseminate the protocol to staff members

The new VSW is encouraged to stagger their hours during the first 3–4 months so that his or her hours can overlap with those of the majority of staff, some of whom work during the day, while others may work during evenings or on week-ends. The VSW should try to meet and speak with as many staff as possible in the beginning.

In addition, the new VSW will want to provide as much education as possible about the human-animal bond, pet loss, euthanasia, quality of life conversations, the education and training journey of veterinarians and veterinary specialties, and other topics unique to this population. When a new VSW has experience in the human medical field or in mental health, or if they have completed the VSW Certificate at the University of Tennessee or comparable program, they are already very knowl-edgeable about many questions about the new program's services. The experienced

VSW can help the new VSW to arrange their office space and, if needed, the euthanasia space as well.

Training to create and implement documentation may also be offered. During the first 2 months, the provision of support, education, and consultation for the new VSW is essential. Much of the time can be spent discussing client cases and staff interventions, and exploring successful methods of dealing with each. In addition, much of the discussions may also revolve around organizational difficulties related to organizational hierarchy, and if and what a VSW may do to ameliorate those types of difficulties. As an example, there may be a doctor or owner who is suffering from burnout who displaces negative emotion onto staff. Or, perhaps the human resources department is unresponsive when multiple staff members report harassment by a manager. During the COVID-19 pandemic, clients' verbal abuse of veterinary staff became a regular occurrence, so discussions about if and when a VSW could help were frequent at that time.

Boundary Issues, Dual Relationships, and Developing Rapport

As noted earlier, veterinary social workers working within in-hospital settings play a unique role. One distinctive aspect of veterinary social work is the dual relationship that arises within the hospital setting as VSWs provide services to both the veterinary staff and the client/pet caregivers. A dual relationship is a nontraditional role for social workers, and at times it can be complicated to navigate (National Association of Social Workers, 2008; Reamer, 2003).

Ethical navigation of a dual relationship requires boundaries and a conscientious thought process. It is important when beginning a relationship with staff in an in-hospital setting for the VSW to explain his or her role. For a strong foundation, it is critical to educate hospital staff including owners, administration, managers, veterinarians, and technical and support staff so that they can understand the role of the VSW. In many hospitals, the VSW consultant introduces the role, but ultimately it will be the hired social worker that is responsible for assisting staff to understand the day-to-day routine of a social worker.

Once a VSW begins at the hospital, they will immediately start building relationships with each staff member to develop trust and rapport. The rapport-building phase is important to develop trust so that each staff member feels comfortable approaching the VSW with a variety of concerns, in addition to referring other staff members and pet owners. During the rapport-building phase, the VSW must identify their title and license. Sometimes the social worker may find it beneficial to explain the education and licensing process within their state to help staff members understand their expertise, experience, and educational background. Author Pepe found that during the early stages of adjusting to the in-hospital setting, she observed staff members referring to her as having various titles, such as psychologist or grief counselor. She used handouts to provide education to staff members to delineate titles of other professional mental health roles to avoid further confusion.

As the rapport-building phase continues, staff members may develop questions or concerns. It is important for the VSW to provide a transparent way of communicating and posting his or her schedule. Pepe found that posting her schedule for each month on her door using a whiteboard was effective. The VSW and interns may also find it helpful to use their hospital's communication method and/or create a standard operating procedure (SOP) to add to the hospital policies for best methods of communication. From our experience, the best methods of communication include in-person discussion as part of an open-door policy, pre-arranging mutually convenient meeting times via email, and using a locked mailbox solely for paper referrals/notes that the VSW and interns can access. It should be noted that not all electronic platforms and associated email addresses comply with the confidentiality and privacy requirements of the Health Insurance Portability and Accountability Act of 1996 (HIPAA) and, accordingly, detail should be limited in the emails. Furthermore, it is best policy to explain the various methods of communication, including the best style for certain questions or topics.

As the VSW is developing relationships with staff, the team will become more comfortable approaching him or her. The social worker provides support for work-related matters such as burnout or compassion fatigue, processing difficult cases, and managing conflicts among staff members. As rapport builds, his or her involvement with staff may deepen. The VSW can also develop trust by frequently being present in the treatment area and intensive care unit (ICU) to demonstrate involvement with the team. The VSW may find it helpful to provide psychoeducational materials through handouts, presentations, and posters which will be discussed in another section.

As the relationship progresses with staff members, individuals will begin to feel comfortable approaching the VSW and interns for personal support. It is the VSW's responsibility to explain confidentiality and the role of the veterinary social worker. Because the veterinary social worker is not working in the capacity of a therapist or counselor, he or she must advise staff members that they can come to the social worker with their concerns and be heard, but that the VSW can only provide them with resources and assist in the process of connecting them with long-term providers. As a key point, in-hospital VSWs should not meet with a staff member on an ongoing long-term basis. Once the VSW notices a pattern or ascertains that the staff member's concern is long term and/or severe in nature, the VSW should begin a discussion about seeking support within their community. From experience, hospitals with local Employee Assistance Programs (EAP) can directly refer a staff member to a therapist/counselor for three to four visits at no cost. Once a staff member uses their visits through the EAP, the EAP counselor will assist them in linking with a more long-term counselor/therapist. The EAP counselor will be familiar with their situation and may help them find services that are suitable for their needs, insurance plan, and location.

Some situations may arise in which the VSW needs to make a judgment call to further support their staff members by assisting them into treatment. This should be reserved for situations where safety concerns exist. An example would be when a social worker may need to leave the office with a staff member to assist in their evaluation or admission for psychiatric care if they are experiencing suicidal ideation or require admission to recovery and/or inpatient services for a substance use disorder. The staff member should be informed that hospital administration or management may need to be aware of some information so that time off of work for an extended period can be granted. It can be helpful for the VSW to develop a plan with the hospital owner(s) or administrator prior to a difficult situation arising so that there is a plan of action for the social worker to follow with the employee. In situations where there is a true emergency or psychiatric crisis, emergency personnel should be contacted through 911.

Working with Hospital Administration

Hospital administration, including the owner(s), administrator, and managers, may find it helpful for the VSW to be involved in difficult discussions or in addressing concerns among staff members. The VSW should ensure they have permission from the staff members when joining these discussions. Social workers can also be an asset to management/administration in helping them problem solve, identify supports for specific situations, and plan for difficult interactions. From our experience, hospital management may find it helpful if the VSW develops a resource binder available to staff that provides a listing of community resources, including crisis support, domestic violence support, and other hotlines that staff may need when the social worker is not available.

Working Alongside the Team

The dual relationship is again noted as the VSW will also be working alongside the veterinary staff to provide support. The VSW or interns may attend daily doctors' rounds as discussed earlier in the chapter. The VSW may also provide debriefings with the staff among all departments to offer support in battling compassion fatigue due to difficult cases, challenging clients, or employee conflicts.

As the relationship within the hospital and among staff is established, the VSW receives referrals for client support and counseling. It is the social worker's duty to provide clarification and communicate the best practice to receive referrals. Social workers who previously worked in more traditional settings may find that this process can take time to develop. It is important for the VSW to remember it will take time for staff to become comfortable and familiar with the services and understand the role of the VSW. Once staff understand the social work role and trust the VSW, they will become more comfortable in explaining information and referring clients. At this time, the social worker will notice a natural escalation of referrals as staff members see the positive outcomes in client support.

VSWs working within in-hospital settings must remember the dual relationship, including boundaries with their co-workers. Boundaries must include events outside of work activities and friendships. Due to the dual relationship, it is imperative to be aware of interactions with staff members that could be potentially harmful to them, such as implying friendship or spending time with an employee outside of the workplace. Social workers in in-hospital situations should use care in their decision-making process about off-site events for employees, such as happy hours, in-home gatherings, and social media.

Interns and Staff Support

As a requirement for licensure, social work interns must be supervised by a licensed social worker who holds the level of licensure required by the particular state to provide supervision. The number of supervision hours required of a social work intern prior to licensure varies across states. The VSW will provide supervision to the social work interns, utilizing the NASW Code of Ethics. Supervision provides students with an opportunity to learn, grow, and reflect on their experience and skill set. VSW should use supervision and the NASW Code of Ethics (National Association of Social Workers, 2008) when discussing dual relationships with their students. To ensure thorough communication, it is best practice for social work interns to use supervision and/or a daily communication log to inform the VSW lead of any interactions with management or staff members. The VSW intern should also follow the same procedures for referrals that are in place for the supervising social worker or social work team at the hospital.

Confidentiality Concerns

While the nature of an in-hospital VSW position is unique, the social worker is still held to high standards relating to confidentiality and compliance with the HIPAA statute and associated regulations. As previously discussed in this chapter, managing a dual relationship can be challenging. The VSW and interns must ensure that the methods of communication used with staff and clients protect protected health information (PHI). The referral system should also protect the information as well. In addition to the social worker explaining their role, he or she is also responsible for developing a referral process to provide a transparent method of communication that meets the criteria for safeguarding personal health information. For example, staff members may use a message system within the veterinary medical record which is documented in the patient chart that may not protect the client's information. The VSW may decide to work with hospital administration and possibly the technology department to develop ways of safeguarding information.

During the development of an in-hospital veterinary social work program, the VSW will choose a documentation system used to record complaints while protecting PHI. The VSW will work with their hospital administration and technology team to educate about these concerns and choose software/cloud-based system that meets requirements. The VSW will also need to consider a way to collect data while safeguarding client information.

Over time, in-hospital VSWs gain the trust of staff. Transparency about confidentiality is essential to building trust. Staff members are more likely to visit the social work office once they are aware of confidentiality and feel that the social work office is a safe place. The social worker will explain that the discussion will be safeguarded by the social work team unless it is learned that:

- There is risk to the individual or others, whether human or animal
- They know of someone that is at risk of hurting themselves or someone else
- There is a need to report abuse, neglect, or maltreatment of a child or other, i.e. an elder or an animal
- They know of a situation that is jeopardizing patient care in the hospital and/or of an animal in an abusive, or unsafe, environment

Furthermore, staff should be informed that the social worker will not share personal discussions with hospital administration, management, or other staff members unless patient care is jeopardized or meets one or more of the criteria indicated above. In situations in which the staff member or the VSW determines a need for advocacy, or that management or human resources involvement is warranted, a discussion should happen first with the staff member to maintain transparency and obtain their permission if at all possible.

The system for documentation of staff interaction or staff intervention should be kept privately from other documentation. It is best practice to have a discussion with hospital owners or administration to develop a plan and help them understand that the notes will remain confidential. Notes should not be kept on the hospital computer as the hospital owns that property. Some VSWs may choose to keep a written log and safeguard it in a private, locked place to which others outside of the social work team do not have access. It is necessary to be aware of laws based on your state that may allow records including notes to be subpoenaed.

Identifying Mental Health Supports

As discussed earlier in the chapter, the veterinary medicine profession struggles with mental health concerns such as depression, anxiety, and even suicidal ideation. Accordingly, the implementation of mental health supports within the hospital setting should be considered a priority. (For further discussion about the need for mental health supports and the challenges faced by the veterinary profession, see the chapter by Volk in this volume.) It is the authors' opinion that in larger hospitals, having an on-site social worker that has established rapport and relationships with the employees is by far the gold standard.

The VSW should have an open-door policy and provide consultation with employees for a wide variety of reasons to promote emotional wellness. All team members, from doctors, technicians, client care staff, and administration, can seek out support for case-related debriefings, processing of difficult client encounters or even family issues, conflict resolution with peers, communication issues with supervisors, and community resources (food pantry, intimate partner violence, housing, parenting, medical bills, support groups, and so forth). Just as often, employees may be looking for a confidential place, with someone they know and trust, to disclose symptoms of anxiety and depression. The authors hold space for team members to express their feelings and can conduct screeners (Shin et al., 2019; Spitzer et al., 2006; Wu et al., 2020) as an informative tool to help them gain insight on the severity of their depression/anxiety symptoms. Descriptive handouts on different diagnoses and forms of therapeutic treatment approaches are also used for discussion and education. The VSW should always have been trained and comfortable in assessing for suicidal ideation and putting an action plan in place for connecting employees with the help that they need, including referrals for counseling or more intensive treatment. Hacker has reached out to several mental health practitioners in the local community to provide specific education surrounding the issues that veterinary staff may face. Employees have preferred to use these connections as the therapists already have a base knowledge of life in veterinary medicine easing the anxiety of initially meeting with a counselor. The VSW assists in finding providers that take the employees' insurance, are accepting new patients, and have experience with their specific needs.

In addition to one-on-one employee mental health support, the authors find in-house group workshops highly beneficial for their hospital teams. By either bringing in outside speakers or presenting themselves, topics have ranged from grief education, de-escalation skills, working with challenging clients, suicide prevention, compassion fatigue, cognitive distortions, coping techniques, psychologically safe environments for communication, work/life integration and wellness, setting boundaries, and open forums for ethical consultations. The authors find these educational sessions to be much more engaging in-person than when they are provided through an online forum, and they allow lengthy question and answer times and ongoing rapport-building among team members.

Furthermore, it is helpful to integrate into the hospital's residency/intern program monthly psychosocial rounds that cover some of the abovementioned topics. Additional topics may include "imposter syndrome," which young doctors often face, the development of resiliency during strenuous training, and the practice of coping techniques, such as meditation, yoga, distraction, art therapy, thought challenging, and others. Psychosocial rounds can also include case discussions/debriefings where everyone presents a case but provides no medical details; rather, the focus is on difficulties related to communication or emotional aspects of the case. The VSW may offer expertise as appropriate; however, it has been observed that the team rallying around one another and providing compliments, support, and suggestions to each other is what ultimately boosts the training doctors' morale and camaraderie with one another.

Summary and Statistics

The authors emphasize and underscore the strong evidence indicating that on-site social workers who engage with clients reduce the stress levels for staff and increase overall well-being by taking over difficult or time-consuming conversations with clients. Moreover, in-hospital social workers free up time for the veterinarians and technical teams to focus on the medicine and treatment needed for the patients. By providing hospital clients with general support and assistance, education, updates about their pet, and resources, and dedicating their time to helping clients process diagnoses and make decisions, a VSW program alleviates the daily strain and emotional toll for the entire veterinary team. Additionally, the team also is relieved of lingering worry about a client's distress in that the VSW and interns continue to offer support and pet loss counseling to clients as per need after the death of a pet.

Regular, consistent, and frequent client interaction with the VSW and VSW interns results in much greater client satisfaction which can easily be measured in reviews on social media for each hospital who employed the authors. During the COIVD-19 pandemic of 2020, VSWs were also able to intervene with clients who were prevented due to safety protocols from accompanying their pets into the hospitals. The authors observed that, for many clients, this situation greatly increased client anxiety and concern for their pet, and many clients projected or displaced their distress onto staff members. The training that all social workers receive in de-escalation was inordinately helpful in these situations.

Over time, on-site work by the authors with clients and employees has resulted in great growth and usage of social work within the hospitals. In terms of client interventions performed in each hospital, the number of VSW interns working in the hospital seems to greatly influence the number of clients receiving social work support. Tabulations by authors Brackenridge and Hacker reveal that any VSW or VSW intern will offer an average of 109–230 services to clients during the duration of their work at the hospital. For example, five VSW interns and a lead VSW will then provide a minimum of 545 services to clients of the hospital in any given year. Because VSW interns may spend as little as one semester completing their hours at the hospital, it is common to count ten or more interns per year.

Hacker has been able to enhance the social work program each year by maintaining statistics that demonstrate the frequent utilization of VSW services. In the first year of her program, 26 percent of employees met with a social worker for personal reasons, and, in the second year, with further connection building, 61 percent of employees reached out for assistance from social work personnel for individual needs. During the pandemic, this number grew to 73 percent of employees having at least one consultation with a social worker for confidential discussions that required emotional support and/or resources or referrals. Brackenridge also reports that average employee consultation with the VSW or interns ranged from 20 percent to 30 percent over a number of years, and this percentage increased also when the COVID-19 pandemic began in 2020. The authors argue that these growing numbers are attributable to their on-site presence and being present with the employees to build rapport and sincere relationships. This rapport and these relationships cannot be developed to the same extent by remote social workers or employee assistance programs.

References

Cima, G. (2020). Emergency, specialty practices hiring to counsel staff members, clients. *JAVMA*, 1–7.

Cohen, S. P. (1985). The role of social work in a veterinary hospital setting. *The Veterinary Clinics of North America. Small Animal Practice, 15*(2), 355–363. https://doi.org/10.1016/s0195-5616(85)50307-1

Crocken, B. (1981). Veterinary medicine and social work: A new avenue of access to mental health care. *Social Work in Health Care, 6*(3), 91–94. https://doi.org/10.1300/J010v06n03_09

Goldberg, K. J. (2019). Goals of care: Development and use of the serious veterinary illness conversation guide. *Veterinary Clinics of North America: Small Animal Practice, 49*(3), 399–415.

Hart, L. A., Hart, B. L., & Mader, B. (1990). Humane euthanasia and companion animal death: Caring for the animal, the client, and the veterinarian. *Journal of the American Veterinary Medical Association, 197*(10), 1292–1299.

Holcombe, T. M. Strand, E. B., Nugent, W. R., & Ng, Z. Y. (2016). Veterinary soocial work: Practice within veterinary settings. *Journal of Human Behavior in the Social Environment, 26*(1), 69–80.

Lagoni, L. (2011). Family-present euthanasia: Protocols for planning and preparing clients for the death of a pet. In C. Blazina (Ed.), *The psychology of the human-animal bond* (pp. 181–202). Springer Science+Business Media, LLC. https://doi.org/10.1007/978-1-4419-9761-6

Lagoni, L., Butler, C., & Hetts, S. (1994). *The human-animal bond and grief*. W.B. Saunders Co.

Larkin, M. (2016). For human needs, some veterinary clinics are turning to a professional. *Journal of the American Veterinary Medical Association News, 248*(1), 8–12.

Leary, S., & Johnson, C. (2020). AVMA GUIDELINES FOR THE EUTHANASIA OF ANIMALS: 2020 EDITION AVMA Guidelines for the Euthanasia of Animals: 2020 Edition* Members of the Panel on Euthanasia AVMA Staff Consultants.

Leary, S., Underwood, W., Anthony, R., Cartner, S., Corey, D., Grandin, T., Greenacre, C., … & Yanong, R. (2013). *AVMA guidelines for the euthanasia of animals: 2013 edition.* Schaumburg, IL: American Veterinary Association.

Morgan, D. L. (1997). *Focus groups as qualitative research.* Sage. https://doi.org/10.4135/9781412984287

Morgan, D., & Lobe, B. (2011). Online focus groups. In S. N. Hesse-Biber (Ed.), *Handbook of emergent technologies in social research* (pp. 199–230). New York: Oxford University Press.

Morris, P. (2009). *Encounters with "death work" in veterinary medicine: An ethnographic exploration of the medical practice of euthanasia.* Unpublished dissertation, Northeastern University, Boston, MA. http://hdl.handle.net/2047/d20000068

Morris, P. (2012). *Blue juice: Euthanasia in veterinary medicine.* Temple University Press.

National Association of Social Workers. (2008). *Code of ethics*. National Association of Social Workers. Available at https://www.socialworkers.org/About/Ethics/Code-of-Ethics/Code-of-Ethics-English. Accessed 19 February 2021.

Reamer, F. G. (2003). Boundary issues in social work: Managing dual relationships. *Social Work, 48*(1), 121–133.

Sharma, A., Lanum, M., & Suarez-Balcazar, Y. (2000). *A community needs assessment guide: A brief guide on how to conduct a needs assessment.* Available at https://t7-live-yfar2.nyc3.cdn.digitaloceanspaces.com/cyfar.org/files//Sharma%202000.pdf. Accessed 19 February 2021.

Scriven, M., & Roth, J. (1978). Needs assessment: Concept and practice. *New Directions for Program Evaluation, 1978*, 1–11.

Shin, C., Lee, S. H., Han, K. M., Yoon, H. K., & Han, C. (2019). Comparison of the usefulness of the PHQ-8 and PHQ-9 for screening for major depressive disorder: Analysis of psychiatric outpatient data. *Psychiatry Investigation, 16*(4), 300–305. https://doi.org/10.30773/pi.2019.02.01

Skipper, G. E., & Williams, J. B. (2012). Failure to acknowledge high suicide risk among veterinarians. *Journal of Veterinary Medical Education, 39*(1), 79–82.

Sleezer, C. M., Russ-Eft, D. F., & Gupta, K. (Eds.). (2014). *A practical guide to needs assessment.* Wiley. https://doi.org/10.1002/9781118826164

Spitzer, R. L., Kroenke, K., Williams, J. B. W., & Löwe, B. (2006). A brief measure for assessing generalized anxiety disorder: The GAD-7. *Archives of Internal Medicine, 166*(10), 1092. https://doi.org/10.1001/archinte.166.10.1092

Spitznagel, M. B., Jacobson, D. M., Cox, M. D., & Carlson, M. D. (2018). Predicting caregiver burden in general veterinary clients: Contribution of companion animal clinical signs and problem behaviors. *Veterinary Journal, 236*, 23–30. https://doi.org/10.1016/j.tvjl.2018.04.007

Spitznagel, M. B., Ben-Porath, Y. S., Rishniw, M., Kogan, L. R., & Carlson, M. D. (2019). Development and validation of a burden transfer inventory for predicting veterinarian stress related to client behavior. *Journal of the American Veterinary Medical Association, 254*(1), 133–144. https://doi.org/10.2460/javma.254.1.133

Spitznagel, M. B., Jacobson, D. M., Cox, M. D., & Carlson, M. D. (2017). Caregiver burden in owners of a sick companion animal: A cross-sectional observational study. *Veterinary Record, 181*(12), 321–321. https://doi.org/10.1136/vr.104295

Spitznagel, M. B., Marchitelli, B., Gardner, M., & Carlson, M. D. (2020). Euthanasia from the veterinary client's perspective: Psychosocial contributors to euthanasia decision making. *Veterinary Clinics of North America: Small Animal Practice, 50*(3), 591–605. https://doi.org/10.1016/j.cvsm.2019.12.008

Tomasi, S. E., Fechter-Leggett, E. D., Edwards, N. T., Reddish, A. D., Crosby, A. E., & Nett, R. J. (2019). Suicide among veterinarians in the United States from 1979 through 2015. *Journal of the American Veterinary Medical Association, 254*(1), 104–112.

Toseland, R. W., & Rivas, R. F. (1995). *An introduction to group work practice* (2nd ed.). Allyn & Bacon.

Volk, J. O., Schimmack, U., Strand, E. B., Lord, L. K., & Siren, C. W. (2018). Executive summary of the Merck animal health veterinary wellbeing study. *Journal of the American Veterinary Medical Association, 252*(10), 1231–1238.

Volk, J. O., Schimmack, U., Strand, E., Vasconcelos, J., & Siren, C. W. (2020). Executive summary of the Merck animal health veterinarian wellbeing study II. *Journal of the American Veterinary Medical Association, 256*(11), 1237–1244.

Wu, Y., Levis, B., Riehm, K. E., Saadat, N., Levis, A. W., Azar, M., Rice, D. B., & Thombs, B. D. (2020). Equivalency of the diagnostic accuracy of the PHQ-8 and PHQ-9: A systematic review and individual participant data meta-analysis. *Psychological Medicine, 50*(8), 1368–1380. https://doi.org/10.1017/S0033291719001314

Chapter 9
Conflict Management and Veterinary Social Work

Elizabeth B. Strand, Addie Reinhard, and Bethanie A. Poe

Introduction

Social workers wear many hats. They can be advocates, therapists, counselors, program developers, protectors, brokers, researchers, professors, lobbyists, and community organizers, to name a few. Veterinarians also wear many hats—they can be in private practice, government, the armed forces, academia, the biomedical sciences, pharmaceuticals, or public health agencies, to name a few. When social workers and veterinarians work side by side, this can be called "veterinary social work." A veterinary clinic is an obvious place where this occurs, but veterinarians and social workers can also cross professional paths in settings such as animal shelters, government, nonprofit associations, and even in conservation settings. Across all these work environments, one aspect of human functioning that will inevitably arise is conflict. Another unique hat that social workers wear is that of mediator, and this hat can be extremely valuable in veterinary social work settings.

Right now, in the United States, animals are considered property, but if you ask people who live with animals as companions, most will tell you that their animal is a family member. On a micro level, this mismatch between how many people experience animals living in their homes and how the law treats these animals can create circumstances that are ripe for human-to-human conflict, both within families and within organizations that care for animals. Moreover, on a macro level, there are

E. B. Strand (✉) · B. A. Poe
University of Tennessee, Knoxville Colleges of Veterinary Medicine and Social Work,
Knoxville, TN, USA
e-mail: estrand@utk.edu

A. Reinhard
MentorVet, Lexington, KY, USA

Lincoln Memorial University College of Veterinary Medicine, Harrogate, TN, USA

© The Author(s), under exclusive license to Springer Nature Switzerland AG 2022
S. Loue, P. Linden (eds.), *The Comprehensive Guide to Interdisciplinary
Veterinary Social Work*, https://doi.org/10.1007/978-3-031-10330-8_9

disagreements about how people think animals should be treated. People who self-identify as vegans or vegetarians, or in some other way connect with the interests of animal rights, are in real conflict with people who see animals as a source of livelihood and sustenance in the food system. In this chapter, we cover the types of conflicts that can arise in settings where veterinary professionals and social workers may work hand in hand as well as various conflict management techniques. Lastly, case scenarios are presented that can be used to apply the information presented in the chapter.

Common Ethical Conflicts Veterinarians Face

Some of the primary responsibilities of veterinarians in clinical practice are to diagnose and treat animal diseases. Commonly reported veterinary identity traits include placing a high emphasis on the diagnosis and treatment of animals and being technically competent (Armitage-Chan & May, 2018; Page-Jones & Abbey, 2015). Veterinarians take an oath to use their skills and knowledge to benefit society through "the protection of animal health and welfare, the prevention and relief of animal suffering, the conservation of animal resources, the promotion of public health, and the advancement of medical knowledge" (American Veterinary Medical Association, 2021). Veterinarians often strive to provide gold-standard care for their patients, but they must also practice medicine to satisfy the desires and needs of the pet owners as well as the welfare of the animal. It is this unique triad of care—the relationship between the veterinarian, client, and animal—that can sometimes result in ethical conflict in veterinary practice.

These ethical conflicts can occur in many veterinary contexts. For instance, some public health or large animal veterinary professionals must assist with the depopulation of many animals, and conflicts may often arise between the best interests of the animal and protecting human and animal health (American Veterinary Medical Association, 2019). In private practice settings, the veterinarian may feel as if he or she must advocate for the best care for the animal but may not be able to provide gold-standard care if the owner does not have adequate resources or the desire to pursue this level of care. Alternatively, the veterinarian may advocate for the humane euthanasia of an animal that they feel has a grave prognosis and is suffering, yet the owner may have the desire and resources to continue care despite the grave prognosis.

The veterinarian's role of providing care for patients while meeting the needs and desires of the client may conflict, and this can result in a moral dilemma, which has been defined as "a conflict between responsibilities or obligations of exactly equal moral weight . . . with no obvious way to prioritize one responsibility over the other" (Morgan & McDonald, 2007). In these scenarios, some veterinarians may choose to prioritize the needs and desires of the human client, while others may prioritize what is in the best interests of the animal patient. Around half of veterinarians reported prioritizing the needs of the patient when a conflict arose between the needs and interests of the client and the patient (Kipperman et al., 2018).

Ethical conflicts occur frequently within veterinary practice. Approximately one-half of veterinarians reported experiencing ethical dilemmas at least weekly, and around one in five veterinarians experienced ethical dilemmas at least once per day (Kipperman et al., 2018). Similarly, in a small sample of veterinarians in the United Kingdom, approximately half of veterinarians reported facing ethical dilemmas once or twice per week, and a third of the veterinarians reported facing ethical dilemmas three to five times per week (Batchelor & McKeegan, 2012). Moses et al. (2018) found that there were conflicts with pet owners about how to proceed with the medical care of a pet often or sometimes for 84 percent of veterinarians sampled, and half of the veterinarians were asked sometimes or often to do something in the course of clinical practice that felt like the wrong thing to do.

Perhaps the most frequently encountered ethical dilemma in veterinary practice is client financial limitations, which restrict the veterinarian's ability to provide care to patients (Batchelor & McKeegan, 2012; Kipperman et al., 2018). Other commonly encountered ethical dilemmas include requests to euthanize a healthy animal, clients wanting to continue treating a pet with poor quality of life, clients requesting harmful or unnecessary procedures, and clients unable or unwilling to provide resources to treat patients (Batchelor & McKeegan, 2012; Kipperman et al., 2018; Morgan & McDonald, 2007). These ethical dilemmas may arise for a variety of reasons, including differing views regarding the role or moral value of the animal or legal considerations (Morgan & McDonald, 2007). Table 9.1 provides a summary of common ethical conflicts faced in veterinary medicine and the reasons these ethical conflicts may arise.

Often, ethical conflict can contribute to the stress, burnout, and moral distress experienced by veterinarians. *Moral distress* has been defined as "one or more negative self-directed emotions or attitudes that arise in response to one's perceived involvement in a situation that one perceives to be morally undesirable" (Campbell et al., 2016). *Moral distress in the workplace* has been further defined as "the experience of psychological distress that results from engaging in, or failing to prevent, decisions, or behaviors that transgress, or come to transgress, personally held moral or ethical beliefs" (Crane et al., 2013). When faced with financial limitations to pet

Table 9.1 Ethical conflict in veterinary medicine

Common ethical dilemmas faced By veterinarians	Reasons ethical dilemmas may arise
Clients requesting harmful or unnecessary procedures (e.g., tail docking, ear cropping, etc.)	Differing views regarding the role of the animal
Clients unable to afford veterinary care	Cultural differences
Clients unwilling to treat patient	Differing views regarding the moral value of the animal
Requests for euthanasia of a healthy animal	
Clients wishing to continue treating a pet with a poor prognosis or poor quality of life	Legal considerations (e.g., animals as property)
Veterinarian working with another veterinarian they believe is providing substandard care	Contextual limitations (e.g., limited client finances
Animal abuse	

care, over half of veterinarians experienced moderate to very high stress, and many veterinarians reported that client financial limitations were a moderate or primary contributor to their level of burnout (Kipperman et al., 2018; Kipperman et al., 2017). Approximately three out of four veterinarians reported that they had moderate to severe distress when they were unable to do what they felt was right for the patient (Moses et al., 2018).

Conflicts Within Teams

Conflict within medical teams has been explored in both human and veterinary medicine. Findings suggest that conflictual interpersonal interactions can negatively impact patient care (Riskin et al., 2017) as well as be contagious throughout organizations (Foulk et al., 2016). A qualitative analysis of written responses from a survey of a large sample of practicing US veterinarians generated a comprehensive list of veterinary practice stressors (Vande Griek et al., 2018). Many of the common stressors faced by the veterinarians identified in this study included interpersonal conflict within the veterinary team, including a lack of support from coworkers and management, and bullying or abuse from coworkers or management. In a study exploring rudeness, researchers found that one person's rudeness in an organization has a contagion effect. When person one was rude, person two—the recipient of that rudeness—was likely to be rude to person three (Foulk et al., 2016), and this contagion occurred by priming individuals to notice rudeness more after witnessing it.

These types of interactions influence the bottom line of patient care. For instance, in a randomized controlled trial exploring rudeness among colleagues in neonatal intensive care unit simulations, Riskin et al. (2015) found that rude behavior among colleagues had a negative impact on both asking for help within the team and sharing important medical information. Team conflict can also be associated with a hierarchy within the team, with those lower on the totem pole experiencing more rude behavior (Bradley et al., 2015).

Power dynamics can also affect how conflict is addressed. Less help-seeking behavior was seen between individuals from varying levels of hierarchy, and employees with less power may feel more uneasy about bringing up thoughts and concerns if the work environment is deemed unsafe or does not foster a high level of intragroup trust (Janss et al., 2012). In veterinary teams, this can manifest in younger veterinarians or support staff being apprehensive about voicing concerns to practice managers and experienced veterinarians. This has the potential to harm patient care. For example, if a veterinary technician makes a mistake, they may be reluctant to tell anyone because of worry that their superiors will yell at them. The patient may suffer because of the delay or absence of the veterinarian mitigating the mistake. These negative outcomes can also affect the mental health of the veterinary team. Bradley et al. (2015) found that 40 percent of individuals who reported experiencing rude, dismissive, or aggressive behavior in the medical environment stated that it negatively impacted their well-being throughout their entire day. These negative outcomes are hypothesized to relate to what rude, dismissive, or aggressive behavior does to the brain. Essentially, when people experience it, the working memory is engaged in trying to understand why the behavior happened or regulate the emotions that arise because of the conflict instead of focusing on providing medical care. This is not volitional; it simply is how the brain processes the stress of interpersonal conflict. Moreover, when the working memory is engaged in trying to manage the effects of a rude interaction, it can rob professionals from remaining present in their more restorative activities, such as eating a pleasant lunch outside or spending time with family and friends after work.

Conflicts Between Clients and Veterinary or Other Animal-Related Professionals

Conflicts between clients and veterinary professionals commonly occur in veterinary practice and can affect patient care and the well-being of the veterinary team. Conflict can arise from client complaints or expectations of clients (Nett et al., 2015) as well as miscommunication, noncompliance, or differing views of how to treat the animal. Clients may even make formal complaints about veterinarians to the state licensing boards, which can also cause stress for the veterinarian involved. In the small animal veterinary workplace, the frequency of experiencing stressful client interactions and behaviors has been positively correlated with burnout and stress levels among veterinarians (Spitznagel et al., 2019). In large animal settings, there can be conflict between producers and veterinarians about the care of animals (Wojtacka, Grudzień, et al., 2020) as well as extreme conflict when there is a disease outbreak and veterinarians and others are forced to depopulate large numbers of animals (Broekema et al., 2017). In fact, 92 percent of veterinary food inspectors in a recent study in Poland reported experiencing conflict in the course of their daily work (Wojtacka, Wysok, & Szteyn, 2020).

Vicious online reviews, cyberbullying, and being bullied through electronic communication (e.g., social media, Google reviews, Yelp, etc.) were considered critical issues faced by the veterinary profession. About one in five veterinarians reported receiving a cruel review over a period of 1 year (Volk et al., 2020). Negative online reviews and cyberbullying have the potential to cause severe distress among veterinarians and their staff by harming the practice's reputation, hurting the business, and taking an emotional toll on the individuals involved.

Viciousness can sometimes even extend beyond painful reviews or cyberbullying to actual threats to safety. For instance, in the 2001 foot-and-mouth disease outbreak in the Netherlands, farmers not only took hostage veterinary inspectors with whom they disagreed with the need to cull their animals but also hung dead animals in trees with the names of inspectors as a threat to their safety (Broekema et al., 2017). These types of conflicts over food animal depopulation also occur in the United States. For instance, in Southern California, there has been an outbreak of a deadly virus called virulent Newcastle disease that affects birds. This virus is extremely contagious and, therefore, influences not only the poultry industry to produce food but can also affect backyard chickens. This virus has caused significant conflict in the community, and there have been threats of lawsuits against government officials, public outcry, and blaming some chicken owners for being "overly sentimental" because of their chickens being culled (Cosgrove, 2019). These types of macro conflicts also occur around differences of opinions about animal welfare. There are animal rights organizations that stage protests against animal production facilities to influence food production practices (Animal Rights Extremists: Trespassing to Rescue Chickens, 2019). Many food animal producers feel deeply misunderstood by the public and animal rights organizations (Ekakoro et al., 2019).

Conflicts Within Client Systems

Veterinarians must also manage conflicts within client systems. These client systems can exist within a family or a company for whom the veterinarian is providing medical care. Within family systems, issues such as treatment and end-of-life decision-making for animals can cause conflict. There may be spouses who have very differing views about how long an animal should live with a condition before the choice of euthanasia is made. There may be strong differences in the amount of money that should be spent on the treatment of a medical condition. Moreover, at times, when spouses have divorced, there may even be joint custody of the pet, causing the veterinary team to be in the middle of a family situation where the conflict stalls the medical team from making progress on patient care due to divorced family power struggles (Rook, 2014). Moreover, there are times when adult children are caring for the animals of aging parents, and there is a conflict between what the animal owner (the parent) wants and what the caregiver (the adult child) can handle. As veterinarians often receive little formal training in conflict management (Moses et al., 2018), they may be unaware of how to approach these situations.

In more macro settings, there can be conflicts between large systems that affect animals. For instance, in Nigeria, there are intense conflicts between nomadic tribes and agrarian settlements that result in emotionally painful and financially costly attacks on cattle for both sides (Ajibo et al., 2018). These conflicts ultimately affect patient health and become a concern for veterinarians' capacity to care for and protect it. There can also be conflicts within client organizational systems related to animal welfare that result in news articles that expose farming practices that animal rights organizations and perhaps the public disagree with (Eller, 2020; Greenwald, 2020).

Conflict Management as Stress Management

Conflict management as a stress management tool within work environments has gained more application-based and scholarly attention (Bingham, 2012; Jones, 2019; McKenzie, 2015; Tallodi, 2015). These efforts have focused on resolving morally ambiguous and distressing medical conflicts (Emran, 2015; Fawcett & Mullan, 2018; Olmstead & Dahnke, 2016) as well as conflicts that occur due to miscommunications, financial constraints, treatment decision-making, differences in values, issues of justice and power, and workload, to name only a few (Bingham, 2012; Jones, 2019). There is even growing attention to the power of conflict management specific to animals (Charles, 2012; Jones, 2019; Voda-Hamilton, 2015).

Two major ways of understanding the source of occupational stress are interactional and transactional in nature (Tallodi, 2015). *Interactional* refers to the structural effects in occupational settings that are associated with stress and conflict, such as role confusion, role status, the goodness of fit between an employee and their work environment, salary levels, and the presence or lack of skills that someone has or lacks to complete a job responsibility. An example of interactional stress can be found in Wallace and Buchanan's (2020) mixed-methods study exploring animal health-related professionals' experiences with the client and interpersonal strain based on work and gender status differences. They found that female veterinarians (considered higher in work role status) reported more client strain than male veterinarians or veterinary technicians. They also found that female gender status was associated with less perceived autonomy and authority in the work environment for veterinarians and veterinary technicians. Last, they found that there was less interpersonal strain, the more autonomy an animal health professional reported in their work.

Transactional refers to the ways in which individuals experience (cognitive appraisal) and manage (emotion-focused or cognitive-focused problem-solving) the stress of the job. Some conflict management strategies can be particularly helpful with this type of stress, as they allow people who conflict with each other to reappraise how they are experiencing the other person through talking and gaining a new perspective of the other person's viewpoint. For instance, one well-known example in the non-veterinary sector is the Resolve Employment Disputes, Reach Equitable Solutions Swiftly (REDRESS) program created by the United States Postal Service (McKenzie, 2015). This program was founded in 1994 to manage a culture of conflict and discrimination in the USPS. This was a free voluntary conflict management service that used outside mediators to develop healthier ways to manage conflict in the workplace. The program was so successful that it was expanded to include formal complaints with legal representation by both USPS attorneys, and non-USPS-representing disputants were included. Outside evaluators found that REDRESS was associated with disputants having an improved perspective of the "other person" in workplace disputes (Bingham, 2012).

In addition to the sources of occupational stress, there are seed sources of conflict. Dana (2001) identified five underlying emotional issues that drive conflict: (1) power, the need to influence others and for the social status deriving from power differences; (2) approval, the need for affection, to be liked by others; (3) inclusion, the need to be accepted as a member of social groups, such as teams at work; (4) justice, the need to be treated fairly, equally, and equitably; and (5) identity, the need for autonomy, self-esteem, and affirmation of personal values. Similarly, researchers identified conflict stemming from experiences of injustice and change (Tallodi, 2015; Watson et al., 2019; Wiedner et al., 2020).

Conflict Management Methods

There are many forms of conflict management that social workers may use to solve problems and help reduce stress. Barsky (2017) identified two main categories in which a social worker may engage. The first is emergent conflict management. This is when a social worker maintains her or his professional hat as counselor, advocate, community organizer, grant writer, executive director, etc. while helping a colleague or client resolve conflicts using basic conflict management skills like active listening, empathy, and problem-solving. The second is contractual conflict management. This is when the social worker wears the formal hat as "mediator" and establishes an agreement to mediate among parties in dispute. There are times when emergent mediation is an acceptable path forward to a conflict presented in animal settings and situations, and there are times when it is more appropriate to engage in a formal agreement to mediate. There will be more discussion of this in the ethics of animal-related conflict management section.

There are several styles of mediation, such as evaluative, facilitative, and transformative. Some argue that these three styles exist on a continuum from most to least "interventionist," and there is a time and place for each. There are also conflict management processes, such as the use of "circles," used by indigenous cultures for centuries (Ito, 1985; Kamana, 2010; Mehl-Madrona & Mainguy, 2014) or models of workplace conflict management methods with and without a peer or boss serving as mediator (Dana, 2006).

Evaluative Mediation

Evaluative mediation is a style in which the mediator offers an expert opinion about the merit and likely legal outcomes of a conflict. From that evaluative position, the mediator works to develop a management approach that considers the likely outcome of a case in court. These mediators often use shuttle diplomacy, where the disputants are never in the same room and never listen to or share their concerns directly with each other. Shuttle mediation occurs when the mediator meets one-on-one (not together) with both parties, listens, evaluates the concerns, and helps generate proposals for coming to a management. The mediator serves as a shuttle going between each of the parties, who do not meet face-to-face. The mediator shares possible solutions between the client and the clinic and ultimately, if successful, generates an agreed-upon management that keeps the dispute out of court. An example of this style can be found in Veterinary Client Mediation Services (VCMS) https://www.vetmediation.co.uk/ in the United Kingdom. Through this program, clients of veterinary clinics can access mediation services to resolve complaints about the care of their pets. The VMS mediator uses shuttle mediation to attain an agreement and management between the client and the clinic.

Facilitative Mediation

The facilitative mediation style is when the mediator creates a structured process for the disputants to follow, and the mediator shepherds the process. The mediator listens to and validates points of view and emotions for the disputants, who are in each other's presence during the process. In this style, the mediator seeks to elucidate the underlying interests of both parties and to create an agreed-upon management that meets the interests of both parties. Disputants are given time to tell their "story" in front of the other party, and then they brainstorm as many ideas as possible that could be included in an agreement. The list includes ideas that fall on a continuum of completely acceptable to completely unacceptable for both parties. The brainstorming allows both disputants to see each party's underlying interests. Next, the mediator helps facilitate discussion about all the ideas, seeing which ones hold interest for both parties. The agreement was created through this final process. In these types of mediations, the mediator may intermittently facilitate a "caucus" whereby the mediator meets privately with both parties individually. The mediator does this if it is clear there is an impasse, emotions are running too high, or parties need to consider options privately, consulting others who may not actually be in the mediation but have an interest in the outcome. Ultimately, however, the goal of this style of mediation is for the solution to be jointly and synchronously generated by and owned by the parties in dispute, instead of decided by the legal system. In the 1960s and 1970s, this was the most prominent style used in community mediation centers (Zumeta, 2000).

Transformative Mediation

Transformative mediation is the least directive of all styles of mediation. Here, the mediator does not structure the process or offer solutions but rather leaves it for the disputants. In transformative mediation, the mediator is solely about empowering the disputants to explore their own solutions, and the intention is that, by doing so, each disputant will transform themselves and their views of the disputant through the process. This is the form of mediation that was ultimately embraced by the United States Postal Services mediation program REDRESS because the goal of that program was to help employees work better together and reduce discrimination in the work environment. It worked. The implementation of REDRESS was associated with a substantial drop (more than 25%) in formal EEO complaints. An evaluative style does not require disputants to work together, and a facilitative style requires third parties to manage conflict. The goal of REDRESS was to improve employee relations and empower employees with the ability to manage conflict; therefore, the transformative mediation style was eventually embraced as the main style for the program. Transformative mediation styles transform the cognitive appraisal of the other party as well as increase emotion-focused and cognitive-focused coping strategies (McKenzie, 2015; Tallodi, 2015).

Talking Circles

The circle process—also called *talking circles* or *circle councils*—has been used by the world's indigenous cultures for centuries. These have more recently been integrated into the justice system (Pranis et al., 2003), schools (Brinson & Fisher, 1999; Lyons et al., 2019), and healthcare (Mehl-Madrona & Mainguy, 2014) by sharing indigenous cultural practices with non-indigenous communities. The social justice system has integrated talking circles, or peacemaking circles, as a form of restorative justice. The goals of the peacemaking circle in social justice are to move (1) from coercion to healing, (2) from solely individual to individual *and* collective accountability, (3) from primary dependence on the state to greater community self-reliance, and (4) from justice as "getting even" to justice as "getting well" (Pranis et al., 2003). These shifts are thought to be possible because of the underlying principles of all indigenous circles, which see the world as holistic, connected, and one in which there is a natural impulse toward harmony and balance, just as nature seeks its own balance and harmony. The American Indian Medicine Wheel, which recognizes the physical, the mental, the emotional, and the spiritual as necessary for harmony and balance, is a core underpinning of why circles are effective. When in a circle, all four parts of each member are recognized within the group and are known as something that all group members share. It is what connects everyone.

The Hawaiian practice of *ho'oponopono* is a circle process that has been integrated into schools and workplaces and is designed to "make things right," the definition of "ho'oponopono." In this process, an elder, or *kahuna*, facilitates the circle and allows circle members to share their perspectives on the conflict or challenge while others listen. This perspective sharing may take several rounds, and at the end, members have completed sharing their perspectives with the elder. The next step is to offer apologies for the parts of the perspectives that each member feels remorse for. The principle is that, by listening to everyone's perspective, remorse will arise in the circle community. Each member is given the chance to share what parts of what they have heard they feel remorse for. The agreement is that, when apologies are offered, forgiveness is granted, and the topic is not to be held in the heart with resentment any longer. This is a process that is transformative in nature and works well with communities that must coexist, such as families, close work, or other community groups, and there is an awareness that the process includes apology and forgiveness. The ho'oponopono process ends with a shared meal.

Conflict Management Models

A multitude of models have been created to help people at work or at home navigate conflict (Christian, 2020; Corr et al., 2015; Dana, 2006; Patterson et al., 2011; Rivers, 2015; Rosenberg, 2015; Scott, 2019). One model of workplace conflict management, created by Daniel Dana, can be both emergent and contractual and can be used by a boss or peer mediator or as a self-mediation between two colleagues. This simple model has cardinal rules for managing workplace conflict: (1) no walking away (or the tendency to distance oneself when there is conflict because of the natural human stress response) and (2) no power plays (or no one-sided solutions where one party is in "the wrong.") Kwame Christian also acknowledges the human stress response in conflict and calls upon us to use our "higher brains" in responding to conflict with compassionate curiosity. His three steps are to (1) acknowledge and validate feelings, (2) get very curious about those feelings with open-ended questions, and (3) mutually brainstorm about possible solutions to the conflict together. In this model, one is always encouraged to go back to step 1 if feelings are strong and seem to be thwarting mutual problem-solving (Christian, 2020). Acknowledging feelings and needs is also a core component of Marshall Rosenburg's nonviolent communication (Rosenberg, 2015). In this model, Rosenburg posits that human beings enjoy giving others what they really need, and the seed of resolving conflict is finding ways to describe universal human needs so others tap into that natural impulse to take joy in helping each other. The four steps include (1) observing and describing what has happened; (2) identifying related feelings; (3) connecting those feelings to core needs, such as a need for peace or freedom, privacy, or clarity, etc.; and (4) making a request to get the need met. All these models acknowledge the stress of conflict, as well as the resources of attending to emotions, identifying needs, and mutual solutions as key ingredients for resolving conflicts.

Ethical Considerations in Conflict Management

There are many ethical considerations in deciding how to proceed with conflict as a veterinary social worker, and there is no overall "code of ethics" for conflict management practitioners as a whole (Barsky, 2017). The reason for this is that many professions can engage in both formal and informal conflict management within the scope of their duties. For our purposes, the conflict management practitioner may be a social worker, but they could just as easily be a veterinary nurse, veterinary practice manager, or veterinarian. Deciding how to handle conflict management requires each professional to follow their own code of ethics (Barsky, 2017). Some general guidelines include confidentiality, conflicts of interest, dual relationships, and legal abuse reporting requirements. McCabe outlines three approaches to conflict management in the workplace: open-door policy, peer review or peer tribunals, and arbitration (McCabe & Rabil, 2002). These three approaches create increasingly more defined boundaries to manage dual relationships and conflicts of interest. For instance, in an open-door policy, any employee can approach the leader in an organization and complain about a conflict he or she may be experiencing. In this circumstance, the leader tries to resolve the problem; however, there can be a tendency for that leader to try to minimize conflicts that may make the employer look bad or, worse, conflicts that interfere with that leader's own success at the organization.

Open-door policies also run the risk of employees breaching information shared in confidence during the conflict management process. The peer-review process increases the sense that a fair decision will be determined for a conflict brought to a committee. However, here, there may also be dual relationships between those in conflict and those on the committee that could affect a committee's decision regarding a conflict or other form of injustice in a workplace. Last, formal arbitration or mediation uses a third-party neutral in resolving conflict. This person is not employed by the organization and is thus likely free from dual relationships. If compensation is provided to the mediator, this will influence the conflict of interest depending on who is covering the fees for services.

A veterinary social worker may find himself or herself in conflict situations handled by all three methods—open door, peer review, and arbitration—and this social worker must carefully consider the ethical path forward. It may be that, at the beginning of a conflict that a social worker learns of through an open-door interaction, the social worker may provide conflict coaching and resources for conflict management tools. If desired, the disputing parties may wish that the social worker support a meeting or a "circle" as a facilitator. If, however, the social worker deems that the nature of the conflict puts them in a conflict of interest because of their role with the organization, it is appropriate for the social worker to help locate a more neutral party to help facilitate conflict management. Moreover, social workers must provide informed consent to the disputants so they are aware of the bounds of confidentiality and reporting requirements, should any information arise that falls into mandated reporting categories. It is important to develop policies and procedures that help an organization where a veterinary social worker is working that outline how decisions will manage conflicts of interest, dual relationships, and mandated reporting.

Case Studies

Each of the following case studies highlights an example of a conflict that a social worker may face within veterinary medicine. The purpose of these case studies is to provide practical examples of scenarios that a social worker may encounter with subsequent questions to apply the knowledge gained within this chapter. The case studies are meant to encourage the reader to consider what they would do as the social worker in each of these scenarios. Questions are provided after each case study to stimulate more in-depth reflection for each case.

Case Study 1

"What are you doing?" You hear the yelling all the way from your office in the back of the veterinary hospital. If you can hear the yelling from the back of the hospital, you are certain that the clients in the lobby can hear the altercation through the thin walls of the practice. Raised voices, shouting, and arguments were very common at Hippopotamus Veterinary Clinic, a small animal veterinary hospital with four full-time veterinarians and a team of around 20 veterinary support staff. This was the exact reason you were hired 3 weeks ago—a veterinary social worker with expertise in conflict management—to help defuse some of the conflict within the practice. Over the past few years, Hippopotamus Veterinary Clinic had a massive turnover among its staff and always seemed to have trouble finding good veterinarians. Upon accepting this position, you were given a tall order. You were hired by Christy, the veterinary practice manager, to establish balance and harmony among the team to reduce employee turnover.

As you rise to investigate the commotion, the yelling continues. "Mrs. Smith has been waiting in the lobby for over an hour. What is taking you so long? You should have been finished with this surgery a long time ago."

You arrive at the scene of the conflict as Dr. Brown, the recent veterinary graduate who had been hired a few months ago, gingerly replies to Christy, the practice manager. "I'm sorry. It usually doesn't take this long. I just had some trouble breaking down the suspensory ligament, but I'm closing now, so I should be done within the next 10 minutes. Please tell Mrs. Smith that I apologize, and I'll be with her as soon as I can."

Christy, seeing your arrival, turns down the volume of her yelling a notch and replies to Dr. Brown, "This is unacceptable. Your efficiency lately has been horrible. We cannot have clients waiting like this. Do you want me to get Dr. Clark? I've seen him do this same surgery in less than 15 minutes."

Dr. Brown, deep in the belly of a Labrador retriever, looks away, tears welling up, and softly replies, "No, I've got this. Please just tell Mrs. Smith I'll be with her soon." Christy exits, leaving you and Dr. Brown alone in the surgery suite.

Case Study 1 Questions
1. What role does power play in this conflict?
2. Workplace conflict can cause stress and emotional distress in the veterinary team. How will you provide support to this veterinarian?
3. What conflict management strategy could be appropriate in this situation, and what steps would you take to address this conflict?

Case Study 2

There has recently been a large outbreak of virulent Newcastle disease in California. Agricultural officials, tasked with the depopulation of chickens infected with this disease, are having trouble because of public outcry about depopulation efforts. There have been public protests and social media campaigns that interfere with and create safety issues for those charged with culling chickens. This is largely due to backyard chicken owners being included in the culling procedures.

California has an agricultural mediation program, and you have just been hired to work there. Although you are an experienced mediator, most of your work has been in civil and family mediation—conflicts such as rental property disputes and family parenting plans during divorce. Agricultural mediation is fairly new to you, but you are excited about working with farmers. You have always loved cows and hoped to have a small hobby farm someday. When you took this job, you thought you would only be mediating issues like disputes over property lines and repayment agreements on default loans.

Your boss has asked you to help resolve a community conflict about whether backyard chickens must be culled. You have read some of the news stories about backyard chickens being culled because they are near poultry farms and are, therefore, exposed to virulent Newcastle disease. You even have a friend who is an active political vegan who invited you to a Facebook page dedicated to "fighting back and saving our chickens" and to resisting agricultural government officials' efforts to quell this disease outbreak. Agricultural officials have invited a group of backyard chicken owners to a town hall meeting to try to reduce enmity and increase understanding about this depopulation.

Case Study 2 Questions
1. What biases do you notice arising in you as you read this case?
2. What knowledge are you lacking, and what impact does that have or not have in responding to your boss's request for you?
3. What form of conflict management strategy might you use and why?
4. Who are all the stakeholders affected by this disease? If you could empathetically put yourself in their shoes, what would you find out?

Case Study 3

"There is no way I'm spending $1000 on that stupid cat!" You just explained to Mr. and Mrs. Johnson that you are the veterinary social worker in the hospital, and you are there to help them navigate their decision of how to proceed with Jelly Bean, their 7-year-old male cat. Jelly Bean had just been diagnosed with urethral obstruction, a life-threatening condition that occurs when a small stone blocks the urethra, preventing the cat from urinating.

Mrs. Johnson pleads, "Please, John, Jelly Bean is suffering, and I don't want to lose him." The veterinarian had explained that one of the only treatment options for this condition was sedation, a procedure to remove the stone, and several days of hospitalization. They had also explained that, without care, Jelly Bean would die soon, and if they did not want Jelly Bean to suffer, another option would be humane euthanasia.

You begin to describe the resources and payment plans available to clients to break up the cost of treatment over the next 6 months. Mr. Johnson interrupts. "I think we should just take him home. We can get you a new cat for free at the shelter if he dies."

Mrs. Johnson begins to cry.

Case Study 3 Questions
1. What are your initial biases and assumptions regarding Mr. and Mrs. Johnson?
2. In your opinion, would this be emergent or contractual conflict management?
3. Conflict often occurs due to conflicting views on how to care for the animal. What will be your first steps in addressing this conflict? Consider what your opening sentence will be.
4. How might the outcome of this case affect the overall well-being of the veterinary team? What might be the underlying emotional issues for the veterinary team?

Case Study 4

The United Egg Producers (UEP) reached out to the Humane Society of the United States (HSUS) to cosponsor a bill on housing for egg-laying chickens. They have agreed on enriched cage housing and have obtained support from the American Veterinary Medical Association to endorse the bill. This collaboration has occurred after years of fighting between the two large organizations that stand for divergent agendas. The United Egg Producers are determined to protect the livelihood of egg farmers, who are increasingly harmed by efforts from animal welfare organizations to disparage their farming practices. To work on stopping this and to reduce the funds lost to fighting the HSUS again, the UEP reached across the aisle to see if there could be a way to create an agreement based on shared interests—better environments for chickens and fiscally sustainable for egg farmers.

You have been an agricultural mediator in Georgia for many years and had grown up on a farm, so you are well aware of animal welfare and animal rights conflicts in the United States. Lately, you have also become increasingly concerned about the well-being of farmers—especially because it seems the suicide rate among farmers continues to increase. You have mediated a few recent cases in which mental illness was a factor in the dispute. You have been approached by HSUS to help resolve a growing conflict that is putting the cosponsored bill at risk: the National Cattlemen's Beef Association (NCBA) has been lobbying against this bill and has determined that if the bill passes, it will open the door for Congress to legislate their animal handling practices. Additionally, you have heard through the grapevine comments that some with the NCBA just do not like HSUS, its tactics, and everything it represents.

Case Study 4 Questions
1. What biases do you notice arising in you as you read this case?
2. What additional information would you need to be able to understand this case more fully? Where would you get such information?

3. Would this be an emergent or contractual approach?
4. What do you think are the needs, interests, and strategies you might use in responding to this conflict?

Conclusion

At both macro and micro levels, social workers face conflict frequently within veterinary medicine. Veterinary medicine includes conflict that arises due to the triad of care resulting from the veterinary-patient-client relationship where the patient cannot speak for him or herself; this is similar to pediatrics with very young children. Unlike pediatrics, however, ethical dilemmas frequently cause conflict within veterinary medicine and may result from contextual limitations or differing views regarding the role or moral value of the animal. Conflict can also occur among teams and within client systems. All conflict has the potential to impact staff morale and overall well-being among the veterinary team. Veterinary social workers may have the opportunity to mediate conflict within these situations, so understanding tools to use in these scenarios becomes vital.

Several approaches to conflict management were presented in this chapter, and these approaches may occur as a more contractual or formal mediation process or as an emergent mediation process. Evaluative mediation, facilitative mediation, transformative mediation, talking circles, and other conflict management models may be beneficial approaches to mediating conflict within veterinary settings. A social worker can use their knowledge regarding these various techniques to select a conflict management strategy that will be most appropriate for each unique situation. Adopting a code of ethics during times of conflict can help ensure the safety confidentiality and of all parties involved in the conflict. Finally, it is important to develop protocols and policies within organizations to prepare the organizations to better navigate conflict when it will inevitably arise.

References

Ajibo, H. T., Onuoha, E. C., Obi-Keguna, C. N., Okafor, A. E., & Oluwole, I. O. (2018). Dynamics of farmers and herdsmen conflict in Nigeria: The implication to social work policy intervention. *International Journal of Humanities and Social Science, 8*(7), 157–163.

American Veterinary Medical Association. (2019). *AVMA guidelines for the depopulation of animals: 2019 edition.* Author.

American Veterinary Medical Association. (2021). *Veterinarian's oath.* https://www.avma.org/resources-tools/avma-policies/veterinarians-oath

Animal Rights Extremists: Trespassing to Rescue Chickens. (2019, February 9). Youtube. https://www.youtube.com/watch?v=Vp8-rYqCAnM

Armitage-Chan, E., & May, S. A. (2018). Identity, environment and mental wellbeing in the veterinary profession. *The Veterinary Record, 183*(2), 68–68.

Barsky, A. (2017). *Conflict management for the helping professions: Negotiation, mediation, advocacy, facilitation, and restorative justice* (3rd ed.). Oxford University Press.

Batchelor, C. E. M., & McKeegan, D. E. F. (2012). Survey of the frequency and perceived stressfulness of ethical dilemmas encountered in UK veterinary practice. *The Veterinary Record, 170*(1), 19.

Bingham, L. B. (2012). Transformative mediation at the United States postal service. *Negotiation and Conflict Management Research, 5*(4), 354–366.

Bradley, V., Liddle, S., Shaw, R., Savage, E., Rabbitts, R., Trim, C., Lasoye, T. A., & Whitelaw, B. C. (2015). Sticks and stones: Investigating rude, dismissive and aggressive communication between doctors. *Clinical Medicine, 15*(6), 541–545.

Brinson, J., & Fisher, T. A. (1999, December). The ho'oponopono group: A conflict management model for school counselors. *Journal for Specialists in Group Work, 24*(4), 369–382.

Broekema, W., van Kleef, D., & Steen, T. (2017). What factors drive organizational learning from crisis? Insights from the Dutch food safety services' response to four veterinary crises. *Journal of Contingencies and Crisis Management, 25*(4), 326–340.

Campbell, S. M., Ulrich, C. M., & Grady, C. (2016). A broader understanding of moral distress. *The American Journal of Bioethics: AJOB, 16*(12), 2–9.

Charles, D. (2012, February 10). *How two bitter adversaries hatched a plan to change the egg business.* National Public Radio. https://www.npr.org/sections/thesalt/2012/02/10/146635596/how-two-bitter-adversaries-hatched-a-plan-to-change-the-egg-business

Christian, K. (2020). *Finding confidence in conflict: how to negotiate anything and live your best life.* American Negotiation Institute LLC..

Corr, A., Sue Kurita, J. M., & Waters, R. (2015). *Empirical analysis of the INACCORD conflict analysis model of alternative dispute management: Mediation and arbitration data from Romania, 2012 to 2015.* https://www.mwbdr.com/publications/

Cosgrove, J. (2019, June 7). To stop a virus, California has euthanized more than 1.2 million birds. Is it reckless or necessary? *Los Angeles Times.* https://www.latimes.com/local/lanow/la-me-ln-virulent-newcastle-disease-outbreak-in-southern-california-20190607-story.html

Crane, M. F., Bayl-Smith, P., & Cartmill, J. (2013). A recommendation for expanding the definition of moral distress experienced in the workplace. *Australian and New Zealand Journal of Organizational Psychology, 6.* https://doi.org/10.1017/orp.2013.1

Dana, D. (2001). *Conflict management* (1st ed.). McGraw-Hill Education.

Dana, D. (2006). *Managing differences: How to build better relationships at work and home* (4th ed.). M T I Pubns.

Ekakoro, J. E., Caldwell, M., Strand, E. B., & Okafor, C. C. (2019). Drivers, alternatives, knowledge, and perceptions towards antimicrobial use among Tennessee beef cattle producers: A qualitative study. *BMC Veterinary Research, 15*(1), 16.

Eller, D. (2020, May 29). Animal activist group secretly tapes euthanization of pigs, alleges they were "roasted alive." *Des Moines Register.* https://www.desmoinesregister.com/story/money/agriculture/2020/05/29/animal-activist-group-secretly-tapes-iowa-pigs-being-euthanized/5272999002/

Emran, S. A. N. (2015). The four-principle formulation of common morality is at the core of bioethics mediation method. *Medicine, Health Care, and Philosophy, 18*(3), 371–377.

Fawcett, A., & Mullan, S. (2018). Managing moral distress in practice. *In Practice, 40*(1), 34–36.

Foulk, T., Woolum, A., & Erez, A. (2016). Catching rudeness is like catching a cold: The contagion effects of low-intensity negative behaviors. *The Journal of Applied Psychology, 101*(1), 50–67.

Greenwald, G. (2020, May 29). Hidden video and whistleblower reveal gruesome mass-extermination method for iowa pigs amid pandemic. *The Intercept.* https://theintercept.com/2020/05/29/pigs-factory-farms-ventilation-shutdown-coronavirus/?fbclid=IwAR1aq6W6RldVIphBv-iKRJewh4A-K8Q0iW7Z6hr9b7_UwZc32dTe-YMZ-XE

Ito, K. L. (1985). Ho'oponopono, "to make right": Hawaiian conflict management and metaphor in the construction of a family therapy. *Culture, Medicine and Psychiatry, 9*(2), 201–217.

Janss, R., Rispens, S., Segers, M., & Jehn, K. A. (2012). What is happening under the surface? Power, conflict and the performance of medical teams. *Medical Education, 46*(9), 838–849.

Jones, J. (2019). How is your client feeling? The power of mediation. *The Veterinary Record, 185*(24), 765.

Kamana, K. P. W. (2010). *Mo'oki'ina Ho'oponopono: The continuity of traditional Hawaiian conflict management at Ke Kula "O Nawahiokalani"opu'u* [University of Hawai'i at Hilo]. http://search.proquest.com.proxy.lib.utk.edu:90/docview/822470192/abstract/12D8EA07EF7948C0PQ/7?accountid=14766

Kipperman, B., Morris, P., & Rollin, B. (2018). Ethical dilemmas encountered by small animal veterinarians: Characterisation, responses, consequences and beliefs regarding euthanasia. *Veterinary Record, 182*(19), 548. https://doi.org/10.1136/vr.104619

Kipperman, B. S., Kass, P. H., & Rishniw, M. (2017). Factors that influence small animal veterinarians' opinions and actions regarding cost of care and effects of economic limitations on patient care and outcome and professional career satisfaction and burnout. *Journal of the American Veterinary Medical Association, 250*(7), 785–794.

Lyons, P., McCormick, K., Sauer, S., & Chamblin, M. (2019). Can conducting a talking circle about a sensitive topic increase participation for elementary aged learners? *Open Access Library Journal, 6*, e5594.

McCabe, D. M., & Rabil, J. M. (2002). Administering the employment relationship: The ethics of conflict resolution in relation to justice in the workplace. *Journal of Business Ethics: JBE, 36*(1), 33–48.

McKenzie, D. M. (2015). The role of mediation in resolving workplace relationship conflict. *International Journal of Law and Psychiatry, 39*, 52–59.

Mehl-Madrona, L., & Mainguy, B. (2014). Introducing healing circles and talking circles into primary care. *The Permanente Journal, 18*(2), 4–9.

Morgan, C. A., & McDonald, M. (2007). Ethical dilemmas in veterinary medicine. *The Veterinary Clinics of North America. Small Animal Practice, 37*(1), 165–179; abstract x.

Moses, L., Malowney, M. J., & Wesley Boyd, J. (2018). Ethical conflict and moral distress in veterinary practice: A survey of North American veterinarians. *Journal of Veterinary Internal Medicine/American College of Veterinary Internal Medicine, 32*(6), 2115–2122.

Nett, R. J., Witte, T. K., Holzbauer, S. M., Elchos, B. L., Campagnolo, E. R., Musgrave, … Funk, R. H. (2015). Risk factors for suicide, attitudes toward mental illness, and practice-related stressors among US veterinarians. *Journal of the American Veterinary Medical Association, 247*(8), 945–955.

Olmstead, J. A., & Dahnke, M. D. (2016). The need for an effective process to resolve conflicts over medical futility: A case study and analysis. *Critical Care Nurse, 36*(6), 13–23.

Page-Jones, S., & Abbey, G. (2015). Career identity in the veterinary profession. *The Veterinary Record, 176*(17), 433.

Patterson, K., Grenny, J., McMillan, R., & Switzler, A. (2011). *Crucial conversations: Tools for talking when stakes are high* (2nd ed.). McGraw Hill Educational.

Pranis, K., Wedge, M., & Stuart, B. (2003). *Peacemaking circles: From conflict to community.* Living Justice Press.

Riskin, A., Erez, A., Foulk, T. A., Kugelman, A., Gover, A., Shoris, I., Riskin, K. S., & Bamberger, P. A. (2015). The impact of rudeness on medical team performance: A randomized trial. *Pediatrics, 136*(3), 487–495.

Riskin, A., Erez, A., Foulk, T. A., Riskin-Geuz, K. S., Ziv, A., Sela, R., Pessach-Gelblum, L., & Bamberger, P. A. (2017). Rudeness and medical team performance. *Pediatrics, 139*(2). https://doi.org/10.1542/peds.2016-2305

Rivers, D. (2015). *The seven challenges workbook cooperative communication skills for success at home and at work* (9th ed.). https://newconversations.net/.

Rook, D. (2014). Who gets Charlie? The emergence of pet custody disputes in family law: Adapting theoretical tools from child law. *International Journal of Law, Policy, and the Family, 28*(2), 177–193.

Rosenberg, M. B. (2015). *Nonviolent communication: A language of life* (3rd ed.). Puddle Dancer Press.

Scott, K. (2019). *Radical candor: Be a kick-ass boss without losing your humanity*, rev. ed. St. Martin's Press.

Spitznagel, M. B., Ben-Porath, Y. S., Rishniw, M., Kogan, L. R., & Carlson, M. D. (2019). Development and validation of a Burden Transfer Inventory for predicting veterinarian stress related to client behavior. *Journal of the American Veterinary Medical Association, 254*(1), 133–144.

Tallodi, T. (2015). Mediation's potential to reduce occupational stress: A new perspective. *Conflict Management Quarterly, 32*(4), 361–388.

Vande Griek, O. H., Clark, M. A., Witte, T. K., Nett, R. J., Moeller, A. N., & Stabler, M. E. (2018). Development of a taxonomy of practice-related stressors experienced by veterinarians in the United States. *Journal of the American Veterinary Medical Association, 252*(2), 227–233.

Voda-Hamilton, D. V. (2015). *Nipped in the bud, not in the butt: How to use mediation to resolve conflicts over animals*. Createspace Independent Publishing Platform.

Volk, J. O., Schimmack, U., Strand, E. B., Vasconcelos, J., & Siren, C. W. (2020). Executive summary of the Merck Animal Health Veterinary Wellbeing Study II. *Journal of the American Veterinary Medical Association, 256*(11), 1237–1244.

Wallace, J. E., & Buchanan, T. (2020). Status differences in interpersonal strain and job resources at work: A mixed methods study of animal health-care providers. *International Journal of Conflict Management, 31*(2), 287–308.

Watson, N. T., Rogers, K. S., Watson, K. L., & Liau-Hing Yep, C. (2019). Integrating social justice-based conflict management into higher education settings: Faculty, staff, and student professional development through mediation training. *Conflict Management Quarterly, 36*(3), 251–262.

Wiedner, R., Nigam, A., & da Silva, J. (2020). GPs are from Mars, Administrators are from Venus: The role of misaligned occupational dispositions in inhibiting mandated role change. *Work and Occupations*. https://doi.org/10.1177/0730888420918643.

Wojtacka, J., Grudzień, W., Wysok, B., & Szarek, J. (2020). Causes of stress and conflict in the veterinary professional workplace – A perspective from Poland. *Irish Veterinary Journal, 73*(1), 23.

Wojtacka, J., Wysok, B., & Szteyn, J. (2020). Analysis of the factors influencing veterinary food inspectors in Poland. *Animals : An Open Access Journal from MDPI, 10*(5). https://doi.org/10.3390/ani10050884

Zumeta, Z. (2000). Styles of mediation: Facilitative, evaluative, and transformative mediation. *National Association for Community Mediation Newsletter, 5*. http://www.rchss.sinica.edu.tw/cibs/law/1.%20Monthly%20Seminar%20Since%202008/Papers/2009/20090211/Chen-Chieh%20Ting_Styles%20of%20Mediation_%20Facilitative,%20Evaluative,%20and%20Transformative%20Mediation.pdf

Chapter 10
Veterinarian Wellbeing and Mental Health

John Volk

Introduction

Veterinary medicine, like human medicine, is a stressful profession. It is a world of sick and injured patients, often requiring rapid-fire life-and-death decisions. In the case of companion animals, many owners are very emotionally bonded to their pets and can be overwrought in emergency situations. Veterinarians may also experience financial stress as well. Fewer than 5 percent of pets are covered by pet health insurance. Pets may require treatment their owners can ill afford, leading to tense discussions about cost. In addition, a vast number of veterinarians, especially young veterinarians, are burdened with oppressive levels of student debt. Veterinarians and their team members work in close quarters, depending on each other for instantaneous cooperation and support. These factors may combine to lead to mental health challenges and a higher rate of suicide among veterinarians compared the general US adult population (Tomasi & Fechter-Legett, 2019).

According to recent research, veterinarians view stress and suicide as two of the three most critical issues facing the profession; the other is student debt. Consequently, fostering good mental health and wellbeing is extremely important to helping veterinarians live healthy, satisfying, productive lives (Volk et al., 2020).

Numerous studies have been conducted on veterinarian mental health in recent years. Two of the most important in providing baseline data are a pair of studies conducted in 2017 and 2019. The Merck Animal Health (MAH) Veterinarian Wellbeing Studies I and II were large scale, quantitative, representative studies of US veterinarians. They were conducted by a team of experts in collaboration with the American Veterinary Medical Association (AVMA) and underwritten by Merck

J. Volk (✉)
Brakke Consulting, Inc, Chicago, IL, USA
e-mail: john@volkonline.com

© The Author(s), under exclusive license to Springer Nature Switzerland AG 2022   229
S. Loue, P. Linden (eds.), *The Comprehensive Guide to Interdisciplinary Veterinary Social Work*, https://doi.org/10.1007/978-3-031-10330-8_10

Animal Health, a supplier of pharmaceuticals, vaccines, and digital technology to the veterinary industry. These studies provided useful comparison data for the US adult general population and, in some cases, comparison data for physicians. This chapter is informed substantially by that research.

Mental Health and Wellbeing Defined

Mental health and wellbeing are two different, but related, constructs, although they may be influenced by common factors. Just like physical health, mental health is defined as optimal functioning of the mind. Wellbeing is defined as having a life that matches an individual's ideal (Diener et al., 1985). Although mental health is necessary for high well-being, it is not sufficient. A good life also depends on actual life circumstances and satisfaction with important life domains such as work and family life. A person who is "suffering" on the wellbeing scale is not necessarily seriously psychologically distressed. In the 2017 Veterinarian Wellbeing Study, for example, only 28 percent of respondents who rated themselves 0–3 in wellbeing were seriously psychologically distressed as measured by Kessler 6 (Volk et al., 2018).

The greatest mental health problems facing veterinarians have been found to be burnout and depression. To assess mental health, the MAH studies used a widely used screening measure, the Kessler Psychological Distress scale (Kessler et al., 2003). The Kessler 6, as the instrument is known, is a validated survey tool that is widely used to determine whether an individual is or is not suffering from serious psychological distress. It involves six questions about feelings such as nervousness, hopelessness, worthlessness, and other attributes. Respondents answer using a five-point frequency scale ("none of the time" to "all of the time"). The minimum score is 0; the maximum score is 24. Those receiving a score of 13 or greater are said to be in serious psychological distress.

Wellbeing was measured with global life-satisfaction judgments. This is the most widely used approach to measure wellbeing and was used in the World Happiness Report (Helliwell et al., 2020). Often just a single item is used. One of the most established and common measures of wellbeing is Cantril's ladder (Cantril, 1965). It asks respondents to imagine a 10-step ladder in which 0 is the worst possible life and 10 is the best possible and to place their life on that ladder. This item was also used in the MAH studies. To increase reliability, two additional items were used that were included in the Panel Study of Income Dynamics (PSID) so that results could be compared to US workers. One item was from the Satisfaction with Life scale (Diener et al., 1985). The other item was created by the PSID research team. The three items are highly correlated and were averaged to create a Wellbeing Index (WBI). Scores on the WBI range from 0 to 10. The WBI was used to create three groups of veterinarians, following Gallup's categories for Cantril's ladder, "flourishing" (7–10), "getting by" (sometimes called "struggling"), and "suffering" (0–3).

Wellbeing of Veterinarians

Data for wellbeing of non-veterinarians was obtained from a special wellbeing study conducted by PSID (Freedman, 2017). Begun in 1968, PSID is the longest-running longitudinal household study in the world. It is a nationally representative study of 18,000 individuals living in 5000 households. In 2016, the PSID conducted a special survey of 8000 members of the panel that answered extensive questions about wellbeing that generally are not included in the biannual survey.

According to the MAH Wellbeing Studies, veterinarians as a whole have levels of wellbeing similar to non-veterinarians. In the 2017 study, 58.3 percent of veterinarians fell into the flourishing category compared to 61.3 percent of the US adult employed population. Likewise, 9.1 percent of veterinarians fell into the suffering category versus 7.3 percent of the general population (Volk et al., 2018) (Fig. 10.1).

Unlike in the general population, there were differences between male and female veterinarians in wellbeing (Volk et al., 2018). A higher percentage (67.8%) of male veterinarians fell into the flourishing category compared to their non-veterinarian counterparts (61.6%), while a smaller percentage of women veterinarians were flourishing (51.3% vs. 60.6%). The greatest variation in veterinarian wellbeing, however, was found to be age related. Only 46.9 percent of veterinarians under 35 were flourishing, while 82.1 percent of veterinarians 65 or older fell into the flourishing group. Veterinarians 55 and older consistently had higher levels of wellbeing than their non-veterinarian counterparts (Fig. 10.2) (Volk et al., 2018).

In both the 2017 and 2019 studies, veterinarians in clinical practice and those veterinarians working in other fields had similar wellbeing profiles. Among those in clinical practice, a higher percentage of food animal veterinarians were flourishing than those in companion animal, equine, and mixed practice (Volk et al., 2020).

So what differentiates veterinarians who were flourishing versus those who were just getting by? There were several factors. Those who were flourishing were more satisfied in all life domains, especially with their job and their financial situation.

Fig. 10.1 Wellbeing of veterinarians vs. wellbeing of US employed adults

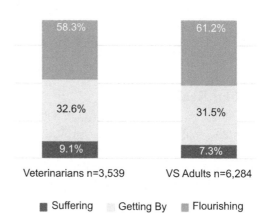

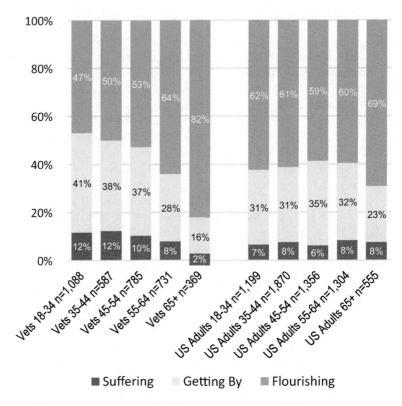

Fig. 10.2 Wellbeing of veterinarians and the general adult population by age

Student debt definitely played a role, too. In multiple regression analysis, student debt was a negative predictor of wellbeing (Volk et al., 2020).

Flourishing veterinarians were found to be more likely to have a healthy method for dealing with stress compared with those in other categories. Flourishing veterinarians were more likely than those with lower levels of wellbeing to spend more time with family and friends, exercise, and spend time away from work reading, traveling, or enjoying a hobby (Volk et al., 2020).

Mental Health

According to the MAH Veterinarian Wellbeing Studies, about 1 in 20 veterinarians suffered from serious psychological distress. This was similar to the level seen in the general employed adult population (Volk et al., 2018). In the veterinary community, those suffering from psychological distress were more likely to be younger and female, although among veterinarians under 45 years of age, there was no statistical significance between males and females in the prevalence of serious psychological distress. From 2017 to 2019, the prevalence of serious psychological distress in women veterinarians increased from 6.2 percent to 8.1 percent, a statistically significant difference (Volk et al., 2020).

Serious psychological distress was also found to be more common in younger veterinarians than their counterparts in the general population. As with wellbeing, serious psychological distress was consistent across practice types except for food animal practice, where it was almost nonexistent. The more hours worked per week, the higher the percentage of those with serious psychological distress. Serious psychological distress was also more prevalent in those working more – or fewer – hours than they desired (Volk et al., 2018).

Without question, a key driver of mental health issues among veterinarians is financial stress. In the 2017 study, serious psychological distress occurred three times more often in those veterinarians with student debt than those without student debt. Interestingly, the *amount* of student debt did not seem to make much difference (Volk et al., 2018).

There is a distinct treatment gap for those suffering mental health issues. About half of those with serious psychological distress had received no treatment within the past year (Volk et al., 2020). Only 30 percent of veterinarians with serious psychological distress said they would be comfortable taking time off work for treatment. While many veterinary organizations provide resources for those experiencing mental health issues, only 12 percent of veterinarians with serious psychological distress had accessed any of those. The most accessed resources were those of the AVMA, but only 40 percent found them useful (Volk et al., 2020).

As in the case of wellbeing, those veterinarians with serious psychological distress were much less likely to have a healthy method for dealing with stress. They were also far less likely to participate in healthy activities outside of work, such as socializing with family and friends, exercising, and participating in other leisure activities. As was seen repeatedly in the research, lack of work-life balance was a key factor in poor mental health and low levels of wellbeing (Volk et al., 2020).

Role of Personality

It's important to recognize that personality may play a significant role in both mental health and wellbeing. The 2017 and 2019 MAH Veterinarian Wellbeing Studies included instruments to measure veterinarians on the Big 5 Personality traits (Mccrae & John, 1992). The traits are as follows:

- *Openness* to experience (inventive/curious vs. consistent/cautious). Appreciation for art, emotion, adventure, unusual ideas, curiosity, and a variety of experience
- *Conscientiousness* (efficient/organized vs. easy-going/careless). A tendency to be organized and dependable, show self-discipline, act dutifully, aim for achievement, and prefer planned rather than spontaneous behavior

- *Extraversion* (outgoing/energetic vs. solitary/reserved). Energy, positive emotions, surgency, assertiveness, sociability and the tendency to seek stimulation in the company of others, and talkativeness
- *Agreeableness* (friendly/compassionate vs. challenging/detached). A tendency to be compassionate and cooperative rather than suspicious and antagonistic toward others
- *Neuroticism* (sensitive/nervous vs. secure/confident). The tendency to experience unpleasant emotions easily, such as anger, anxiety, depression, and vulnerability

Longitudinal studies suggest that these characteristics are stable over long periods of time.

Two of the characteristics are highly associated with wellbeing. Neuroticism is a strong negative predictor of wellbeing (Steel et al., 2008), and extraversion is a consistent positive predictor of wellbeing (Schimmack, 2008). Openness and agreeableness tend to be weak predictors of wellbeing.

In the Veterinarian Wellbeing Studies, veterinarians on average scored substantially lower in extraversion (−28% SD) – i.e., they were more introverted – and substantially higher in neuroticism (+38% SD) than non-veterinarians (Volk et al., 2017). In fact, veterinarians were almost twice as likely to score high in neuroticism than non-veterinarians (17% vs. 9%). Veterinarians as a group scored slightly lower than their non-veterinarian counterparts in openness and agreeableness, and about the same in conscientiousness (Fig. 10.3).

In multiple regression analysis, neuroticism was the factor most associated with serious psychological distress in veterinarians, followed by student debt. Both neuroticism and debt were also closely associated with wellbeing of veterinarians (Volk et al., 2018).

No doubt the tendency to score high in agreeableness is useful for veterinarians. Individuals with that characteristic tend to be compassionate and cooperative (Schimmack, 2008), useful traits in a medical profession requiring teamwork.

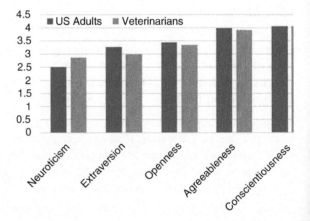

Fig. 10.3 Mean scores of US veterinarians and non-veterinarians on the Big 5 Personality traits

However, the fact that many are introverted and also worriers (neurotic) can be challenging in a profession with a very high level of client contact.

Financial Stress

As mentioned at the beginning of this chapter, high student debt is one of the most critical issues facing the veterinary profession. According to the AVMA, in 2019 more than 80 percent of students graduating from veterinary college had student debt. Their average amount of debt was more than $183,000, with some individuals burdened with more than $400,000 in student debt! At the same time, the mean starting salary for 2019 graduates was only $70,045, far less than many other professions requiring similar levels of education (Bain et al., 2020).

Financial stress was a prominent issue in the MAH Veterinary Wellbeing Studies. The largest gaps in satisfaction with life domains between veterinarians with serious psychological distress and those without were in personal financial situation, personal income, and household income. In the multiple regression model, student debt and a personality high in neuroticism were the two greatest predictors of serious psychological distress as well as low levels of wellbeing (Volk et al., 2020).

One of the most alarming findings of the wellbeing studies was that a majority of veterinarians (52%) would *not* recommend the profession to a friend or family member (Volk et al., 2020). This compares to 70 percent of US college-educated, employed adults that *would* recommend their profession, and 51 percent of physicians (Volk et al., 2018). The two most frequent reasons given by veterinarians for not recommending their profession were student debt (50%) and low pay (45%).

Burnout

Burnout is a common complaint of veterinarians. Burnout and compassion fatigue are terms that are often used interchangeably and sometimes are viewed as two separate but highly related conditions. Some consider burnout an umbrella term and compassion fatigue a type of burnout. Others view burnout as a chronic condition, whereas compassion fatigue is more acute.

Burnout was first recognized in 1974 by Freudenberger, who described it as "exhaustion, disillusionment and withdrawal resulting from intense devotion to a cause that failed to produce the expected result" (Coles, 2018). Symptoms can include anxiety, depression, and decreased commitment to clients and patients. The term "compassion fatigue" was first coined in 1992 and was defined as a unique form of burnout that affected caregivers and resulted in a "loss of the ability to nurture" (Coles, 2018).

For purposes of the wellbeing studies, burnout and compassion fatigue were grouped together as a single condition. In the 2017 Wellbeing Study, 50 percent of respondents indicated that they had felt burnout or compassion fatigue within the past year. Of those with serious psychological distress, 88 percent said they had experienced burnout or compassion fatigue (Volk et al., 2017).

To measure burnout more precisely and to compare burnout in veterinarians with physicians, the 2019 Wellbeing Study included a burnout assessment tool, the Mayo Clinic Physicians Wellbeing Index (Shanafelt et al., 2019). The instrument includes seven yes-or-no questions and the score is the sum of the "yes" answers. Veterinarian burnout scores averaged 40 percent higher than physician burnout scores: 3.10 vs. 2.24. Mean burnout score for adults in the US general population was lower, 2.00. Interestingly, the difference between burnout in veterinarians and burnout in physicians was not a function of hours worked. In their respective studies, 41.8 percent of physicians worked more than 60 hours per week compared with 19.6 percent of veterinarians. In the general population, only 6.4 percent of employed adults worked 60 or more hours per week (Volk et al., 2020).

It's not totally clear why a higher percentage of veterinarians experienced burnout than physicians. In multiple regression analysis, high burnout scores were associated with poor work-life balance, not enjoying work, not finding work invigorating, and having a conflict with one or more work associates.

There are other factors that could be involved. For example, veterinarians not only deal with the medical condition of their patients but also often confront highly bonded pet owners who may become overwrought when their beloved pet is injured or has a serious illness. Veterinary medical procedures are client-paid rather than insurance-paid, unlike in human medicine. Hence, veterinarians often have to deal with uncomfortable financial negotiations with pet owners. The high level of introversion of veterinarians may also play a role; they may simply feel worn out after a day filled with interaction with co-workers and clients.

Substance Use

Given the levels of stress, burnout, and serious psychological distress, especially among younger veterinarians, it raises the question: are veterinarians prone to self-medicating with alcohol or drugs? In the 2019 MAH Veterinarian Wellbeing Study, substance use among veterinarians was compared with results of the National Survey on Drug Use and Health (NSDUH) conducted for the National Institutes of Health (NIH). The NDSUH study has been conducted annually since 1971 (NSDUH, 2019). Information from NSDUH is used to support prevention and treatment programs, monitor substance use trends, estimate the need for treatment, and inform public health policy. The 2018 NDSUH study used for comparison was based on 71,000 respondents.

Illicit drug use among veterinarians was almost nonexistent; 2 percent had used opioids without a prescription in the previous 30 days compared to 1 percent of non-veterinarians. No other drugs (e.g., cocaine, hallucinogens) were mentioned at all.

Even use of marijuana was lower among veterinarians – 7 percent in the last 30 days compared to 10 percent in the general population (Volk et al., 2020).

Likewise, alcohol use among veterinarians was consistent with that of the general population. Binge drinking occasions were uncommon; 73 percent of veterinarian had experienced no binge drinking episodes in the past month, versus 68 percent of non-veterinarians. For women binge drinking is defined as consuming four drinks on any one occasion; for men, five drinks. The average number of binge drinking episodes for veterinarians in the previous month was 1.19 versus 1.26 for non-veterinarians (Volk et al., 2020).

Suicide

As mentioned at the beginning of this chapter, veterinarians view suicide as one of the three most critical issues facing the profession (Volk et al., 2020). The suicide rate among veterinarians is higher than in the general population, to be sure. Tomasi and Fechter-Legett (2019) reported that male veterinarians were 2.1 times more likely to die by suicide and female veterinarians were 3.5 times more likely to die by suicide than their general population counterparts. This was based on an analysis of death records for veterinarians who died from 1979 through 2015. There was some indication that the suicide rate may be increasing over time. The leading methods of suicide were firearms (45%) and pharmaceuticals (39%). The use of pharmaceutics was higher (42%) for veterinarians in clinical practice, and much higher for women (64%) than men.

The findings of the MAH Veterinarian Wellbeing Studies were consistent with the Tomasi report. As surveys, the wellbeing studies provided no information about suicide rate, but they did provide insights on attitudes, intentions, and attempts. In addition, the NDSUH study also provided comparative data for the general population.

In the 2019 Veterinarian Wellbeing Study, 21.9 percent of veterinarians indicated that they had thought about killing themselves at some point in the past, including 7.5 percent within the past year. That's more than twice the incidence among US adults in the NSDUH study. Further, 1.4 percent of veterinarians said they went so far as to plan to kill themselves in the past year, and 0.2 percent had actually attempted suicide. Suicide attempts among veterinarians were nearly three times that of the general population (Volk et al., 2020).

Among those veterinarians suffering from serious psychological distress, 41 percent had seriously thought about ending their life in the past year, and 25 percent had made plans to kill themselves. Three percent said they had attempted suicide. While female veterinarians were twice as likely to consider suicide as male veterinarians, a higher percentage of men were likely to actually attempt it. That said, the rate for male veterinarians attempting suicide is about twice that of non-veterinarians and for female veterinarians, three times the rate (Volk et al., 2020).

In the MAH Veterinarian Wellbeing Studies, multiple regression analysis demonstrated that serious psychological distress as measured by Kessler 6 was the single strongest predictor of suicide planning (Volk et al., 2020). Higher levels of distress were found to be associated with higher neuroticism, more debt, and long work hours. Female veterinarians may be at an increased risk because on average they were found to have higher levels of neuroticism. Younger veterinarians also appear to be at an increased risk due to higher scores in neuroticism, high debt, and longer work hours. Clearly, counseling and suicide prevention are critical services in veterinary school environments, as well as throughout the profession, especially for young veterinarians.

Improving Mental Health and Wellbeing of Veterinarians

There are many ways that veterinary social workers can assist veterinarians and veterinary organizations in their efforts to foster mental health and wellbeing.

Creation of a healthy work-life balance A consistent theme throughout the Veterinarian Wellbeing Studies was the need for better work-life balance. Fifty-one percent of veterinarians said they were working more hours than they wished. In an analysis of 14 factors contributing to job satisfaction, the greatest gap between those with serious psychological distress and those without was "I have good work-life balance" (38% vs. 70%). The same attribute was an important differentiator between those veterinarians in the "getting by" category compared to those who were "flourishing" (53% vs. 84%) (Volk et al., 2020). When asked about their participation in a list of nonwork, healthy activities, those with serious psychological distress, and those with lower levels of wellbeing, consistently participated substantially less often than those without serious psychological distress or higher levels of wellbeing (Volk et al., 2020) (Fig. 10.4).

Interestingly, some of the largest gaps between those with and without serious psychological distress are in "spending time with family" and "socializing with friends." Yet, these may be the single biggest contributors to mental health and wellbeing. Ruth Whippman, an author who has written extensively on mental health, including *America the Anxious, How Our Pursuit of Happiness is Creating a Nation of Nervous Wrecks*, said:

> Study after study shows that good social relationships are the strongest, most consistent predictor there is of a happy life, even going so far as to call them a "necessary condition for happiness," meaning that humans can't actually be happy without them. This is a finding that cuts across race, age, gender, income and social class so overwhelmingly that it dwarfs any other factor. (Whippman, 2017, p. 1)

Development of a personal stress management plan In the Veterinarian Wellbeing Studies, another major differentiator between those with serious psychological stress and those without was the existence of a personal stress management

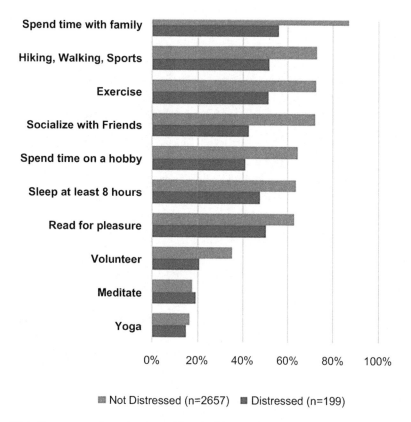

Fig. 10.4 Percentages of veterinarians with and without serious psychological distress who participate frequently in various activities

plan. It was also a differentiator in the level of wellbeing of veterinarians (Fig. 10.5) (Volk et al., 2020). Veterinary social workers providing support to veterinary personnel will want to be aware of these strategies and encourage their clients to utilize them, as appropriate.

Such a plan includes activities a person commits to doing daily or after experiencing a particularly stressful event.

Some examples[1]:

- High-intensity interval training (HIIT). HIIT generally involves a brief warm-up followed by 5—7 minutes of physical activity (e.g., fast walking, jogging, jumping jacks, stair climbing) followed by a brief cool-down period. The idea is to have a 2:1 ratio of work to recovery. HIIT works not only to reduce stress and improve condition but also to improve glucose metabolism.

---

[1] Drawn from Volk and Strand (2018); used with permission

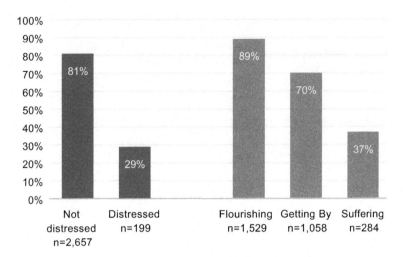

Fig. 10.5 Percentages of veterinarians who said they had a healthy method for dealing with stress in their lives

- Breathing exercises such as 4-7-8 are also useful. The individual breathes in through their nose for four counts, holds their breath for seven counts, and breathes out for eight counts; repeat. This can help individuals to calm down during the day, or fall back asleep at night by engaging the parasympathetic nervous system.
- Eating yogurt. Getting enough probiotics in one's diet can help the central nervous system manage stress (Davis et al., 2016).
- Snacking on fruits, veggies, and nuts. Eating plenty of fruits, veggies, and nuts is good for one's body and they also support positive improvement in mood (Mujcic & Oswald, 2016; Pribis, 2016).
- Practicing 5 minutes of mindfulness. Here's how:

  (a) The individual sit in a chair or cross-legged on the floor with his or her back straight. If on the floor, the individual may wish to sit on a pillow to raise their hips off the floor.
  (b) The individual breathes in and while breathing out, counts "one."
  (c) The individual counts their breaths out until they have reached "five."
  (d) The process is begun again.
  (e) If the individual gets to "ten," it is likely that their mind has wandered. That is not unexpected and the individual should be encouraged to begin again.
  (f) The client may wish to consider downloading a mindfulness app; "Insight Timer" is an example. It's free with many resources for learning to practice mindfulness.

Suggesting that the client call a friend In this day and age when we spend so much time emailing and texting, it's good to actually have a conversation. The social worker may want to suggest that the client call a personal friend or family member or another individual with whom the client has a connection outside of work, someone positive who can help lift the client's spirits. Even a 10-minute conversation can help put work stress into perspective.

Limiting time on social media In the Veterinarian Wellbeing Studies, time spent on social media, e.g., Facebook and Instagram, was negatively associated with mental health and wellbeing. Respondents who spent more than 2 hours a day on social media were more than twice as likely to have serious psychological distress (Volk et al., 2018). There are several reasons why this might be the case. Ironically, time spent on social media isn't socializing. Instead, it's sitting at a computer reading instead of real-time interaction with family or friends. Excessive time spent on social media takes time that could otherwise be spent on healthier activities such as exercise, a hobby, or reading a book for pleasure. And much of the content on social media are reports of happy experiences of acquaintances – vacations, parties, good food – that by contrast can make a person feel even more distressed about their stressful, overworked life.

Engaging a financial planner Given the role that debt and other financial pressures play in veterinarians' lives, it's important for them to seek professional help in managing finances. A financial planning professional can help work out a plan to manage student debt, provide for purchases such as a home, and manage investments for retirement or perhaps purchasing a practice in the future. In the 2019 MAH Veterinarian Wellbeing Study, those respondents who, regardless of age, engaged a financial planner were a third less likely to experience serious psychological distress and had much higher levels of wellbeing than those who did not work with a financial planner (Volk et al., 2020) (Fig. 10.6).

The National Association of Personal Financial Advisors (https://www.napfa.org) provides information about, and links to, fee-based financial advisors. Those are professionals that do not sell stocks, bonds, or other financial products but instead work only for the financial interests of the client for a fee. NAPFA also has a foundation that helps provide financial planning assistance for those unable to pay.

Veterinary organizations such as the AVMA (https://www.avma.org/resources-tools/personal-finance) and the VIN (Veterinary Information Network) Foundation Student Debt Center (vinfoundation.org/resources/student-debt-center/) provide online information and resources to assist veterinarians in managing student debt and other financial issues.

Seeking mental health counseling As mentioned earlier in this chapter, about one-half of those veterinarians with serious psychological distress had not received treatment within the past year, and very few had accessed mental health and wellbeing resources available through professional organizations. As one would expect, one obstacle is the perceived societal stigma attached with mental illness. In the 2019 Wellbeing Study, respondents with serious psychological distress were less comfortable discussing mental health topics with other veterinarians than those without serious psychological distress (44% vs. 61%), and even fewer would be comfortable taking time off for treatment (30% vs. 55%) (Volk et al., 2020).

Fig. 10.6 Percentages of seriously psychologically distressed veterinarians who did or did not work with a financial planner

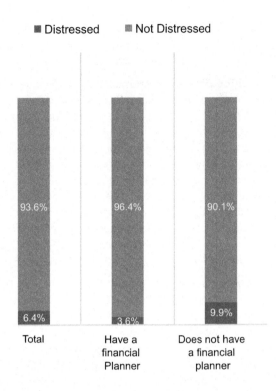

There is some evidence that the stigma associated with mental illness may be subsiding a bit. In the 2017 Veterinary Wellbeing Study, only 24 percent of respondents agreed that "veterinarians are caring toward those with mental illness." However, in the 2019 study, 57 percent of respondents agreed with the statement (Volk et al., 2017, 2020).

Ideally, every person experiencing serious psychological distress should seek professional help to address it. Where professional help isn't readily available, or where the person doesn't feel comfortable taking time off work to visit a counselor, tele-behavioral health resources may be available. They can make mental healthcare more time-efficient and inexpensive. Examples include resources available at sites such as e-counseling.com and 7cups.com.

There are many steps that organizations can take to promote mental health and wellbeing among employees. The following primarily address the needs of veterinary practices, but many can apply to other organizations as well.

Provision of an Employee Assistance Program (EAP) An Employee Assistance Program is a program that helps assist employees with personal problems and/or work-related problems that may impact their job performance, physical or mental health, or emotional wellbeing. An EAP is part of an organization's employee benefit program, and often the employer pays for part or all of the services provided under the program. EAPs are relatively common in large companies and other organizations, less so in small retail organizations such as veterinary practices. However, that may be changing. One veterinary organization, the Veterinary Hospital

Managers Association (VHMA), has worked with an employee benefits service provider to offer EAP services even to small, independent veterinary practices.

Encouraging discussion about stress Veterinary practices commonly hold weekly or monthly meetings to discuss cases, workload, and organizational issues, celebrate birthdays, recognize outstanding performances, and the like. These are ideal venues to periodically discuss the very real daily stresses of veterinary work and the mental and emotional toll it can take from time to time. By discussing it in the open, perhaps even sharing some of the mental health and wellbeing research findings, it acknowledges the universality of stress and the impact that it has on individuals. Open discussion can help remove the stigma of mental health issues and help those in distress realize that they are not alone in experiencing it. It's easy for individuals to feel "it just must be me" if no one else is verbalizing their concerns.

Occasionally, team meetings involve outside speakers. It would be prudent to invite local mental health professionals and financial planners to talk about resources available in the community. That helps employees learn firsthand about assistance that is readily available. While the Merck Animal Health Veterinarian Wellbeing Studies were conducted among veterinarians, there is every reason to believe that the same stresses affect non-veterinarian staff members as well. Consequently, making these topics important components of team meetings will build awareness among all employees.

Encouraging preparation for crises While most veterinary organizations will never face a life-or-death mental health crisis, some may. It's important to be prepared in case one occurs. Here are several suggestions.

- The National Suicide Prevention Lifeline poster should be placed in the break room. This makes the lifeline number readily available to anyone that may wish to call it.
- Individuals should be encouraged to dial 9-1-1 any time that they think someone may be a danger to themselves or others.
- Appropriate resources can be accessed in any community in the USA by typing "mobile crisis" into the search engine on a computer or smartphone.
- Texting "Hello" to 741,741 will provide immediate access to a trained counselor.

Summary

Although the average level of wellbeing among veterinarians is similar to the US adult population, the issues facing veterinarians are different. This starts with the profile of veterinarians in distress. Younger practitioners who work as employees (not owners) with high student debt are particularly vulnerable to poorer wellbeing and mental health. They work longer hours than their peers, perhaps in part to pay down debt. It is currently unknown whether, like their older peers, they will exhibit better wellbeing than the US population at an older age or whether systemic changes in the profession have put them on a path of permanent lower wellbeing.

Veterinary work also requires constant interaction with clients and co-workers, which can be especially stressful for the majority of veterinarians, who are introverts.

The majority of veterinarians also score higher than average in neuroticism, which makes them vulnerable to experiencing unpleasant emotions. The vast majority of new graduate veterinarians are women, who tend to score higher in neuroticism than men.

Veterinarians should strive to develop good mental health defenses early; veterinary social workers can provide assistance in this regard. First, veterinarians should be encouraged to develop a stress management plan that works effectively for them. Ideally, that should be developed while still at university; it will be extremely helpful whether studying for an anatomy exam, preparing for the licensing boards, or facing a personal crisis. Second, veterinarians should develop good work-life balance habits early, including a focus on building healthy personal relationship with friends and family, e.g., spending time with them frequently, going for a short walk, and spending a few minutes on the phone. Additional strategies to promote good mental health include avoiding excessive time on social media, developing hobbies, and reading for pleasure.

Veterinary practices and other organizations that employ veterinarians should be alert to the challenges that veterinarians face, especially young veterinarians. They should discuss mental health and wellbeing in employee meetings, encourage those who feel overwhelmed to seek professional counseling, help to reduce the stigma associated with mental illness, and provide an Employee Assistance Program that makes it easier for employees to access help.

Psychologists and social workers can be especially valuable resources to veterinarians. Understanding veterinarians' vulnerabilities and the environments in which they work can make counseling more productive. Also, professional counselors can be especially useful in helping young veterinarians develop habits that can help reduce the risk of serious psychological distress throughout their careers.

Veterinary medicine is not just a profession; it's a calling. In the second MAH Veterinarian Wellbeing Study, when respondents were asked to rate 14 different dimensions of veterinary work, the 2 receiving the highest agreement were "I am invested in my work and take pride in doing a good job" (8.9/10) and "My work makes a positive contribution to other people's lives" (8.3/10) (Volk et al., 2020). That suggests a very high level of emotional involvement in their profession and makes good mental health and wellbeing especially important.

References

Bain, B., Hansen, C., Ouedraogo, F., Radich, R., & Saloi, M. (2020). *Economic state of the veterinary profession*. American Veterinary Medical Association. https://ebusiness.avma.org/ProductCatalog/product.aspx?ID=1905. Accessed 25 January 2021.

Cantril, H. (1965). *The pattern of human concerns*. Rutgers University Press.

Coles, T. (2018). *Introduction to professional wellbeing with overview of compassion fatigue and burnout*. Presentation to the American Association of Veterinary Laboratory Diagnosticians, Kansas City, MO, 20 October 2018.

Davis, D. J., Doerr, H. M., Grzelak, A. K., Busi, S. B., Jasarevic, E., Ericsson, A. C., & Bryda, E. C. (2016). Lactobacillus plantarum attenuates anxiety-related behavior and protects against stress-induced dysbiosis in adult zebrafish. *Scientific Reports, 6*, 33726.

Diener, E., Emmons, R. A., Larsen, R. J., & Griffin, S. (1985). The satisfaction with life scale. *Journal of Personality Assessment, 49*, 71–75.

Freedman, V. A. (2017). The panel study of Income Dynamics' Wellbeing and Daily Life Supplement (PSID-WB) user guide: Final release 1. Institute for Social Research, University of Michigan.

Helliwell, J., Layard, R., Sachs, J., & De Neve, J-E. (2020). *World happiness report 2020*. https://happiness-report.s3.amazonaws.com/2020/WHR20.pdf. Accessed 25 January 2021.

Kessler, R. C., et al. (2003). Screening for serious mental illness in the general population. *Archives of General Psychiatry, 60*, 184–189.

Mccrae, R. R., & John, O. P. (1992). An introduction to the 5-factor model and its applications. *Journal of Personality, 60*(2), 175–215.

Mujcic, R., & Oswald, A. J. (2016). Evolution of well-being and happiness after increases in consumption of fruit and vegetables. *American Journal of Public Health, 106*(8), 1504–1510.

Substance Use and Mental Health Services Administration. (2019). *Key substance use and mental health indicators in the United States: Results from the 2018 national survey on drug use and health*. (HHS Publication No. PEP19-5068, NSDUH Series H-54). Rockville, MD: Center for Behavioral Health Statistics and Quality, Substance Abuse and Mental Health Services Administration. Available at https://www.samhsa.gov/data/sites/default/files/cbhsq-reports/NSDUHNationalFindingsReport2018/NSDUHNationalFindingsReport2018.pdf. Accessed 25 January 2021.

Pribis, P. (2016). Effects of walnut consumption on mood in young adults—A randomized controlled trial. *Nutrients, 8*(11). Available at https://doi.org/10.3390/nu8110668. Accessed 25 January 2021.

Schimmack, U. (2008). The structure of subjective wellbeing. In M. Eid & R. J. Larsen (Eds.), *The science of subjective well-being* (pp. 97–123). Guilford.

Schimmack, U., Schupp, J., & Wagner, G. G. (2008). The influence of environment and personality on the affective and cognitive component of subjective well-being. *Social Indicators Research, 89*, 41–60.

Shanafelt, T. D., West, C. P., Sinsky, C., Trockel, M., Tutty, M., Satele, D. V., … Dyrbye, L. (2019). Changes in burnout and satisfaction with work-life integration in physicians and the general US working population between 2011 and 2017. *Mayo Clinic Proceedings, 94*(9), 1681–1694.

Steel, P., Schmidt, J., & Shultz, J. (2008). Refining the relationship between personality and subjective well-being. *Psychological Bulletin, 134*(1), 138–161.

Tomasi, S., & Fechter-Legett, E. (2019). Suicide rate among veterinarians from 1979 through 2015. *Journal of the American Veterinary Medical Association, 254*(1), 104–112.

Volk, J. O., Schimmack, U., Strand, E., Lord, L. K., & Siren, C. W. (2017). *Merck animal health veterinarian wellbeing study*. Unpublished research available from the author.

Volk, J. O., Schimmack, U., Strand, E., Lord, L. K., & Siren, C. W. (2018). Executive summary of the Merck Animal Health veterinarian wellbeing study. *Journal of the American Veterinary Medical Association, 252*(10), 1231–1238.

Volk, J. O., Schimmack, U., Strand, E., Vasconcelos, J., & Siren, C. W. (2020). Executive summary of the Merck Animal Health veterinarian wellbeing study II. *Journal of the American Veterinary Medical Association, 256*(11), 1237–1244.

Volk, J. O., & Strand, E. (2018). 3 steps to a healthier team. *DVM360, 49*(10), 34–35.

Whippman, R. (2017). Happiness is other people. *New York Times*, October 29, sec. SR, p. 1.

Chapter 11
Veterinary and Other Animal-Related Practice Management and Veterinary Social Work

Pamela Linden

Introduction

What do veterinary social workers need to know about animal-related practice settings? How can veterinary and other animal-related practice managers learn how veterinary social workers can add value to their settings? How can practice managers and veterinary social workers collaborate to improve the experiences of pet owners or clients, as well as enhance the animal-related practice setting?

To achieve optimal outcomes, an interprofessional team is created between veterinary social workers, veterinarians, and other professionals in animal-related settings who work together to achieve goals. Each team member should be aware of the knowledge, values, and skills of their interprofessional partners. Nancarrow et al. (2013) state "interdisciplinary teamwork is a complex process in which different types of staff work together to share expertise, knowledge, and skills to impact on patient care" (p. 1). They provide ten principles of high-functioning interdisciplinary teamwork: positive leadership and management attributes; communication strategies and structures; personal rewards, training, and development; appropriate resources and procedures; appropriate skill mix; supportive team climate; individual characteristics that support interdisciplinary teamwork; clarity of vision; quality and outcomes of care; and respecting and understanding roles. This chapter explores the veterinary social work scope of practice and discusses typical veterinary social work activities performed within veterinary and other animal-related settings. In addition, common challenges in veterinary settings are explored along with a review of typical roles of veterinary team members working in a variety of veterinary settings.

P. Linden (✉)
University of Tennessee, College of Social Work, Knoxville, TN, USA
e-mail: plinden@utk.edu

Who Are Veterinary Social Workers?

Veterinary social workers support and strengthen interdisciplinary partnerships that attend to the intersection of humans and animals (International Association of Veterinary Social Work, 2020). The term "veterinary social worker" refers to licensed social workers who have completed a standardized training program in veterinary social work. Dr. Elizabeth Strand is credited with having founded the field of veterinary social work in 2002 as a collaboration between the University of Tennessee-Knoxville (UTK) College of Social Work and the College of Veterinary Medicine, and, in 2010, she created the first veterinary social work certificate training program. At the time of this writing, several other institutions of higher education in the USA and Canada are developing programs based on the UTK model. Veterinary social work certificate training programs prepare social workers to intervene in four areas of veterinary social work practice: animal-related grief and bereavement, animal-assisted interventions, the link between human and animal violence, and compassion fatigue and conflict management.

Veterinary social work certificate students independently complete online modules in each of the four areas, participate in group supervision sessions, and complete a 250-hour service learning keystone practicum whose topic falls within one or more of the four areas of veterinary social work. Each student at the time of their VSW certificate graduation ceremony declares the Veterinary Social Work Oath, originally penned by Dr. Elizabeth Strand. The oath, reproduced below, provides context and definition to veterinary social worker aims:

> Specializing in veterinary social work, I pledge my service to society by tending to the human needs that arise in the relationship between humans and animals. From a strengths perspective and using evidence-based practice, I will uphold the ethical code of my profession, respect and promote the dignity and worth of all species, and diligently strive to maintain mindful balance in all of my professional endeavors.

The oath acknowledges the graduate's training in veterinary social work concepts and practices, identifies the veterinary social worker as a specialist, and prioritizes the veterinary social worker's service to others above self-interest. Notably, the oath unequivocally identifies the human, not the animal or pet, as the target client system of veterinary social work interventions. Neither traditional social work education curricula nor veterinary social work training include content on how to help animals. Veterinary social work is an interdisciplinary practice area that focuses on human needs, and their veterinary and other animal-related setting partners attend to the needs of the animals.

The Veterinary Social Work Oath reinforces the central role of the Strengths Perspective (Saleebey, 1992) as the guiding practice framework for veterinary social workers. This perspective suggests that targets of social work intervention be "see in the light of their capacities, talents, competencies, possibilities, visions, values, and hopes" (Saleebey, 1996, p. 296). Key concepts of the Strengths Perspective include empowerment, resilience, and membership to a viable group or community. The oath directs veterinary social workers to employ evidence-based strategies to address individual, group, and organizational challenges to promote the health and well-being of individuals in veterinary or other animal-related settings. Further, veterinary social workers are aware that significant disparities exist for workers in animal-related settings based on race, ethnicity, gender, sexual identity, romantic preference, age, ability, and socioeconomic status. Veterinary social workers bring attention to these disparities and work to ameliorate them by expanding access to veterinary care and working to increase the diversity of veterinary professionals entering and staying in the field. Ethical guidelines promulgated by the National Association of Social Workers (NASW) in its *Code of Ethics* (2017) further inform social work practice. The *Code* sets forth broad ethical principles that are based on social work's core values of service, social justice, dignity and worth of the person, importance of human relationships, integrity, and competence. Reflecting a focus on the intersection of humans and animals in veterinary social work practice, the Veterinary Social Work Oath extends the *Code*'s reach to include the core value of dignity and worth from "the person" to "all species." Lastly, veterinary social workers pledge to maintain mindful balance in their professional endeavors to prevent compassion fatigue and promote well-being through self-care strategies. The next section provides a brief review of the various types of settings in which veterinary care services are performed.

Veterinary Medicine and Practice Settings

Veterinarians provide preventive/wellness, sick or injury, and emergency medical care to nonhuman animals. The American Veterinary Medical Association (AVMA) (2019) provides a unifying definition of veterinary medicine:

> to diagnose, prognose, treat, correct, change, alleviate, or prevent animal disease, illness, pain, deformity, defect, injury, or other physical, dental, or mental conditions by any method or mode; including the: i. performance of any medical or surgical procedure, or ii. prescription, dispensing, administration, or application of any drug, medicine, biologic, apparatus, anesthetic, or other therapeutic or diagnostic substance, or iii. use of complementary, alternative, and integrative therapies, or iv. use of any procedure for reproductive management, including but not limited to the diagnosis or treatment of pregnancy, fertility, sterility, or infertility, or v. determination of the health, fitness, or soundness of an animal, or vi. physical rehabilitation, meaning the use of therapeutic exercise and the application of modalities intended to restore or facilitate movement and physical function impacted by disease, injury, or disability. vii. rendering of advice or recommendation by any means including telephonic and other electronic communications with regard to any of the above.

Veterinary care may be provided in a variety of settings, and the setting name denotes the type of veterinary practice that is conducted. Veterinary social workers should be prepared to provide services specific to the host setting and be able to discern similarities and differences between types of veterinary settings. The American Veterinary Medical Association (2021a) offers the following description of types and functions of common veterinary settings (Table 11.1).

Table 11.1 Veterinary settings and associated functions

Setting	Functions
Veterinary teaching hospital	A facility in which consultative, clinical, and hospital services are rendered and in which a large staff of basic and applied veterinary scientists perform significant research and teach professional veterinary students (doctor of veterinary Medicine or equivalent degree) and house officers
Hospital/clinic	A facility in which the practice conducted typically or may include in-patient as well as out-patient diagnostics and treatment
Outpatient clinic	A facility in which the practice conducted typically or may include in-patient as well as out-patient diagnostics and treatment
Mobile practice	A veterinary practice conducted from a vehicle with special medical or surgical facilities, or from a vehicle suitable for making house or farm calls. Regardless of mode of transportation, such practice shall have a permanent base of operations with a published address and telecommunication capabilities for making appointments or responding to emergency situations
Emergency facility	One with the primary function of receiving, treating, and monitoring of emergency patients during its specified hours of operation. A veterinarian is in attendance at all hours of operation and sufficient staff is available to provide timely and appropriate care. Veterinarians, support staff, instrumentation, medications, and supplies must be sufficient to provide an appropriate level of emergency care. A veterinary emergency service may be an independent, after-hours service, an independent 24-hour service, or part of a full-service hospital
Specialty facility	A veterinary or animal facility that provides services by board-certified veterinary specialists
Referral facility	Provides services by those veterinarians with a special interest in certain species or a particular area of veterinary medicine
Center	Center—The word "center" in the name of a veterinary or animal facility strongly implies an advanced depth or scope of practice, e.g., Animal medical center, veterinary imaging center, canine sports medicine center

Source: American Veterinary Medical Association (2021a)

Just as settings vary, so too do roles and responsibilities of individuals working within veterinary host settings. Veterinary social workers should be familiar with the roles and responsibilities of individuals commonly found in veterinary settings.

Roles and Responsibilities in Veterinary Settings

Many diverse roles can be found in veterinary and other animal-related settings. Depending on the type and size of the practice or organization, most will likely employ one or more licensed veterinarians, licensed veterinary technicians or nurses, veterinary assistants, kennel workers, front desk/reception clerks, maintenance workers, and practice managers. Veterinarians are trained to examine animals to assess their health and diagnose problems; treat and dress wounds; perform surgery on animals; test for and vaccinate against diseases; operate medical equipment, such as x-ray machines; advise animal owners about general care, medical conditions, and treatments; prescribe medication; and euthanize animals. Veterinarians must complete a Doctor of Veterinary Medicine (DVM or VMD) degree at an accredited college of veterinary medicine (United States Department of Labor, 2021b).

Veterinary technicians carry out medical orders prescribed by a supervising veterinarian and may perform a variety of functions to assist veterinarians and help the animals in their care. They may prepare and give medications; take x-rays; collect blood, urine, and fecal specimens for lab analysis; induce and maintain anesthesia; and assist with medical, dental, and surgical procedures (United States Department of Labor, 2021c). They are required to pass the Veterinary Technician National Examination (VTNE). The National Association of Veterinary Technicians in America (NAVTA), 2016 member survey reported that animal nursing, anesthesia, client communication, and client education are the primary functions of veterinary technicians (National Association of Veterinary Technicians in America, 2016).

Veterinary assistants require training, but not formal education to perform the skills of restraining pets during examinations and treatment, feeding, bathing, and exercising the animals. Veterinary assistants may assist veterinarians and veterinary technicians to draw blood and collect urine samples. They feed and monitor pets, clean kennels and operating and examination rooms, and sterilize surgical equipment. Veterinary assistants may assist in euthanasia procedures with or without the pet owners present and may be responsible for the disposition of the animal's remains. Veterinary assistants, who may have a high school diploma or equivalent and on-the-job training, may apply for the Approved Veterinary Assistant (AVA) designation from the National Association of Veterinary Technicians in America (NAVTA). This voluntary certification requires graduation from a NAVTA-approved training program and passing an exam.

Additional personnel are needed to ensure the care of the animals, to address the needs of the human clients, and to attend to the business aspects of the practice. Kennel workers are responsible for cleaning and sterilizing animal cages and runs. They work with the maintenance staff to identify and address issues to ensure that the facility is safe and clean for animals, clients, and staff. Front desk receptionists provide customer service such as greeting customers, answering questions, processing incoming patients, and handling payments. They answer phone calls and manage the appointment schedule. Generally, front desk receptionists update and manage patient charts. Some veterinary practices also employ practice managers. Veterinary practice management refers to the business skills, budgeting, leadership, teamwork, marketing, and other strategies necessary to build and sustain successful veterinary practices.

The American Veterinary Medical Association (2021b) recognizes that veterinary practices "need to create supportive, healthy workplaces that nurture individual and workplace wellbeing." The American Animal Hospital Association (AAHA) reported in 2016 that "workplace culture and relationships may have a significant impact on key business metrics at veterinary clinics." The AAHA is the only organization that accredits veterinary practices in the USA and Canada. As of 2021, only

12 percent to 15 percent of veterinary practices in the USA and Canada hold the "AAHA-accredited" designation (American Animal Hospital Association, 2021).

To improve veterinary workplace culture and build successful teams, the AVMA offers resource toolkits to practice managers on topics such as new hire training, employee performance feedback, effective team meetings, and team-building activities. In an effort to recognize the specialized skills and experiences of veterinary practice managers, the Veterinary Hospital Managers Association, Inc. offers the Certified Veterinary Practice Manager (CVPM) certification to qualified managers. Veterinary practice managers perform key human resource functions. Generally, these include overseeing employee relations, securing regulatory compliance, and administering employee-related services such as payroll, training, and benefits. They typically plan and coordinate an organization's workforce to best use employees' talents; link an organization's management with its employees; plan and oversee employee benefit programs; serve as a consultant to advise other managers on human resources issues, such as equal employment opportunity and sexual harassment; coordinate and supervise the work of specialists and support staff; oversee an organization's recruitment, interview, selection, and hiring processes; and handle staffing issues, such as mediating disputes and directing disciplinary procedures (United States Bureau of Labor Statistics, 2021a).

Veterinary social workers may be called upon to assist individuals in a variety of other animal-related roles. These groups include students of veterinary medicine and veterinary nursing, pet parents/animal owners, zookeepers, animal rescue workers, animal-assisted therapy and service/guide animal trainers, volunteers and service recipients, service and guide animal handlers and volunteers, farmers, animal laboratory workers, animal shelter workers, animal food production workers, first responders (firefighters, law enforcement), municipal animal control officers, and pet crematory and cemetery workers. Veterinary social workers also interact with pet-owner clients, and representatives of unowned animals, such as animal control officers, rescue and shelter groups, and good-willed individuals who bring in found injured animals for veterinary care.

Students enrolled in colleges of veterinary medicine and veterinary technician or nursing programs may be integrated into a veterinary setting to fulfill educational requirements for a degree program. They may be performing in a practicum, internship, or other short-term training experience.

Contemporary Challenges in Veterinary and Other Animal-Related Settings

The human side of veterinary medicine has received little attention. However, recent research has shed light on the types of individual and group challenges that are commonly found in veterinary settings. These challenges include compassion fatigue (Stoewen, 2020), burnout (Ouedraogo et al., 2021), moral distress (Moses et al.,

2018), conflict (Wojtacka et al., 2020), and others. (For an in-depth discussion of each of these issues, see in this volume Chaps. 3, 9, and 10)

Surveys of veterinarians and veterinary technicians have illuminated significant ongoing challenges that impact individual well-being and job satisfaction. The 2016 National Association of Veterinary Technicians in America survey reported an estimated turnover rate of 22 percent for veterinary technicians and 31 percent for other veterinary staff. They found that low pay, and compassion fatigue and burnout, and lack of recognition and career advancement remain ongoing concerns in the veterinary technology profession.

Veterinary technicians identified office dynamics and communication, client noncompliance, and lack of resources within the clinic as the greatest challenges they face in practice (National Association of Veterinary Technicians in America, 2016). Hayes et al. (2020) surveyed 256 US- and Canada-based veterinary technicians and found associations between burnout and frequency of self-reported medical error, resilience, and depression and job-related risk factors, including factors related to the physical work environment, workload and schedule, compensation package, interpersonal relationships, intellectual enrichment, and exposure to ethical conflicts. They found that burnout, characterized by high emotional exhaustion, depersonalization, and low sense of personal accomplishment, was common, together with compassion fatigue. Although 70 percent of surveyed veterinary technicians indicated that the topic of compassion fatigue was discussed at their practice, only 23 percent of practices offered support for team members experiencing compassion fatigue. Almost 2 percent said a fellow co-worker had committed suicide because of compassion fatigue, yet only 3 percent of those respondents had had grief counseling provided to the team (National Association of Veterinary Technicians in America, 2016).

Recently, veterinary student mental health and well-being has received widespread attention. Strand et al. (2017) investigated adverse childhood experiences (ACEs) among 1118 veterinary medical students. They found that students who had experienced four or more ACEs had an approximately threefold increase in signs of clinical depression and higher than average stress when compared to students who had experienced no ACEs. They found that veterinary students are no more at risk of poor mental health due to ACEs than the general population. Nahm and Chun (2020) examined stressors leading to depression, stress, and anxiety in a sample of veterinary students studying in ten veterinary colleges in Korea. They found that female and preclinical students are more vulnerable to depression, anxiety, and stress. Drake et al. (2012) found elevated scores of anxiety and depression in a sample of 142 veterinary medical students across 4-year cohorts, with students in their second and third years having the highest anxiety and depression scores. The higher prevalence was attributed to physical health, unclear expectations, difficulty fitting in, heavy workload, and homesickness. Karaffa and Hancock (2019) investigated mental health experiences and rates of mental health service use in a sample of 573 veterinary students from multiple institutions. They found that approximately one-third of participants reported levels of depression or anxiety above the clinical cutoff, and depression and anxiety were associated with prior engagement in non-suicidal self-injury (NSSI), suicidal ideation, and prior suicide attempts. Nearly 80 percent of participants who scored above the clinical cutoff for depression or anxiety reported seeking some form of mental health services currently or in the past, and a majority reported having positive experiences with services. Results also indicated a higher than typical rate of NSSI among veterinary medical students. (See Chap. 12 in this volume and Karaffa, Bradtke, and Hancock (2020) for a detailed discussion of embedded university counseling services in colleges of veterinary medicine.)

Veterinary Social Work Service Delivery Models

There are a variety of service delivery models for veterinary social work services. A veterinary social worker can be embedded in a veterinary setting full time or part time with an office on-site or off-site. Veterinary settings can contract with a veterinary social worker to be on-call. This model allows the veterinary social worker to work with more than one veterinary practice and be available for crisis debriefing, emergencies, and consultations with veterinary staff regarding the non-veterinary medical needs and concerns of pet owners. The work that a veterinary social worker performs may contribute to improvement in employee turnover rates by improving the setting culture, increasing teamwork, and reducing the likelihood that employees experience compassion fatigue and burnout.

Veterinary social workers may work with only veterinary staff, only pet owners, or both. Although the veterinary social work service and the practice management/human resource department may be involved in employment-related issues, only practice management/human resource representatives directly affect the individual's employment status, performance review, and compensation.

Establishing the Veterinary Social Work Practice

Veterinary social workers use their specialized knowledge and expertise to enhance human-to-human interactions in animal-related settings. Although each veterinary or animal-related setting is different based on type, size, location, and business model, there are a number of standardized policies and procedures that veterinary social workers should address to begin a veterinary social work practice.

The VSW should establish the scope of their practice in the veterinary or animal-related setting based on the activities reflected in the level of their social work licensure. One of the social work values provided in the NASW's *Code of Ethics* is competence. VSWs should practice within the scope of their experience and expertise and engage in professional development activities to expand their knowledge base. The veterinary social worker should request time during a regular staff meeting or special meeting to describe the role, function, and policies of the veterinary social work service.

A client agreement should be provided to individuals and group participants that describes, at a minimum, the scope of practice, terms of services, cost of service, and limits of service. VSW referrals may be initiated by veterinarians, veterinary technicians, reception/admitting service, and practice managers. Animal-related professionals, students, and volunteers may self-refer to the VSW practice. The VSW referral protocol should be conveyed to anyone referring a pet-owner client. In keeping with the social work value of self-determination, employees and pet-owner clients should not be mandated to participate in the VSW service.

Veterinary social workers should develop aesthetically appealing material that conveys the nature of the services being provided. Informational pamphlets describing the VSW service should be printed and posted on the practice or organization's website. Promotional material may include brochures, business cards, and informational handouts on a variety of relevant topics targeted to specific populations. Topics appropriate for clients/pet owners may include understanding feelings associated with pet loss, end-of-life decision-making, self-care for the caregiver, living with a pet with a chronic medical condition, and locating low-cost/no cost pet-related community resources. Helpful materials with topics designed for veterinary professionals may include setting and maintaining boundaries, creating a self-care routine, fundamentals of teamwork, managing conflict at home and in the workplace, how to ask for help, techniques to manage stress, and improving active listening and communication skills. Veterinary and other animal-related staff may find information useful on topics of mindfulness, sleep and health, choosing healthy foods, successful budgeting strategies, boundary setting, and negotiating and asking for what you need. The VSW should include their contact information and a brief description of how to request services on all materials. Promotional materials can be posted outside the VSW office and positioned prominently in the lounge/break area.

The ethical value of confidentiality should be maintained at all times. As such, VSWs should refrain from confirming or denying if an employee or pet-owner client contacts or received VSW services. In situations in which a pet owner requests that the VSW discuss information about their pet with the veterinarian or other animal-related professional, the VSW should gain consent in writing beforehand.

Client notes, or documentation of services provided, are used to facilitate the delivery of services, ensure continuity of care, protect clients' privacy and ensure reasonable future access to client treatment history. Notes are an important part of maintaining professional practice standards and should only be accessible by the VSW. Social workers should store records following termination of services. The VSW should document activities with and on behalf of the client and be in a Subjective, Objective, Assessment, and Plan (SOAP) format. Notes should indicate the date and time of interaction, the client name, and the VSW name. VSWs should protect time in their schedule to write case notes. Notes should be documented as soon as possible following the interaction to ensure accuracy. Timely note writing is important for professional accountability. This offers the opportunity for the VSW to reflect on the client interaction and develop goals of care, thus improving client outcomes.

Documentation should protect clients' privacy and should only include information relevant to the delivery of the social work service. To protect client confidentiality, VSWs should avoid noting client interactions in the animal medical record or chart. Client forms, such as agreements and informed consent for release of information, should be stored in the client's file. Paper files should be locked when not in use, and electronic systems should be password protected and utilize whatever other safeguards may be necessary to ensure the confidentiality of the information as required by the Health Information Portability and Accountability Act (HIPAA).

In order to further ensure confidentiality and privacy, thoughtful consideration should be given to the location, entryway, and privacy of the office. The practice should avoid placing the veterinary social worker's office in a high traffic volume area to increase the likelihood that individuals will seek help when they need it without being concerned that others in the setting will see them going into and out of the veterinary social worker office. Ample space should be available to conduct educational groups, wellness activities, or other small or large group activities. Veterinary social workers should have a separate telephone line and email to ensure confidential communications with people seeking and utilizing the veterinary social work service.

Applied VSW: Four Areas of Veterinary Social Work

Veterinary and other animal-related settings provide opportunities for VSWs to address concerns related to the four areas of veterinary social work. The following section details the strategies veterinary social workers may engage in to address these important human aspects of veterinary and other animal-related settings.

The Link between Human and Animal Violence

The link between human and animal violence may involve the welfare of companion animals affected by violent interpersonal relationships, animal neglect, abandonment, intentional harm, dog fighting, backyard breeding, and animal hoarding. VSWs should be familiar with local, state, and federal laws on animal abuse and collaborate with local animal control officers and law enforcement personnel involved in cases of alleged animal abuse and neglect. The VSW can provide assessment and treatment, make referrals, and coordinate services for the people involved in the case, while animal-related organizations address the health and welfare needs of the affected animals. Veterinary social workers can provide training to veterinarians and hospital staff on what to look for and how to respond when they suspect abuse. They can establish mutually beneficial partnerships with domestic violence shelter organizations, and if they don't already provide safe shelter for pets of those seeking shelter, they can assist in creating community-based resources to keep families safe together. Veterinary social workers can consult with courts on interpersonal violence (IPV) cases when pets are involved, and with governing bodies like local and state legislatures to draft policies that protect pet owners and pets involved in interpersonally violent relationships. Community abuse prevention programs can mobilize like-minded people to change policies and save lives. The veterinary social worker adds value to the team by raising awareness of the link between IPV and animal abuse, creating mutually beneficial linkages with law enforcement, and linking potential victims of IPV with helpful resources to keep them, their loved ones, and pets safe. For a detailed discussion of the link between human and animal maltreatment and violence, see the chapter authored by Susan Hatters Friedman and colleagues in this volume.

Animal-Related Grief and Bereavement

Because pets are unable to communicate their wants, needs, and preferences, pet owners must act in the capacity of surrogate decision-maker for their pets. A grave or terminal prognosis, or the sudden onset of severe illness or injury, places pet owners in the position of making end-of-life decisions for their pets. Veterinary social workers can help families make difficult decisions regarding palliative or hospice care, and euthanasia. Working alongside the veterinarian, the veterinary social worker can assist in end-of-life decision-making with the pet owner. When veterinary social workers are available, veterinarians and other practice staff can attend to the patient's needs while the veterinary social worker supports the pet owner.

Veterinary social workers can assist pet owners in asking veterinary providers direct questions or voicing their concerns so that they can make informed end-of-life decisions jointly with the treating veterinarian to minimize their pet's suffering or distress.

When a beloved pet dies, many pet owners' feelings of grief are referred to as disenfranchised because there is no socially sanctioned ritual to acknowledge the painful loss. Disenfranchised grief is experienced when a loss cannot be openly acknowledged, socially sanctioned, or publicly mourned (Doka, 1989). Offering pet loss grief and bereavement veterinary social work services may convey to pet owners that the practice acknowledges the strength and value of the bond people have with their animals. Feelings of goodwill can be generated by offering opportunities for pet owners to process their grief with veterinary social workers. Veterinary social workers can add value to an animal-related practice by offering emotional support and sharing resources to help them understand and cope with the death of their pet. Veterinary social workers may contact families after the loss and validate feelings of grief. This can be a relief to process their thoughts and feelings with a social worker with specialized training in pet-related grief and bereavement. Some families may gain comfort by sharing their loss with other pet owners grieving the loss of a pet. Veterinary social workers may offer pet loss support groups to facilitate resolution of pet owner grief. These groups provide opportunities for pet owners to explore their thoughts and feelings surrounding their pet's life and the meaning of the loss of their pet. Pet owners experiencing complicated, or prolonged grief, may be referred to grief specialists for continued treatment.

When requested, veterinary social workers can provide in-person support during the euthanasia procedure. The word "euthanasia" has a Greek origin, *eu* meaning "good" and *thanatos*, meaning "death." In-home euthanasia veterinary service may be an option, depending on the availability of veterinarians in the area who are credentialed in home euthanasia procedures. Veterinary social workers may discuss with the client post-euthanasia options, including disposition of their pet's remains, including individual cremation, group cremation, pet cemetery burial, or, if allowed in their municipality, home burial. Veterinary social workers may explore with families meaningful ways to memorialize their pet and the bond that they shared. Memorials, which can be homemade or purchased, help people cope with the death of their pet by honoring the bond they shared. Families can repurpose a pet's food or water bowl into a plant container decorated with the departed pet's collar or leash. A shadow box with the pet's favorite toys and photos of the pet can be created and displayed in the home. Pet owners can purchase personalized stones or plaques, etched crystal mementos with the image of the pet and their name, and jewelry containing pet cremains. These items can be purchased online or through the pet crematory who handled the pet's remains. The availability of veterinary social work service can create goodwill between veterinarians and their clients by acknowledging, valuing, and honoring the bond between people and their pets.

Compassion Fatigue and Conflict Management

Compassion fatigue describes a "work-related stress response in healthcare providers that is considered a 'cost of caring' and a key contributor to the loss of compassion in healthcare" (Sinclair et al., 2017, p. 9). First used to describe a cluster of signs and symptoms exhibited by individuals who provide care to others, compassion fatigue has been identified as a major concern in veterinary practice environments (Stoewen, 2020). Veterinary social workers can help those employed in animal-practice settings to address and prevent compassion fatigue through individual, group, and organizational interventions. On the individual level, veterinary social workers can offer debriefing following crises or stressful events and provide supportive counseling to veterinary staff. Some practices offer on-site veterinary social workers; practice staff can drop in or make appointments to talk confidentially about their concerns.

At the group level, veterinary practices can provide education to practice staff on the topics of wellness, emotional regulation, conflict management, and mindfulness. (For an additional discussion of these topics, see in this volume Chaps. 3 and 10.) These sessions can build teamwork and improve the culture of the work environment and positively impact staff morale. Helping veterinary staff improve communication skills can reduce conflict in the workplace and improve teamwork. Working with a veterinary social worker can increase self-awareness, build cohesive teams, identify common stressors, and find ways to manage stressors. Some veterinarians and animal-related staff may find it useful to participate in Veterinary Social Work Grand Rounds to process thoughts and feelings about stressful cases or interactions. Dr. Elizabeth Strand's "How to Conduct Veterinary Social Work Grand Rounds" guide can be found at the end of this chapter as Appendix A. Incorporating "Ten guidelines for making conversations with emotional charge productive," found at the end of this chapter as Appendix B may enhance the efficacy of these and other group conversations.

Animal-Assisted Interventions

Veterinary social workers are trained to provide education to organizations and communities about the various species and breeds of animals that are commonly employed to benefit people, training, and laws involving a wide variety of assistance animals. Veterinary social workers may assist with interviewing, training, and supporting owner/handler teams. As proponents of evidence-supported interventions, veterinary social workers may advocate that organizations providing service animals are accredited by Assistance Dogs International Standards for Service Animals (Assistance Dogs International, 2021).

Volunteers and handlers who provide comfort visits to congregate care facilities may find it challenging to directly observing people who are incarcerated (jails), actively dying (hospice), or ill/injured (hospitals/rehab centers). Recipients of animal-assisted intervention visits may talk with owners/handlers about their pain, loneliness, fear, and/or anxiety. Veterinary social workers can debrief teams following challenging visits and provide disability etiquette training to owner/handler teams to prepare them to interact with people with disabilities with dignity and respect. Veterinary social workers may be called upon to assess potential owner/handler motivation to volunteer with their trained companion animal. They can also create opportunities to build volunteer camaraderie and strengthen teamwork. These activities may generate goodwill between volunteers and organizations that host animal-assisted intervention teams. For an in-depth discussion of animal-assisted interventions, see Chap. 5.

Emotional support animals are companion animals that are not required to have any special training. The need for the emotional support animal must be denoted in writing by a licensed mental health professional to be a therapeutic necessity for someone living with chronic mental health symptoms and who has a condition that meets the legal definition of a disability. Emotional support animals (ESA) are recognized within federal disability legislation, with limited rights to those who have emotional support animals as accommodations for their disabilities. "Under current federal legislation, people seeking to own an ESA must have a disability that can be alleviated or ameliorated through emotional support provided by an animal" (Fine et al., 2019, p. 199). The letter of verification should include the professional's license, the state or jurisdiction of the license, date(s) of the license, the individual's clinical diagnosis, and a statement that the individual is under the care of this professional and that the animal is necessary for the individuals' functioning/treatment (Hoy-Gerlach et al., 2019).

Special Topics in Veterinary Social Work

Financial Barriers to Access to Veterinary Care

Temporary and chronic poverty affects every aspect of human life—social, physical health, mental health, housing stability, educational achievement, opportunities for gainful employment, and enjoyment of social relationships. Pet-related consequences of human poverty result in inequitable access to veterinary care for pets, insufficient nutritional pet food, and delay in accessing needed pet medication. Lack of preventive care (heartworm prevention, vaccinations, examinations) often result in more serious medication conditions or death. Poverty and associated consequences like eviction, homelessness, illness, and disability may lead to the relinquishment or surrender of pets to shelters and pet abandonment.

In 2018, the Access to Veterinary Care Coalition (AVCC) at the University of Tennessee surveyed pet owners and found that the overwhelming barrier to veterinary care is financial "with 80.0 percent unable to obtain preventative care due to financial constraints, 73.8 percent unable to obtain sick care, and 55.7 percent unable to obtain emergency care. Most at risk for not receiving recommended care are cats and dogs living in lower-income households with younger pet owners" (pp. 14–17). Pet owners may become distressed when they cannot afford to pay for diagnostics (e.g., radiographs, bloodwork) or treatment (surgery, medications) that could save their pet's life. Many animal rescue groups, shelters, and other animal welfare organizations can help with wellness (prevention and vaccinations) and spay or neuter surgeries. There are few options for families who cannot pay for sick, injury, and emergency veterinary care, and sometimes pets are euthanized because their owners cannot afford to pay for care for treatable medical conditions. In such instances, veterinary social workers may provide crisis intervention, suicide assessments, and referrals for mental health treatment for pet owners in need.

There is a stark contrast in perspectives regarding barriers to access to care between providers of veterinary services and consumers of veterinary services. In 2018, the Access to Veterinary Care Coalition (AVCC) commissioned a study that found among veterinarians, factors impacting their provision of financially accessible care include personal finances (e.g., student debt), concerns about standard of care, workplace policies, and devaluing professional services (p. 80). Among pet owners, socioeconomic and financial factors are significant barriers to accessing veterinary care along with transportation challenges, not having appropriate equipment (e.g., carrier), geographic barriers, and not knowing where to get care (p. 14).

Initiatives like the Humane Society of the United States Pets for Life program and the University of Tennessee Program for Pet Health Equity AlignCare program are creating national large-scale approaches to increase healthcare equity for pets. VSWs should be knowledgeable about a wide range of pet and non-pet-related resources in the local community to assist pet owners experiencing financial hardship. At a minimum, a local resource list should include referrals for pet food and supply pantry; low-cost/free spay/neuter providers; low-cost/free vaccination sites; affordable general veterinary and vet surgical care providers; vet care voucher sources, e.g., animal welfare organizations, like humane societies, rescue groups, and shelters; pet-friendly domestic violence shelters; grant programs to pay for boarding for safe escape from domestic violence; pet-friendly hotels for emergency/evacuation stays; and volunteer programs that help seniors and people with disabilities care for their pets. Appendix C to this chapter provides a listing of national organizations that may be able to provide pet-related assistance to pet owners in need of help (active at time of publication).

Lack of Diversity in Veterinary Medicine

The concepts of cultural competence and cultural sensitivity figure prominently in social work education, as do issues related to diversity, cultural sensitivity, and cultural competence. To address the lack of diversity in the veterinary profession, veterinary social workers can partner with veterinary exploration programs for high school students in geographically, racially, and economically diverse communities to expose young learners to careers in veterinary and affiliated careers. These programs allow underrepresented students to network with other students and professionals with similar interests. Veterinary social workers can contribute to national and international initiatives with governing and leadership coalitions that are aimed at increasing diversity, equity, and inclusion (DEI) industry-wide. Recently, industrial and educational leaders have partnered with associations such as the National Association for Black Veterinarians (NABV) and the Multicultural Veterinary Medical Association (MCVMA) to set target DEI goals of increasing diversity, equity, and inclusion in veterinary medicine.

Conclusion

Veterinary social workers (VSWs) attend to the human needs that arise in the intersection of veterinary medicine and social work. Collaborations with interprofessional partners in host settings create opportunities to address a wide range of issues, including the provision of support for and psychoeducation about animal loss, grief, and bereavement, strategies for coping with common life concerns and stressors, and the presence and impact of employment-related stressors. VSWs may refer clients for longer-term or specialized treatment of mental health concerns. Veterinary social work services may have a positive impact on employee turnover, resulting in savings in staff recruitment, orientation and training, and overtime for remaining staff due to staff vacancies. Veterinary professionals' time with patients is increased when veterinary social workers are available to provide direct nonclinical client services, such as end-of-life decision-making support. A veterinary social worker can provide communication assistance and provide emotional support to families instead of families' sole reliance on the veterinary professional and other veterinary team members. Additionally, veterinary staff can call for a veterinary social work consultation when they are concerned about the well-being of a pet.

Appendix A

How to conduct veterinary social work rounds

1. Gather your group together
2. Set the guidelines
(a) Affirm that the purpose of the group is to process the "human side of things" in providing medical care
(b) Everyone is invited to share or NOT share according to what would feel helpful to them at that time
(c) Review Ten Guidelines for Making Conversations with Emotional Charge Productive (Strand, n.d.)
(i) If you meet with a group in an ongoing way and they already know the eight guidelines you can summarize the guidelines by restating:
1. Everyone speaks for themselves
2. Avoid giving unasked advice
3. Be open, receptive, and supportive as you listen by noticing how you would feel in the situation being described
(d) Show your support for people nonverbally by drumming the table if you have empathy or resonate with what a person is saying
(e) State or re-state the structure of the group
(i) Short body scan and relaxation practice
(ii) Share challenges
(iii) Share victories
3. Invite participants to share a case that was a challenge
(a) Useful questions are as follows:
(i) What case lingered in your heart/mind?
(ii) What case did you have negative feelings about after the fact?
(iii) What case made you feel unsure or afraid?
(iv) What case caused you trouble sleeping?
(v) Was there a particular day or constellation of cases that was particularly stressful for you?

4. Invite participants to share what they were feeling throughout the case
(a) Angry, sad, afraid, guilty, disgusted, shocked, grateful, happy, secure, proud, etc.
(b) Role model drumming on the table if you would have shared those feelings
5. Invite participants to share what they did well in the case
6. Invite participants to share what they wish they had done better in the case
7. Invite participants to share what they learned from the case
8. Repeat steps 3–7 with others who have a case to share
9. Invite participants to share victories
(a) Useful questions are as follows:
(i) What was a case this week that was very satisfying?
(ii) What case made you feel great about being a veterinarian (or other animal-related professional?
(iii) What did you do this week as a veterinarian that was exciting?
1. Here let participants tell you cool medical things that were rewarding
10. If time and appropriate to the group you could end with going around the room and sharing
(a)What self-care activity have you done in the past week?
(b) What self-care activity do you commit to doing in the next week (or month or whatever time frame)?
(c) What have you learned most in the past year/month, etc., (this is particularly goof for residents and interns)?

Used with permission from Dr. Elizabeth Strand

Notes:

- Describe that veterinary social work rounds are a way to process emotions that get stuck when we handle a stressful case. Processing these emotions by giving them a little attention in a supportive group helps with learning from and letting the stressful event go. This is particularly important for handling moral stress.
- Watch free online videos on the work of Dan Siegel and teach participants the hand = model of the brain so they understand how stress affects them and their clients.
- The non-verbal show of support helps to address the emotional brain subcortical part of the brain that is a key part in processing moral stress.
- Occasionally you can, if appropriate, ask others in the group to put into words how they would feel in the situation described if they were the DVM, the technician, the front desk staff, the client—this is to support perspective taking after the fact. Be sure to do this in such a way that is supportive and not blaming of the person sharing the case.

Appendix B

Ten guidelines for making conversations with emotional charge productive

Speak for yourself	Avoid making statements like "I am sure we would all agree." Inevitably there will be someone who does not agree with you who will be offended by your assumption
Do not interrupt	Allow people to fully share their perspectives by not interrupting
Be concise	Be mindful to express your opinion, interest, or position in a manner that is clear and concise. Saying too much without coming to a point can harm people's ability to listen to you
Really listen	Listen completely to what is being said. Listening is compromised when you are mentally focused on your rebuttal instead of the speaker's comments
Acknowledge what has been said	Letting a person know you understand their perspective, does not mean that you agree. It is simply a sign of respect, not a show of agreement
Agree where you can	Highlighting the areas in which you do agree makes the places where you differ less difficult
Be courteous	Avoid labels like "that is stupid" or "he's an idiot." These types of labels of person or position inflame emotion and conflict and reduce productivity
Give and receive olive branches	Admit your mistakes or misunderstandings and outwardly acknowledge such admissions from others
Keep an open mind	Conversations about topics where people have differing opinions and positions have the greatest possibility of teaching something new. Allow yourself to be open to the possibility that your perspective may change through participation
Express gratitude and growth	Share the ways your connection with others helps you feel grateful and grow in your life

Used with permission from Dr. Elizabeth Strand

Appendix C

National organizations providing pet owner services

National program	Website
Pets of the Homeless	https://www.petsofthehomeless.org/
The Humane Society of the United States	https://www.humanesociety.org/resources/are-you-having-trouble-affording-your-pet

National program	Website
Veterinary Care Charitable Financial Assistance	https://www.vccfund.org/
Bow Wow Buddies Foundation (for seriously ill/injured dogs and urgent care) financial assistance	https://www.bowwowbuddies.com/
Canine Cancer Awareness (offers support forums, articles, and contact form for support)	https://caninecancerawareness.org/category/therapy-&-support/
Frankie's Friends Fund (providing financial assistance for emergency and specialty medical conditions)	https://www.frankiesfriends.org/national-frankies-friends-fund
Program that donates wheelchairs to pets	https://hpets.org/
Provides financial assistance for veterinary services, supplies, medications, etc.	https://www.help-a-pet.org/apply.html
Land of Pure Gold— financial assistance for cancer treatment for working dogs	http://landofpuregold.com/grants/index.htm
Financial assistance for dogs and cats with cancer (National Program)	https://themagicbulletfund.org/https://waggle.org/
Offers financial assistance for veterinary care, food, medicine, supplies, spay and neuter services, and helps dogs of veterans suffering from PTSD	https://www.onyxandbreezy.org/
Offers financial assistance for spay and neutering, cancer treatment, and critical veterinary care	https://www.themosbyfoundation.org/
Provides financial support for cancer treatment	https://wagglefoundation.org/riedelcody/
Provides financial assistance for veterinary care	https://waggle.org/

References

Access to Veterinary Care Coalition (AVCC). (2018). *Access to veterinary care: Barriers, current practices, and public policy.* https://pphe.utk.edu/wp-content/uploads/2020/09/avcc-report.pdf. Accessed July 5, 2021.

American Animal Hospital Association (AAHA). (2021). *AAHA standards of accreditation.* https://www.aaha.org/accreditation%2D%2Dmembership/aaha-standards/. Accessed July 5, 2021.

American Veterinary Medical Association (AVMA). (2021a). *Guidelines for classifying veterinary facilities.* https://www.avma.org/resources-tools/avma-policies/guidelines-classifying-veterinary-facilities. Accessed July 5, 2021.

American Veterinary Medical Association (AVMA). (2021b). *Setting up a workplace wellbeing program.* https://www.avma.org/resources-tools/wellbeing/setting-workplace-wellbeing-program. Accessed July 14, 2021.

American Veterinary Medical Association (AVMA). (2019). *2019 Model Veterinary Practice Act.* https://www.avma.org/sites/default/files/2021-01/model-veterinary-practice-act.pdf. Accessed July 5, 2021.

Assistance Dogs International (ADI). (2021). *ADI standards.* https://assistancedogsinternational.org/standards/summary-of-standards/. Accessed July 5, 2021.

Doka, K. J. (1989). Disenfranchised grief. In K. J. Doka (Ed.), *Disenfranchised grief: Recognizing hidden sorrow* (pp. 3–11). Lexington Books/D. C. Heath and Com.

Drake, A. A. S., Hafen, M., Jr., Ruch, B. R., & Reisbig, A. M. J. (2012). Predictors of anxiety and depression in veterinary medicine students: A four-year cohort examination. *Journal of Veterinary Medical Education, 39*(4), 322–330. https://doi.org/10.3138/jvme.0112-006R

Fine, A., Knesl, O., Hart, B., Hart, L., Ng, Z., Patterson-Kane, E., Hoy-Gerlach, J., & Feldman, S. (2019). The role of veterinarians in assisting clients identify and care for emotional support animals. *Journal of the American Veterinary Medical Association, 254*(2), 199–202. https://avmajournals.avma.org/doi/pdf/10.2460/javma.254.2.199

Hayes, G. M., LaLonde-Paul, D. F., Perret, J. L., Steele, A., McConkey, M., Lane, W. G., et al. (2020). Investigation of burnout syndrome and job related risk factors in veterinary technicians in specialty teaching hospitals: A multicenter cross-sectional study. *Journal of Veterinary Emergency and Critical Care (San Antonio), 30*(1), 18–27. https://doi.org/10.1111/vec.12916

Hoy-Gerlach, J., Vincent, A., & Lory Hector, B. (2019). Emotional support animals in the United States: Emergent guidelines for mental health clinicians. *Journal of Psychosocial Rehabilitation and Mental Health, 6*(2), 199–208.

International Association of Veterinary Social Work (IAVSW). (2020). www.veterinarysocialwork.org. Accessed July 5, 2021.

Karaffa, K. M., & Hancock, T. S. (2019). Mental health experiences and service use among veterinary medical students. *Journal of Veterinary Medical Education, 46*(4), 449–458.

Karaffa, K. M., Bradtke, J., & Hancock, T. (2020). Embedded student counseling services: Insights from veterinary mental health practitioners. *Journal of College Counseling, 23, 276–288.* https://doi.org/10.1002/jocc.12171

Moses, L., Malowney, M. J., & Boyd, J. W. (2018). Ethical conflict and moral distress in veterinary practice: A survey of North American veterinarians. *Journal of Veterinary Internal Medicine, 32*(6), 2115–2122. https://doi.org/10.1111/jvim.15315

Nancarrow, S. A., Booth, A., Ariss, S., Smith, T., Enderby, P., & Roots, A. (2013). Ten principles of good interdisciplinary team work. *Human Resources for Health, 11,* 19. https://doi.org/10.1186/1478-4491-11-19

National Association of Social Workers. (2017). *Code of ethics of the National Association of Social Workers.* https://www.socialworkers.org/About/Ethics/Code-of-Ethics/Code-of-Ethics-English. Accessed July 5, 2021.

Nahm, S.-S., & Chun, M.-S. (2020). Stressors predicting depression, anxiety, and stress in Korean veterinary students. *Journal of Veterinary Medical Education.* https://doi.org/10.3138/jvme-2019-0031

National Association of Veterinary Technicians in America (NAVTA). (2016). *NAVTA demographic survey results.* https://cdn.ymaws.com/www.navta.net/resource/resmgr/docs/2016_demographic_results.pdf. Accessed July 14, 2021.

Ouedraogo, F. B., Lefebvre, S. L., Hansen, C. R., & Brorsen, B. W. (2021). Compassion satisfaction, burnout, and secondary traumatic stress among full-time veterinarians in the United States (2016–2018). *Journal of the American Veterinary Medical Association., 258*(11), 1259–1270. https://doi.org/10.2460/javma.258.11.1259

Saleebey, D. (1996). The strengths perspective in social work practice: Extensions and cautions. *Social Work, 41*(3), 296–305.

Saleebey, D. (1992). *The strengths perspective in social work practice.* Longman.

Sinclair, S., Raffin-Bouchal, S., Venturato, L., Mijovic-Kondejewski, J., & Smith-MacDonald, L. (2017). Compassion fatigue: A meta-narrative review of the healthcare literature. *International Journal of Nursing Studies, 69,* 9–24. https://doi.org/10.1016/j.ijnurstu.2017.01.003

Stoewen, D. L. (2020). Moving from compassion fatigue to compassion resilience Part 4: Signs and consequences of compassion fatigue. *The Canadian Veterinary Journal – La revue veterinaire canadienne, 61*(11), 1207–1209.

Strand, E. B., Brandt, J., Rogers, K., Fonken, L., Chun, R., Conlon, P., & Lord, L. (2017). Adverse childhood experiences among veterinary medical students: A multi-site study. *Journal of Veterinary Medical Education, 44*(2), 260–267.

United States Department of Labor, Bureau of Labor Statistics. (2021a). *Occupational outlook handbook, human resources managers.* https://www.bls.gov/ooh/management/human-resources-managers.htm. Accessed June 07, 2021.

United States Department of Labor, Bureau of Labor Statistics. (2021b). *Occupational outlook handbook.* Veterinarians, at https://www.bls.gov/ooh/healthcare/veterinarians.htm. Accessed June 27, 2021.

United States Department of Labor, Bureau of Labor Statistics (2021c). *Occupational outlook handbook, veterinary technologists and technicians.* https://www.bls.gov/ooh/healthcare/veterinary-technologists-and-technicians.htm. Accessed June 02, 2021.

Wojtacka, J., Grudzień, W., Wysok, B., & Szarek, J. (2020). Causes of stress and conflict in the veterinary professional workplace – A perspective from Poland. *Irish Veterinary Journal, 73*(23). https://doi.org/10.1186/s13620-020-00177-9

Part IV
Veterinary Social Work Education

Chapter 12
Veterinary Social Work in Veterinary Colleges

Athena Diesch-Chham

Working with Veterinary Students

In 2019, there were over 13,000 students enrolled in colleges of veterinary medicine in the United States (American Association of Veterinary Medical Colleges, 2020). The college of veterinary medicine (CVM) where this author works has over 430 students pursuing a doctoral degree in veterinary medicine (DVM), and over 60 percent of the students are female. More recently, many colleges of veterinary medicine have prioritized issues of diversity and inclusion, a demanding task given that the veterinary profession has historically been made up of white males (Lofstedt, 2003). In 1985, for the first time, the proportion of men and women entering a veterinary medicine education were equal. Now, the current graduating classes in the United States and Canada reflect an 80/20 ratio, 80 percent women and 20 percent men (American Association of Veterinary Medical Colleges, 2020).

Many veterinary students report that they decided on a career in veterinary medicine at a young age, oftentimes between 5 and 8 years old. Admissions data indicate that many students reflect a typical Type A personality profile. Elite performers are known to have a laser-sharp focus to reach the top of their field. Colleges of veterinary medicine are highly competitive. For example, students that entered the veterinary curriculum in the fall of 2019 at Purdue University had 17 applicants per 1 open seat. Students at Texas A & M University had 4 applicants per 1 open seat (American Association of Veterinary Medical Colleges, 2020). Veterinary college tuition is expensive. In 2021, with resident status in the respective state, a student could gain a veterinary education at a cost per year that ranged from $19,000 to $60,000. For students who are accepted to programs in which they are a nonresident, the range is $32,000 to $63,000. These numbers only account for tuition and

A. Diesch-Chham (✉)
University of Minnesota, Minneapolis, MN, USA
e-mail: Diesc009@UMN.edu

© The Author(s), under exclusive license to Springer Nature Switzerland AG 2022   271
S. Loue, P. Linden (eds.), *The Comprehensive Guide to Interdisciplinary Veterinary Social Work*, https://doi.org/10.1007/978-3-031-10330-8_12

do not consider the costs of books and living costs. The academic pressure can lead to mental health difficulties including depression, anxiety, obsessive-compulsive disorders, and suicidal thoughts and behaviors.

Research shows that DVM students enter their professional programs with some form of mental disorder. Of these mental disorders, anxiety and depression are the most common. Within the student population, 19.2% struggled with moderate to severe anxiety symptoms, and 33.9% of students struggled with moderate to severe depression symptoms (Karaffa & Hancock, 2019).

Accordingly, social workers in veterinary colleges can be incredibly beneficial by providing mental health services on-site. This was the entire reason most mental health professionals within colleges of veterinary medicine were hired. In 2013, the first data were published on suicide among veterinarians. From this research, the Veterinary Wellbeing Summit was born. This meeting has been held annually and has allowed for each VMC to have representatives present to conceptualize and address the issues leading to the suicide crisis within veterinary medicine. From the Wellbeing Summits, a number of the colleges of veterinary medicine have addressed mental health concerns and quickly hired a mental health professional for their individual programs.

Due to the size of the populations and the demand for social work assistance, it has been determined that the brief treatment model is the most effective treatment. This model addresses in fewer than 12 sessions the reason the client is pursuing therapeutic intervention. Social workers engage client systems by utilizing open-ended questions, using reflective listening skills and asking clarifying questions. Engagement is enhanced by taking note of nonverbal communication like voice tone and inflection, body positioning, and eye contact. The social worker's use of these skills with veterinary students serves as a model for those students when they later enter veterinary practice; these are the same skills veterinarians need to effectively utilize when interacting with clients and colleagues.

Social workers in veterinary colleges should advocate for the opportunity to teach classes on mental and physical health, emotional coping skills, interpersonal communication, and human emotional dissection. Veterinary social workers can teach veterinary students about the complex human emotional processes of grief and bereavement. Pet death, either due to natural causes or euthanasia, occurs frequently in veterinary settings. The ways in which people process death are individual and based on previous experience and the ability to regulate emotions.

After veterinary students complete coursework, they move from the classroom to a variety of hospital, clinic, field, farm, and laboratory learning settings (See Crocken, 1981). In this phase, they are no longer learning from professors lecturing in front of them, but instead are engaging in individual interactions with clinicians, veterinary nurses, laboratory staff, farmhands, and support individuals.

The traditional pedagogy for veterinary clinical education involves "rounds." Rounds are conducted each morning and often led by one or more faculty members, the chief of service or the treating clinician with the purpose of giving clinicians, veterinary nurses, and support staff the opportunity to discuss goals and trajectory for the patient and client. As active participants in rounds, veterinary students practice case management under the guidance of instructors.

The CVM where the author practices social work has started social work rounds. These interactions are often scheduled for the same day and time each week and give a predictable opportunity for the entire team to sit down and discuss cases, concerns, and ethical conundrums without rushing. During social work rounds, veterinary students and the social workers debrief and process challenging or difficult situations. Ethical issues are explored, including animal abuse reporting, effective communication about finances, working with families with small children, and managing difficult clients.

As life in a college of veterinary medicine and a veterinary teaching hospital goes, not all important or crucial learning situations happen in a predictable or scheduled way like rounds. More often than not, learning and teaching are spontaneous. Case consultation with students and all team members within the hospital is valuable. These students have spent at least 3 years studying science and medicine. Thus, the ability to consult with a veterinary social worker or other helping professionals cannot only help round out how one might approach a case, but also helps students understand the human experience and perspective more deeply (Crocken, 1981).

Case debriefing is similar to case consultation. There are some components of veterinary medicine and the long held culture that lean away from case debriefing. As an example, the profession has not traditionally engaged in discussions regarding the ways in which repeated trauma is perpetrated within veterinary medicine as a result of the practice of euthanasia, despite clear evidence for the usefulness of debriefing and social support as noted by Bennett and Rohlf (2005). Social workers and mental health professionals have practiced and known the usefulness of relating one's vicarious trauma, processing it, and then continuing to move forward with self and career. Debriefing allows for the individual, and hopefully the team, to talk about how they were impacted by the case and the components with which they may be struggling. By talking through the trauma, veterinary social workers not only give the individuals an opportunity to share their experience with their colleagues but also give them time and space to work through and process through where this lives within them from this point on. More often than not, students would not otherwise engage in this process with the whole team, as frequently they believe that they are the only one struggling. This is a great opportunity for the veterinary social worker to engage with the whole team, as there is value in all of the perspectives that may be offered. Additionally, this process provides the student with an opportunity to learn and practice what are often referred to as the "softer skills."

Clinical year students are not the only group that can benefit from these processes. As the pressure and desire to specialize within veterinary medicine grow, so does the rising number of veterinarians who decide to enter into a yearlong internship program. By all accounts, these individuals are veterinarians, as they have graduated their DVM program, and are fully licensed to practice. However, because of their drive to specialize, and significant self-doubt about their skills, they enter into a program where they are yet again student learners, but different from students.

Veterinary interns may be confronted with challenging power dynamics. These doctors often have just graduated and are now finding themselves teaching and engaging with clinical year students as though they are seasoned practitioners. So frequently though, these new professionals struggle with incredible levels of impostor syndrome as they believe they should know more than they do and often expect high levels of perfection from themselves as found by Appleby et al. (2020). They may experience additional stress if they have relocated to complete this year, often far away from their well-developed support network, and must now adjust to a new city, potentially new state, and new career. The internship likely requires that they participate in rotating blocks through multiple specialties, with varying hours, including overnights through the emergency department, and often 50- to 60-hour workweeks. Many of the individuals seek out academic internships as there is the greater likelihood that they will see and treat cases to which they would not otherwise be exposed. Additionally, internships provide exposure to exemplary people in the field.

Addressing Veterinary Mental Health

Veterinarian mental health has received attention in recent years, largely in response to the 2014 suicide of a well-known veterinarian, Dr. Sophia Yin. Important topics that have been found to be associated with mental health in the veterinary profession are compassion fatigue, burnout, moral injury, and moral distress.

Compassion fatigue is "the emotional residue or strain of exposure to working with those suffering from the consequences of traumatic events" (American Institute for Stress, 2020). Burnout has been defined as:

A syndrome conceptualized as resulting from chronic workplace stress that has not been successfully managed. It is characterized by three dimensions:

- Feelings of energy depletion or exhaustion;
- Increased mental distance from one's job, or feelings of negativism or cynicism related to one's job; and
- Reduced professional efficacy (World Health Organization, 2021).

Moral injury is "the damage done to one's conscious or moral compass when one perpetuates, witnesses, or fails to prevent acts that transgress one's own moral beliefs, values or ethical codes of conduct" (Syracuse University, 2019). Lastly, moral distress as it relates to veterinary medicine occurs when ethical principles are at stake, but external factors prevent the individual from pursuing an action (Kahler, 2014). These issues should be part of the core veterinary curriculum because they directly impact veterinarians' mental health and job satisfaction. Veterinary social workers can be instrumental in facilitating discussions about these topics and in helping students develop skills to proactively reduce the occurrence of burnout and compassion fatigue.

A survey of more than 11,000 US veterinarians in 2014 found that 9 percent had current serious psychological distress, 31 percent had experienced depressive episodes, and 17 percent had experienced suicidal ideation since leaving veterinary school. The data suggest that nearly one in ten US veterinarians might suffer from serious psychological distress, yet only half are seeking help (Tomasi et al., 2019). This same study found that female veterinarians have a higher prevalence of risk factors for suicide, including depression, suicidal ideation, and previous suicide attempts (Tomasi et al., 2019). A recent study published by the Centers for Disease Control and Prevention indicated that female veterinarians are 3.5 times as likely to die by suicide compared to the general populations; their male counterparts are 2.1 times as likely to commit suicide as the general population (Tomasi et al., 2019). Additionally, 7 percent of these veterinarians' deaths were veterinarians practicing in small animal practices (Tomasi et al., 2019) Although the proportion of female veterinarian deaths by suicide has remained at about 10 percent since the early 2000s, the number of deaths is steadily rising (Tomasi et al., 2019).

Despite these data, there has not been one solidly held view on what a helping professional's role should be across all institutions. As mentioned previously, many of the institutions took a reactive approach to bringing on helping professionals like social workers after the first round of research was published on veterinary mental health. It is because of this that many colleges of veterinary medicine have a very deliberate divide between who helps their students and who helps their clients. Currently, almost every college of veterinary medicine has either an embedded mental health professional to work with their students, or they have formed an alliance with their campus counseling centers. These alliances allow the two entities to ensure that the students of the college of veterinary medicine have the resources needed to address their mental health and well-being with as few barriers as possible.

While the institutions are doing whatever is needed to address the student population, there are also many schools that have other professionals on staff to work with the hospital client population. There are very few institutions that have social workers available to assist everyone, i.e., the client population, the student population, faculty, and staff. To be clear, this is an unsustainable model and one that should not be considered. It is recommended that there be multiple social workers on staff to address student, faculty, staff, and hospital client needs.

Preparing Students for Interprofessional Practice

The Veterinary Oath, sworn to by graduates of accredited veterinary colleges, states:

Being admitted to the profession of veterinary medicine, I solemnly swear to use my scientific knowledge and skills for the benefit of society through the protection of animal health and welfare, the prevention and relief of animal suffering, the conservation of animal resources, the promotion of public health, and the advancement of medical knowledge.

I will practice my profession conscientiously, with dignity, and in keeping with the principles of veterinary medical ethics.

I accept as a lifelong obligation the continual improvement of my professional knowledge and competence (American Veterinary Medical Association, 2020).

As the oath states, veterinarians are advocates obligated to alleviate suffering for animals. The primary focus for the veterinarian is the patient and the patient's symptoms. As a practice owner or co-owner of a veterinary clinic, there are challenges that arise. As Sacco-Bene and Roseman (2020) have noted, veterinarians face numerous pressures inherent in managing the business side of a clinical practice. Thus, veterinarians do not have the resources or education to supply the same services to their clients that a social worker can. While students may have gained some insight or information about these additional roles within their professional development courses, it is oftentimes not enough training to be able to attend to all the roles that veterinarians may encounter.

The social worker serves as a great resource to be a liaison between the veterinarian and the client (Crocken, 1981). It's essential that students enrolled in veterinary medicine are educated about the benefits of teaming with social workers within a veterinary setting. The social worker's client-centered approach models the value of client self-determination. By facilitating effective veterinarian-client communication, crises, conflicts, and dilemmas can be avoided. As veterinary social workers have joined in veterinary settings, veterinary professionals are able to concentrate their time and focus on providing medical care to their patients and interacting with the pet owner. The availability of social workers on site relieves the veterinarian of the responsibility to attend to human needs. The veterinarian/social worker team provides a holistic and collaborative approach to the professional service and care the patients and the pet owners experience. Clinical students who are on their rotations have access to firsthand experience and can come back to the classroom with tangible experiences like challenging communications with clients, overtly emotional response, or delivering hard news. Giving veterinary students the skills and autonomy to determine if this client could benefit from social work intervention could give more patients access to the social work care they need.

As noted earlier, students proceed from their college-based learning to a rotating internship, where they are practicing veterinarians, but are also active learners. They have mentors, and clear criteria that must be achieved to successfully complete that 1-year internship. After the internship comes a 3-year residency. In residency, they continue to be practicing veterinarians, but they spend the majority of their time within the specialty that they are pursuing. Because interns and residents are not students, and not faculty, they may experience additional challenges. First, interns and residents are still learning how their academic institution works interprofessionally. Second, interns and residents in a particular practice or hospital may be coming from an institution that did not have a social work department and thus may have no concept of how social workers can be beneficial to them and their clients. Third, interns may be preoccupied with other work and building relationships with the social worker may not be a priority for them. Therefore, it is often up to the social worker and long-term faculty to reiterate and model how beneficial this working relationship can be not only for the client, but for the entire team. Ultimately, maintaining a strong working relationship with multiple specialties in a major veterinary teaching hospital can ensure that students benefit from understanding and having access to social workers.

Modeling Skills

A Strengths-Based Approach

Social work adopted the strengths-based perspective in the 1980s. In strengths-based practice, social workers see the person first, not the etiology of the pathologic or problematic patterns. Social workers place higher value on the person and their talents, experiences, feelings, abilities, and resources. In this practice, social workers give their clients the space and voice to determine the appropriate path for moving forward so they are as involved as the professional in their treatment plan (Corcoran, 2017; Council on Social Work Education, 2015). This approach is in stark contrast to the medical model, which is a problem-based approach (observe, diagnose, treat) (Engel, 1979). Thus, the strengths-based model is more suited for veterinary social work purposes, considering clients need emotional and psychological support.

Veterinary social workers can both instruct veterinary students about this approach and model its implementation in the context of their interprofessional internships and residencies. Veterinary social workers can help veterinarians and their staffs approach clients from a strengths-based perspective, rather than seeing only their clients' deficiencies and difficulties.

Critical Values

The critical social work values of competence, confidentiality, and self-determination, enunciated in the *Code of Ethics* of the National Association of Social Workers (2017), are also relevant to the practice of veterinary medicine. The value of competence suggests that social workers should actively seek out additional training in areas that need more support. Similarly, veterinary students, interns, and residents should continue to pursue further education, not only for their licenses, but to enhance their abilities to address their patients' situations.

NASW has very specific and detailed guidelines on privacy and confidentiality for social workers. Although veterinary medicine does not require adherence to the same privacy and confidentiality mandates, within the context of education, veterinary faculty, mentors, and supervisors may be required to adhere to the provisions of the Family Educational Rights and Privacy Act (FERPA), which was enacted in

1974 to protect the privacy of students' educational records (United States Department of Education, n.d.). The social workers' familiarity with confidentiality and privacy concerns and protections may help veterinary faculty and students understand their rights and obligations under this law.

In all 50 states, animals are considered personal property. As a consequence, their medical information is not protected by confidentiality regulations. However, people's mental and physical health information is protected as Personal Health Information (PHI) under the Health Insurance Portability and Accountability Act of 1996 (HIPAA) (Centers for Disease Control and Prevention, 2018). Sharing PHI without consent from the patient could result in criminal and civil penalties. In the spirit and practice of effective interprofessional practice, social workers in veterinary settings should make veterinarians aware that information about clients cannot be shared without informed consent. As an example of a situation in which this may be raised as an issue, the veterinary team might refer a client to the social worker. The social worker must have the support and trust of the veterinary team when they make the client referral, but the veterinary team must understand that the social worker cannot divulge confidential information back to the other team members.

Because social workers have a professional obligation to create a safe, professional environment for clients, the office placement in this interprofessional setting is important. Social workers need to be intentionally and strategically placed in a space that allows them to work directly with the clients, students, staff, and veterinarians and facilitates ease of interaction and healthy communication. It is helpful if social workers are placed near an exit, so that grieving owners don't have to walk through a busy hospital or lobby to exit the building. The social workers also need to be placed a bit off the beaten path in order for the faculty, staff, and students to feel as though the space has enough anonymity such that their peers, colleagues, and superiors don't see them coming and going. This anonymity is essential to a strong and trusting relationship between the social worker, the client, and the veterinary team members. The offset of the social worker's office space helps to reinforce the requirements for privacy and confidentiality.

Self-determination is one of the most basic ethical standards for social workers. As defined in the *Merriam-Webster Dictionary*, self-determination is "free choice of one's own acts or states without external compulsion" (Self-determination, 2021). However, the veterinary team, the social worker, and the client may have different ideas about what self-determination looks like. As an example, a veterinarian suggesting that a client authorize euthanasia of their animal may discourage the client from being present, or may not offer the client the option of being present for the euthanasia. Now, as a result of more collaboration between veterinary social workers, veterinarians, and the client, it's more likely that the client will have input into how the last moments with their companion animal will occur. As a result of the collaboration between veterinarians and veterinary social workers, hospitals, clinics, and teaching institutions have built special rooms that are warm, comforting, and inviting for clients to sit in and process their loss in a less sterile environment. With the help of the social worker, the clients can receive space, support, and the ability to dictate what the death of their companion animal will look like, and the veterinarian and veterinary technicians will have support in their efforts to address the needs of both their patient and their client.

Self-Care: Boundary Setting and Self-Care Techniques

Healthy boundary setting leads to the ability to set work-life balance. Seasoned social workers learn that intentional boundary setting is necessary to practice effectively; this skill can be both taught and modeled to veterinary students and members of a veterinary team.

Boundary setting and sustainable practice is relevant for people who choose careers in both social work and for those in veterinary practice. In both of these professions, there are opportunities and expectations that the individual is to give continuously over long periods of time.

Without intentional caretaking practice, the risk of burnout and compassion fatigue is present. A key role of social workers in veterinary colleges is to model self-care behaviors and teach veterinary professionals to care for themselves so that they can continue to provide quality services. Social workers in veterinary colleges should advocate that the veterinary curriculum incorporate self-care techniques. Veterinarians cannot be expected to be experts at caring for anyone other than animals, especially taking care of themselves. Many of them may have worked beyond hard to reach veterinary school and have learned to dismiss their own needs and place themselves behind everyone else.

Social workers need to teach the students to listen to how their bodies may be expressing the early signs of stress or distress and acknowledge them, the importance of sleep and sleep hygiene, and the negative effects of long-term sleep deprivation. Social workers should also teach them the art of processing feelings versus venting about them, and how the difference could impact their overall life and career satisfaction. Ultimately, social workers need to teach them how to recognize someone else's pain and empathize, without carrying it themselves. Veterinary medicine can be a painful and difficult career, especially with respect to euthanasia. It is critical that social workers teach the next generation of veterinarians to see their role as the facilitator, and not as the holder of the grief; this could change the lives of so many veterinarians for the better.

Challenges in Interprofessional Settings

Host settings are arenas where social workers practice that are defined and dominated by nonsocial workers (Dane & Simon, 1991). Host settings can be any work setting where one theoretical lens is utilized with a small subset of individuals whose role is different. Host settings are fairly common within human healthcare and human service agencies, as they are conducive to interprofessional collaboration and a systemic approach. One of the significant challenges for veterinary professionals and social workers in the interprofessional setting is the potential for misunderstandings of each other's role and function in the setting.

Dane and Simon (1991) posit that there are four predictable problems that arise when social workers work within a host setting: discrepancies in values between host and social workers, the marginality of the social workers token status, evaluating social work as women's work in settings that are predominantly male in inspiration and composition, and the role ambiguity and role strain within the cluster of roles those social workers enact as resident guests.

Traditionally, human health professionals, like social workers, were grouped within organizations in offices by discipline. Clients or patients were expected to come to an office to receive services. Most social workers were trained in this service delivery model and therefore many expected that they would be working side by side with other social workers and have ready access to support, supervision, and shared understanding of the work being performed in their work setting. One of the significant challenges for social workers in host settings is that few others in the setting understand their role and function in the setting.

Recordkeeping serves as one example of situations in which the needs of veterinary professionals may conflict with the ethical responsibilities of veterinary social workers. Social workers are required to keep HIPAA-compliant case records. Many veterinary hospitals, private hospitals, and neighborhood clinics are moving from paper records to electronic medical records (EMR). Krone et al. (2014) found in their study focused on small animal veterinary practices in Massachusetts that EMR use either alone or in conjunction with paper records occurred in 80.5 percent of practices. They additionally found that large to medium practices were more likely to utilize an EMR, and most frequently the EMR was used by all clinics for more logistical components like billing, automating reminders, providing effective cost estimates, scheduling, and recording medical and surgical information and tracking patient health (Krone et al., 2014).

These findings suggest that having an EMR within the veterinary teaching hospital is valuable to the veterinary team, and even the social worker, to ensure that the interprofessional team has a complete picture of what the patient and client are experiencing. However, the ease with which the veterinary team does have access makes it the least protective option for the social worker. Therefore, in order to fulfill the professional, ethical, and legal obligations of a licensed mental health practitioner, veterinary social workers practicing in host settings must advocate for a separate, HIPAA-compliant EHR.

Future of Veterinary Social Work in Veterinary Colleges

The number of social workers and other licensed mental health professionals working in veterinary settings is growing. In 2009, there were approximately 20 social workers in this field; in 2021, there are several hundred.

To be effective as both teachers and role models to veterinary students and faculty, social workers and other licensed mental health professionals working in veterinary colleges should be required to demonstrate competency in all of the foundational pieces of veterinary social work including, but not limited to, pet loss and bereavement, conflict management, human-animal bond, animal abuse and neglect, the link between violence toward people and violence toward animals, compassion fatigue, and animal-assisted interventions.

Various organizations offer resources to individuals engaged in interprofessional veterinary practice, including veterinary professionals and veterinary social workers. The AAVMA Academic Veterinary Wellbeing Professionals (AVWP) Group (https://www.aavmc.org/programs/wellbeing) is for veterinary hospital-based mental health professionals working in academic and private veterinary hospitals. The group operates under the American Association of Veterinary Medical Colleges (AAVMC).

The International Association of Veterinary Social Work was incorporated in 2020 and is an interdisciplinary membership organization that supports and promotes professionals who tend to the human needs that arise in the relationship between humans and animals by creating and maintaining professional standards, encouraging research, and advocating for a better world for all species (www.veterinarysocialwork.org).

References

American Association of Veterinary Medical Colleges. (2020, September 22). *Admitted student statistics*. (2020, September 22). https://www.aavmc.org/becoming-a-veterinarian/what-to-know-before-you-apply/admitted-student-statistics/. Accessed February 27, 2021.

American Institute of Stress. (2020). *Compassion fatigue 2019*. Available at https://www.stress.org/military/for-practitionersleaders/compassion-fatigue. Accessed 25 October 2019.

Appleby, R., Evola, M., & Royal, K. (2020). Impostor phenomenon in veterinary medicine. *Education in the Health Professions, 3*(3), 105. https://doi.org/10.4103/ehp.ehp_17_20

Bennett, P., & Rohlf, V. (2005). Perpetration-induced traumatic stress in persons who euthanize nonhuman animals in surgeries, animal shelters, and laboratories. *Society & Animals, 13*(3), 201–220. https://doi.org/10.1163/1568530054927753

Centers for Disease Control and Prevention. (2018). *Health Insurance Portability and Accountability Act of 1996*. https://www.cdc.gov/phlp/publications/topic/hipaa.html. Accessed May 31, 2021.

Corcoran, J. (2017, May 1). Strengths-based models in social work. *Oxford bibliographies*. https://www.oxfordbibliographies.com/view/document/obo-9780195389678/obo-9780195389678-0006.xml. Accessed January 27, 2021.

Council on Social Work Education. (2015). *2015 educational policy and accreditation standards for baccalaureate and master's social work programs*. https://www.cswe.org/getattachment/Accreditation/Standards-and-Policies/2015-EPAS/2015EPASandGlossary.pdf.aspx. Accessed January 27, 2021.

Crocken, B. (1981). Veterinary medicine and social work. *Social Work in Health Care, 6*(3), 91–94.

Dane, B. O., & Simon, B. L. (1991). Resident guests: Social workers in host settings. *Social Work, 36*(3), 208–2013. https://doi.org/10.1093/sw/36.3.208

Engel, G. L. (1979). The biopsychosocial model and the education of health professionals. *General Hospital Psychiatry, 1*(2), 156–165. https://doi.org/10.1016/0163-8343(79)90062-8

Kahler, S. (2014, December 17). *Moral stress is the top trigger in veterinarians' compassion fatigue*. https://www.avma.org/javma-news/2015-01-01/moral-stress-top-trigger-veterinarians-compassion-fatigue. Accessed March 5, 2021.

Karaffa, K. M., & Hancock, T. S. (2019). Mental health experiences and service use among veterinary medical students. *Journal of Veterinary Medical Education, 46*(4), 449–458. https://doi.org/10.3138/jvme.1017-145r1

Krone, L. M., Brown, C. M., & Lindenmayer, J. M. (2014). Survey of electronic veterinary medical record adoption and use by independent small animal veterinary medical practices in Massachusetts. *Journal of the American Veterinary Medical Association, 245*(3), 324–332. https://doi.org/10.2460/javma.245.3.324

Lofstedt, J. (2003). Gender and veterinary medicine. *Canadian Veterinary Journal, 44*(7), 533–535.

National Association of Social Workers. (2017). *Code of ethics*. https://www.socialworkers.org/About/Ethics/Code-of-Ethics/Code-of-Ethics-English. Accessed May 31, 2021.

Sacco-Bene, C., & Roseman, F. (2020, January 13). When the caring is too much [Editorial]. *Counseling Today*. from https://ct.counseling.org/2020/01/when-the-caring-is-too-much/#. Accessed January 28, 2021.

Self-determination. (2021). *Merriam-Webster dictionary*. https://www.merriam-webster.com/dictionary/self-determination#:~:text=1. Accessed March 19, 2021.

Syracuse University. (2019). *The moral injury project*. http://moralinjuryproject.syr.edu/about-moral-injury/. Accessed 25 September 2019.

Tomasi, S. E., Fechter-Leggett, E. D., Edwards, N. T., Reddish, A. D., Crosby, A. E., & Nett, R. J. (2019). Suicide among veterinarians in the United States from 1979 through 2015. *Journal of the American Veterinary Medical Association, 254*(1), 104–112. https://doi.org/10.2460/javma.254.1.104

United States Department of Education. (n.d.). *34 CFR Part 99—Family educational rights and privacy (FERPA)*. https://studentprivacy.ed.gov/node/548/. Accessed January 28, 2021.

World Health Organization. (2021). *International classification of diseases*, 11th ed. https://icd.who.int/en. Accessed May 31, 2021.

Chapter 13
Veterinary Social Work Internships in Veterinary Settings

Janet Hoy-Gerlach, Joelle Nielsen, Jessica Ricker, and Aimee St. Arnaud

Introduction

Approximately 67 percent of households in the United States report having at least one pet, and the majority of those report considering their pets to be family members (American Pet Products Association, n.d.). Social workers have addressed issues related to the bonds people share with their pets for over 30 years; in 1975, a case study about an elderly woman and the importance of her relationship with her dog Lacey was described by a medical social worker (Bikales, 1975). Veterinary social work is an area of social work practice that addresses the human issues that emerge within the human-animal relationship. The four primary areas of focus within veterinary social work are: grief and pet loss, animal-assisted interactions, the link between human and animal violence, and compassion fatigue and conflict management (University of Tennessee, 2021). In 2002, under the leadership of social worker Dr. Elizabeth Strand, the University of Tennessee College of Veterinary Medicine and College of Social Work collaboratively established the first veterinary social work certificate program within the United States (Cima, 2020). Within the University of Tennessee's graduate social work program, veterinary social work is

J. Hoy-Gerlach (✉)
University of Toledo, Toledo, OH, USA
e-mail: janet.hoy@utoledo.edu

J. Nielsen
The Ohio State University, Veterinary Medical Center, Columbus, OH, USA

J. Ricker
Community Pet Care Clinic former intern, Toledo, OH, USA

A. St. Arnaud
Community Pet Care Clinic, Toledo, OH, USA

© The Author(s), under exclusive license to Springer Nature Switzerland AG 2022
S. Loue, P. Linden (eds.), *The Comprehensive Guide to Interdisciplinary Veterinary Social Work*, https://doi.org/10.1007/978-3-031-10330-8_13

offered as a concurrent certificate specialization or as a postgraduate certificate program for social workers who are licensed and practicing in social work.

The need for veterinary social workers within veterinary settings has continued to expand since the formalization of veterinary social work education (Cima, 2020). At least one-half of US colleges of veterinary medicine have a veterinary social worker on staff in their hospital/medical center (Joelle Nielsen, personal communication, March 3, 2021). This role generally is twofold: to address emergent psychosocial issues with human clients who bring their animals in for treatment and to address compassion fatigue and related issues among veterinary staff (Larkin, 2016). Veterinarians face a myriad of stressors in their work and are at disproportionate risk of serious psychological distress and depressive episodes (Nett et al., 2015), as well as suicide (Tomasi et al., 2019), as compared to the general population. Private emergency and specialty veterinary practices and large corporate chain veterinary practices are more frequently hiring veterinary social workers to address such issues (Cima, 2020). While the need for and value of veterinary social workers is increasingly recognized in such settings (Cima, 2020), owners of private companion animal-focused veterinary practices – where many people take their pets for veterinary care – may not be aware of veterinary social work and how to integrate it within their practices, or may be aware of veterinary social work but have not yet determined how to sustainably afford veterinary social work services.

Hence, while there is a need for veterinary social work, most individuals who have companion animals do not have ready access to a veterinary social worker within veterinary settings. Because there are few veterinary social workers currently working in private companion animal veterinary practices (Cima, 2020), internship sites for graduate social work students interested in social work practice within a veterinary clinic setting are likewise generally limited to academic veterinary medical centers and specialty and emergency veterinary practices, for these are where most veterinary social workers are practicing.

The absence of a social worker in a veterinary setting should not be a limitation for hosting a social work intern at a general companion animal practice. An off-site supervision model in social work education already exists. In this model, an off-site social worker collaborates with an on-site nonsocial worker to support and supervise a social work intern at an internship site that does not have an on-site social worker available to supervise. This model has been effectively applied to develop graduate social work internships at an internship site in which human-animal interaction issues were a primary focus; graduate social work internships began at the Toledo Humane Society (THS) in Ohio in 2010 and have continued to the present day (Hoy-Gerlach et al., 2019). Using the strategies for developing a social work internship at a humane society that were delineated by Hoy-Gerlach et al. (2019), together with an off-site MSW supervision model (Abram et al., 2000), the authors of this chapter collaboratively developed and implemented a veterinary social work internship at a private companion animal practice. Within this chapter, authors explain how to develop, structure, and implement a graduate social work internship in a companion animal private practice without an on-site veterinary social worker present. Ultimately, this chapter offers guidance to expand access to veterinary social work through creative partnerships between veterinary practices, veterinary social workers, and social work academic programs.

Social Work Internship in a Veterinary Practice

Whether at a veterinary practice or a human health or social service agency, organizations that host social work students as interns must meet certain obligations determined by the respective student's social work education degree program. The student's social work education degree program must, in turn, meet the standards enunciated by the Council on Social Work Education (CSWE), which is the national accreditation organization for social work degree programs in the United States and its territories. Attending an accredited social work program is crucial in order to obtain licensure and practice social work in the United States. Although licensure varies by state, graduation from an accredited program is a requirement in all 50 states and the District of Columbia (Council on Social Work Education, 2021).

Social work students in accredited social work graduate and undergraduate programs are required to complete internships, which are referred to by social work educators as field placements. Field education – the students' internship experiences and related integrative experiences such as internship supervision and discussion of internships within integrative internship seminars – is the primary method through which a student learns their profession. The purpose of the field placement is to enable social work interns to apply classroom learning and develop skills and mastery of specified social work competency areas, as detailed by CSWE. CSWE has identified nine foundational social work competencies that students must master by the conclusion of their social work degree program (see Table 13.1). In addition to these foundational competencies, there are also advanced competencies that social work graduate programs develop and submit to CSWE for approval. Each

Table 13.1 Competencies identified by the Council on Social Work Education

Competencies	
1	Demonstrate ethic and professional behavior
2	Engage diversity and difference in practice
3	Advance human rights and social, economic, and environmental justice
4	Engage in practice-informed research and research-informed practice
5	Engage in policy practice
6	Engage with individuals, families, groups, organizations, and communities
7	Assess with individuals, families, groups, organizations, and communities
8	Intervene with individuals, families, groups, organizations, and communities
9	Evaluate with individuals, families, groups, organizations, and communities

Source: Council on Social Work Education (2015)

competency has related practice behaviors which further delineate dimensions that need to be developed and mastered.

A typical full-time Master's in Social Work degree program can be completed in 2 years if a person holds an undergraduate degree in a field other than social work. If a person holds an undergraduate social work degree and meets grade and other criteria, they may qualify for advanced standing and be able to complete the program in 1 year by getting the foundation classes waived. Generally, graduate social work interns will complete a required number of weekly hours over the fall and spring semesters during their foundation graduate year, and a higher number of required weekly hours over the fall and spring semesters during their advanced graduate year. For instance, at the University of Toledo in Ohio, foundation graduate social work students complete a 425-hour internship over two semesters, averaging about 16 hours per week; advanced graduate social work students complete a 525-hour internship over the course of two semesters (University of Toledo, 2021).

Upon beginning an internship, the social work intern must collaboratively develop a learning contract (also referred to as a learning agreement or field plan) with the person or people who are supervising their internship. The learning contract lists each of the social work competencies the student must develop, along with specific corresponding learning tasks and activities that will enable the student to build the requisite competencies. While the competencies listed are the same across internship sites for students at a given accredited graduate social work program, the learning tasks and activities are specific to an internship site and must be collaboratively identified by the student and the person who is supervising the student at that internship site.

Social work internships occur in a wide range of settings and include nonprofit, for-profit, and government organizations. Some internship sites have hundreds of employees and multimillion dollar budgets, whereas other sites are small grassroots organizations with very limited budgets. Each site provides various learning opportunities and therefore students and those who supervise their internship experiences can select or create activities/tasks that reflect an agency's unique mission and goals. (Examples of competency-related learning tasks and activities specific to social work internships in veterinary settings are provided further below.)

Social work interns are typically supervised by a social worker who works at the internship site; within social work education, this role is referred to as the field instructor. The field instructor, through the provision of social work-related supervision on a regular basis, helps to ensure the intern is developing the needed social work practice skills at the internship site. Field instructors generally provide this internship supervision to the students without additional compensation from the social work degree program or student, within the parameters of their existing employment.

While most sites that host social work interns, whether large or small, employ social workers in some capacity who can serve as a field instructor, there are service-oriented organizations that do not currently employ a social worker yet offer rich learning environments in which to build social work practice competencies. In such instances, a nonsocial work staff at the internship site who is knowledgeable in operations and tasks related to the internship can be designated as a task instructor through the social work education program. While not a social worker, the on-site task instructor provides daily activity coordination and guidance for the social work intern. CSWE requires that task instruction be supplemented by social work supervision or instruction to ensure the development of required social work professional competencies (Council on Social Work Education, 2015). Many graduate social work programs across the country do this through the identification and designation of an off-site social worker who is willing to provide such supervision on a regular and voluntary basis; such is specified in the respective field education manual of a given social work program, which is reviewed by CSWE as part of the accreditation process.

A social worker who is employed by a social work education program and typically has responsibility for coordination, oversight, and evaluation of a set number of social work internships at an institution will serve in the role of field liaison or field coordinator. The field liaison is the formal linkage between the internship site and the social work degree program and is in addition to the field and task instructor roles.

A social work internship thus operates through coordination between a team of people in various roles as described in previous paragraphs. While most veterinary practices do not have social workers on-site to supervise a graduate social work intern, the range of tasks and activities performed by veterinary social workers to support veterinary staff and human clients are nonetheless available to varying degrees for a social work intern to engage in and build practice competencies through. Using an on-site nonsocial work veterinary staff person as a task instructor, along with an off-site social worker serving as a field instructor, the social work learning opportunities offered at a veterinary practice as well as the benefits of veterinary social work practice can be actualized.

Identifying a Companion Animal Veterinary Practice as an Internship Site

Potential veterinary internship sites can be identified and engaged through a variety of means. Perhaps the simplest way to identify a veterinary practice as a potential social work internship site is through networking. For example, the co-owner of a companion animal veterinary practice (and a co-author of this chapter) was on an advisory committee for a human-animal interaction project co-led by a social work faculty member (another author of this chapter). Through a series of conversations between the veterinary practice co-owner and the social work faculty member about the needs of the practice, the idea of a veterinary social work internship emerged. While "cold calling" could likewise result in potential internship partners, building on existing relationships that span social work and veterinary settings can ease and accelerate the internship development process. Social workers with pets can ask their own veterinarian about their familiarity with veterinary social work and offer to provide information. Another approach would be to talk with colleagues, friends, and family members about making introductions to area veterinary practices that may be receptive to learning more about veterinary social work and/or hosting a veterinary social work intern.

Veterinary practices and social work programs that are interested in exploring social work internships in veterinary settings may contact the University of Tennessee Veterinary Social Work Certificate Program (https://vetsocialwork.utk. edu/) or the International Association of Veterinary Social Work https://veterinary-socialwork.org/). Some veterinary social workers, such as Sandra Brackenridge (https://www.sbrackenridgelcsw.com/), provide consultation services to veterinary practices that are interested in setting up a social work internships or hiring a veterinary social worker. Veterinary practices may also contact the Field Education department at an accredited graduate social work program to explore the option of developing social work internships. (See https://www.cswe.org/Accreditation/Directory-of-Accredited-Programs.aspx.) When contacting a Field Education department, it is important to keep in mind that veterinary social work is an emerging area of practice; field staff may not yet be familiar with the rich social work learning opportunities afforded in a veterinary setting. Referencing this chapter and including links to veterinary social work resources provided in this paragraph can help provide a context for social work internships in veterinary settings for those unfamiliar with veterinary social work.

The social work internship placement mentioned in the previous paragraph was created by chapter authors at the Community Pet Care Clinic (CPCC), a full-service private companion animal veterinary practice located in Toledo, Ohio. CPCC employs three veterinarians and 13 support staff and has served over 10,000 pets since opening in 2017. Support staff roles at CPCC include receptionists, veterinary assistants, veterinary technicians, and a practice manager. CPCC was opened under the belief that all families should have access to affordable care for their dogs and cats; the business model was designed accordingly to maintain a net positive revenue while also building a support system for clients. Various payment plan options are offered at CPCC, and a fund is maintained to assist people who cannot afford to pay for services. One dollar from every healthy pet exam goes into this fund. Partnerships with nonprofit humane organizations and human health and social services are an important element in CPCC's work which uses a One Health approach. As explained by Hediger et al. (2019), a One Health approach is collaborative and transdisciplinary and focuses on leveraging connections between human, animal, and the environmental well-being in order to optimize health outcomes beyond what could be accomplished by focusing on only one of those three domains. The co-owner of CPCC who initiated a veterinary social work internship is a developer of accessible, affordable veterinary service models and has trained and consulted with veterinary social work practices on such nationally. CPCC seeks to help other veterinary practices integrate such tools into their operations to help improve veterinary staff, client, and patient well-being.

Planning the Veterinary Social Work Internship: A Collaborative Process

Once a veterinary practice has been identified as a potential veterinary social work internship site, the nature and scope of activities entailed in the internship needed to be determined. This may be accomplished by identifying how organizational needs can be met through learning activities associated with social work practice competencies. An exchange of knowledge between those familiar with social work education requirements and those familiar with the organization's operations is thus necessary. In cases where a social worker is not present at the internship site and the site is not a traditional human health or social service organization, such collaborative and proactive planning is especially crucial. An organization in which human-animal interactions are a central focus has both unique opportunities and challenges; for starters, most current staff may not be familiar with social workers or the nature of social work practice. In developing graduate social work internships at a humane society, Hoy-Gerlach et al. (2019, p. 9) identified four key questions necessary to collaboratively address the following:

- What is a social worker and what does a social worker do?
- What are the needs and goals of a humane society that could be addressed by a veterinary social work intern?
- How could the humane society meet the social work program's learning objectives/competencies as a field site?
- How would the student be supervised?

A humane society is a private nonprofit organization with a mission focused on animal welfare promotion by addressing issues that include, but are not limited to, companion animal homelessness and overpopulation, reducing and preventing animal abuse, and humane education. As an example of efforts to establish an internship, Hoy-Gerlach and colleagues (2019) described how interested parties from the social work education program and the humane society held an exploratory meeting to discuss and plan the internship. Attendees included the humane society executive director, the director of volunteers at the humane society, the lead animal cruelty investigator, the field director of the social work education program, and the social work faculty member (Hoy-Gerlach et al., 2019). Although the executive director did not assume a supervisory role for the intern, the director acted as an internal champion for hosting the graduate social work internship by conveying enthusiasm and fostering support for the internship among the shelter staff. In adopting and/or implementing something new, a person in a leadership role within the system who is an active proponent of the new endeavor is referred to as an internal champion (Miech et al., 2018). Champions for the development and implementation of a new idea, project, or process are those who:

(1) are internal to an organization; (2) generally have an intrinsic interest and commitment to implementing a change; (3) work diligently and relentlessly to drive implementation forward, even if those efforts receive no formal recognition or compensation; (4) are enthusiastic, dynamic, energetic, personable, and persistent; and (5) have strength of conviction. (Miech et al., 2018, p. 2)

The humane society did not have a social worker on staff, so the assignment of roles of task instructor and field instructor was also discussed during the exploratory meeting. The humane society director of volunteers and the lead cruelty investigator were invited to the exploratory meeting because both were potential task instructors. This internship placement would be the first to take place within a US humane society. Given the novelty of the placement, the university field director and faculty member served as internal champions within the university social work education environment and advocated for the internship. The decision was made for the social work faculty member to serve in the off-site field instructor role for the interns placed at the humane society (Hoy-Gerlach et al., 2019).

In contrast to the role of social workers at humane societies, the role of veterinary social work within veterinary clinics is much more established in both social work and veterinary medicine institutions. As an example, the University of Tennessee offers a postgraduate veterinary social work certificate program and hosts an annual International Veterinary Social Work Summit. Many veterinary professionals are aware of veterinary social work because of several articles published in the *Journal of the American Veterinary Medical Association* that described the scope of practice for veterinary social work. In comparison with larger humane societies, owner-operated veterinary practices also have fewer administrative layers to navigate, which can simplify the hosting and planning of a social work internship.

For the CPCC exploratory meeting, the four key questions were satisfactorily addressed, and the individuals in the key roles (internal champion, on-site task instructor, and off-site field instructor) were involved in discussions. The CPCC co-owner served in the roles of both internal champion and task instructor. The social work faculty member served in the off-site field instructor role. To address the key question "What is a social worker and what does one do" (Hoy-Gerlach et al., 2019), the team consulted an expert in veterinary social work within a veterinary practice setting (another co-author of this chapter). The consultant expanded the answer to include "What does a social worker do in a veterinary setting?"

The second key question posed by Hoy-Gerlach et al., (2019) in internship development calls for identification of the needs and goals of a particular organization/internship setting that could be addressed by a graduate social work intern. The list of needs and goals may be brainstormed within the initial exploratory meeting once a shared understanding of social work and veterinary social work is established. In starting where the veterinary practice is at, it is crucial to foreground the perspective of those in the internal champion and task instructor roles here; these are the priorities *from the veterinary clinic perspective*. The task instructor and internal champion are the experts in the area of veterinary service provision and are by far the best situated to brainstorm a list of needs, goals, and types of activities possible within their veterinary setting. At this juncture, brainstorming without editing or judging is recommended in order to generate as comprehensive a list as possible.

The CPCC co-owner (task instructor) brainstormed a list of needs of the practice, and the student intern and field instructor determined which items were appropriate and attainable for the student within their time in field placement. These items were then written into the student's field contract/agreement. Appendix 1 shows a list of possible tasks and learning activities a social work intern might complete in most veterinary practice settings in order to develop social work practice competencies. Many of the tasks in the table were generated from the CPCC needs list.

Social Work Intern Supervision Model

In the presented model, the CPCC co-owner was the task instructor, located at the veterinary practice. They managed the day-to-day interactions and provided training and orientation to the student, with appropriate staff, at the practice. The social work faculty member served as the off-site field instructor of record and completed formal intern evaluations. The field instructor provided regular social work-focused supervision to the student intern, as required by the CSWE, to ensure that practice competencies were being addressed. To further supplement the social work supervision for this internship with veterinary social work-specific expertise, the field instructor requested the social worker at the Ohio State University (OSU) Veterinary Medical Center to attend supervision sessions as requested. Several of these supervision sessions were in an online group format using web conferencing software and included multiple social work interns who had been placed in a veterinary setting. This supervision model was well received by the students, as well as the field instructor and consulting veterinary social worker.

Selecting a Social Work Intern for a Veterinary Social Work Internship with an Off-Site Field Instructor

The situation of a student placed in a nontraditional internship setting and an off-site field instructor poses significant challenges. Social work internships are intended to provide a type of apprenticeship with opportunities to shadow seasoned social workers as they perform in the role of social worker. Student social workers practice their skills and receive critical feedback to improve performance and hone skills. Since there was no on-site social worker for the student to emulate and learn from, an advanced social work graduate student who held a social work license and a Bachelor's Degree in Social Work was selected for the veterinary social work internship. Earning a BSW degree involves completing one or two field placements in a social work setting. In this case, the student had bachelors-level social work practice experience and a strong understanding of the basic roles of social workers, both of which were essential to the intern being able to function as a social worker in a nontraditional internship setting. In contrast, if a foundation graduate social work student (a student with an undergraduate degree in something other than social work) had been placed in a veterinary practice internship for their foundation year with no on-site social worker, it would be much more challenging for both the student and internship site staff to determine appropriate social work practice activities.

In addition to holding a BSW and post-BSW practice experience, the consulting veterinary social worker and social work faculty member/field instructor identified several additional attributes for the ideal veterinary social work intern candidate: emotional maturity, the ability to work autonomously, comfort with ambiguity, cognitive flexibility in shifting tasks readily based on emergent needs, and the ability to engage easily with clients, including seeking out clients rather than clients seeking them out.

An Overview of a Veterinary Social Work Internship Experience

The student selected for the Community Pet Care Clinic internship, in addition to meeting all of the above attributes, had actually actively sought out a graduate social work internship in the area of human-animal interaction (HAI) and was thus highly motivated. She readily identified her bifurcated client system: the human clientele who were seeking veterinary care, and the veterinary staff of CPCC.

In focusing on building engagement skills and working with CPCC practice to be a mezzo client system, the initial weeks of the internship were spent focusing on relationship-building with the veterinary teams. Specific strategies included crafting an introductory email that explained who she was and a simple overview of how she could be helpful to the staff and clientele: shadowing staff and helping with nonanimal-related tasks (keeping within the scope of social work practice), having informal conversations with them about their work as time allowed, and attending meetings and events. As staff members became accustomed to and comfortable with the intern's presence and role, they began to invite and include her in client situations where they anticipated they might need her assistance.

The COVID-19 pandemic undoubtedly added stressors to both clients and the veterinary team and complicated the seeking and provision of veterinary services. The intern shadowed clinic staff as they went outside to talk with clients in the parking lot, brought pets inside for treatment, and returned them to their people who remained waiting in cars. Clients were often distressed about their animals, upset about the mask mandate, and frustrated at being unable to accompany their animals into the clinic. In some instances, the clients refused outright to wear masks, even when offered them by CPCC. While the staff was accustomed to human clients being worried and distressed about the well-being of their animals, asking people to wait in the car while their animal was examined was a new process for both the staff and clients. Clients would express concern about how their animals would fare without them in the appointment, and anxiety and/or anger at not being permitted to accompany their animal. Such anxious and angry client reactions were unfortunately routinely directed at the staff who would come to a parked vehicle to retrieve an animal for an appointment, and then return the animal to the vehicle afterword. The overall stress level of both clients and staff was also heightened due to the COVID-19 pandemic; veterinary services were essentially being provided in a mass trauma that has affected everyone worldwide to varying degrees. Anecdotal reports from veterinary staff suggest that clients tended to come in with lower distress tolerance thresholds, and more quickly lose their tempers. This constellation of factors led to increased staff-client conflicts, which unsurprisingly in turn led to increased staff reports of frustration and emotional fatigue.

Basic de-escalation skills are valuable for veterinary staff working under typical practice conditions that present a host of routine stressors; for veterinary staff working in a pandemic, such de-escalation skills were vital. To support the staff in addressing and resolving both routine and COVID-related client concerns, the CPCC co-owner/task instructor tasked the intern with a priority assignment: developing a simple training that could assist staff in responding to angry clients and de-escalating conflict situations. Key aspects of such a staff training included creating a safe environment for staff to share situations, explaining barriers to communication and how to reduce them, providing de-escalation and communication tips such as active listening strategies, explaining how to express empathy, and helping people be mindful of tone and body language. Many staff talked about personalizing clients' expressions of anger toward them; working with staff to identify their reactions, debrief, and choose more helpful reactions was another key strategy. Such a de-escalation training can serve as the kick-off to the building of an informal peer support network for veterinary staff, along with providing a shared language and foundation for staff debriefing. Following the training, the social work intern continued to facilitate intermittent informal staff debriefings after the close of clinic and was especially careful to offer to do so after particularly challenging days. Both the de-escalation training and the debriefings were well received by staff; as time went on, the staff increasingly proactively sought the intern out, individually and informally, to share concerns and issues they had experienced and to ask her to assist with client situations.

Assessing staff needs and strengths is another important social work internship task, both from the standpoint of building that social work practice competency and because it is necessary in order to best serve the veterinary practice. Given staff at a veterinary practice often work varying days and shifts, a simple way to access them is through an emailed survey instrument. Google Forms is a simple tool in which one can easily create an assessment survey; other survey tool could certainly also work. The social work intern at CPCC used Google Forms to create an assessment survey which was emailed to all of the staff; they were able to respond anonymously, and the response rate showed the vast majority of the staff completed the survey.

Based on assessment survey results, a veterinary social work intern will be able to better tailor support responses to identified staff needs while building on existing staff strengths. For example, staff expressed both a need for more encouragement and appreciation and a sense that they cared for each other (a strength). In response, the CPCC intern created a "Secret Encourager" program, which functioned much like a "Secret Santa" program; the participation was voluntary, and staff who wish to participate fill out a form about their interests and what helps them feel good. Staff were then matched with a "Secret Encourager" who provided personalized small tokens of encouragement and appreciation while building on the care between staff. Staff feedback on this was overwhelmingly positive. As the CPCC social work internship drew to a close, the staff asked the CPCC intern to help them set up a second round of "Secret Encourager" so that they could continue the process after she left.

The assessment survey results also indicated that a primary stressor for veterinary staff was having conversations with clients about finances. The veterinary staff suggested that one person should be responsible for having the financial conversations with clients and develop expertise in such. The intern recognized that in addition to helping alleviate staff stress, the development, linkage, and coordination of resources for veterinary clients would enhance veterinary access and provide opportunities for her to build practice competencies related to fostering economic justice. The veterinary staff trained and educated the social work intern on the various financial options available. There were two ultimate goals identified in having a social work intern engage in financial conversations with clients: to link the client with financial resources to cover veterinary care costs and to build rapport with the client so that any additional needs could be identified and appropriate resources provided.

It is worth reiterating that the social work intern's initial engagement and assessment efforts focused on supporting the veterinary staff. As gatekeepers to the human clients who bring their animals to a veterinary practice for care, the veterinary staff had significant influence on the social work intern's ability to engage and intervene with the practice clients. As the intern's relationship with the CPCC staff deepened and solidified, she was increasingly viewed as part of the team and began to work with the human clients of CPCC more actively and consistently as her second client system. CPCC staff became more conscious of their clients' unique psychosocial situations and proactively involved the intern to better support clients and their animals. An interaction with a client who was experiencing domestic violence served as a catalyst for the intern to develop a resource for the staff on how to assist clients facing a domestic violence circumstance. At the request of staff, the intern began making routine follow-up phone calls to clients that had euthanized their pets, as well as others they identified as potentially in need of additional bereavement support. After networking with a with a veterinary social worker at the Michigan State University Veterinary Social Work Program, the CPCC intern collaborated with the graduate social work intern at the Toledo Humane Society to establish a virtual pet loss support group. This support group, co-facilitated by both interns, was held via Zoom for a 6-week period. The intern networked with various local animal welfare organizations to publicize the group to the community.

The development and dissemination of a community resource guide for pet owners is another social work internship task in a veterinary practice that can help alleviate stress for human clients who may have animal-related needs other than veterinary care. In response to staff referrals of clients who presented with such additional needs, the CPCC intern developed a community directory of commonly needed animal-related resources; this was widely disseminated in human health and social service organizations in Northwest Ohio. On the CPCC intern's last day at CPCC, she was linked with and helped a client concerned about a family member with a pet who lacked permanent housing and was in dire need of resources. The intern was immediately able to provide this client with the directory of low-cost pet resources, which addressed several of their family member's needs. The client expressed gratitude to CPCC for the information. Such an information guide can be of value not only to the people and pets in need of such supports but also to those who care for them.

Conclusion

In sum, not having a social worker on staff at a veterinary clinic is not an insurmountable barrier to developing a graduate social work veterinary internship. The benefits offered to the staff and clients of a veterinary practice via hosting a veterinary social work internship, in combination with the diverse learning opportunities afforded graduate social work students at veterinary practices, truly make such endeavors a win-win proposition. Through networking, collaboration, planning, and creative innovation when faced with emergent situations, veterinary social work internships can be developed in a range of veterinary practice settings. This chapter offers a simple process that can be readily followed and an appendix list of practice needs/learning activities that can be easily adapted by an owner-operated veterinary practice interested in hosting a social work internship. The response of CPCC staff and owners to having a social work graduate intern was overwhelmingly positive; they have expressed excitement at hosting their next intern and are seeking funds to hire the individual who just completed her veterinary social work internship with them.

Appendix 1: CSWE Competencies and Sample Veterinary Practice-Based Learning Activities

While some of these will not apply to every veterinary practice, the authors wanted to include all possible.

Competency 1: Demonstrate Ethic and Professional Behavior

- Discuss ethical issues that are common to social workers in veterinary host settings (confidentiality and documentation-social work notes separate from animal medical record, dual relationships with providing support to staff).

- Discuss animal abuse reporting (Is it mandated for veterinarians or social workers in your state? If not mandated, how does one deal with it?).

Competency 2: Engage Diversity and Difference in Practice

- Explore diversity, equity, and inclusion efforts in veterinary medicine (American Veterinary Medical Association, American Animal Hospital Association).
- Identify subpopulations in need of differential supports due to emergent needs.

Competency 3: Advance Human Rights and Social, Economic, and Environmental Justice

- Discuss access to pet care for underserved populations.

    - https://pphe.utk.edu/wp-content/uploads/2020/09/avcc-report.pdf

- Research Safe Haven for Pets programs, and determine if the clinic is willing/will able to provide Safe Haven.
- Find out if the agency is involved in advocacy at the local, state, and federal level.
- Design and execute an outreach/low-cost veterinary clinic event.

Competency 4: Engage in Practice-Informed Research and Research-Informed Practice

- Complete evaluation of hospital services in regard to accessibility of services and use of services from the social work perspective.
- Research and develop a lists of best practices conducted by other veterinary.
- Locate and read articles, research studies, and/or book chapters related to veterinary social work, mental health issues in veterinary medicine, etc.

Competency 5: Engage in Policy Practice

- Review policies/procedures in the veterinary setting.
- Develop/update the social work intern training/procedure manual.
- Identify current bills related to animal welfare and the human-animal bond at the local, state, and federal levels.
- Attend policy planning meetings.
- Develop policies (animal abuse reporting, domestic violence suspicion, etc.).

Competency 6: Engage with Individuals, Families, Groups, Organizations, and Communities

- Intern to share introduction letter/bio/photo with staff explaining social work role.
- Meet key members of the team (practice owner, practice manager, etc.).
- Engage with clinic staff through shadowing, observation, and participation in clinic activities to build relationship/rapport.
- Conduct follow-up calls to owners after euthanasia or death of pets.
- Connect with area social service agencies to disperse a pet support guide with local support options for animals (low-cost grooming, pet food banks, temporary boarding, etc.).
- Tour cremation company the clinic uses.

- Develop collaborative relationships with human health and social service organizations that have clients that are pet owners (determine community partners for outreach clinics).

Competency 7: Assess with Individuals, Families, Groups, Organizations, and Communities

- Survey team requesting their input on stressors, strengths, and desired supports.
- Observe reception staff and/or phone staff to get an understanding of both the needs of the clients and the needs of the staff.
- Explore financial options available to clients.
- Conduct a needs assessment, survey, and/or focus group with clinicians and staff re: their training needs.
- Review websites of other veterinary social work and how they serve their clients.
- Assess client needs for referrals to ongoing services.
- Assessment of suicidal tendencies, mental health issues, and domestic violence issues.
- Review data trends within the clinic and develop interventions, e.g., determine how many parvovirus cases the clinic has, whether there is a trend in the geographic area, and whether vaccine clinics should be offered in that area.
- Assist in redesign of the practice's comfort room.
- Design and deliver a survey to determine client's needs regarding pet support. Analyze the data and help develop resources to address needs.
- Assess/connect with local social service agencies to evaluate their client's veterinary care needs and how to assist in providing affordable pet care.

Competency 8: Intervene with Individuals, Families, Groups, Organizations, and Communities

- Interventions with clients:

  - Crisis intervention.
  - Assist in processing difficult treatment decisions and end-of-life and quality-of-life discussions.
  - Support during euthanasia.
  - Grief support.
  - Facilitate a pet loss support group (in person or online).

- Interventions with veterinary clinic team:

  - Consultation about clients, e.g., communication coaching, boundary setting, angry clients, etc.
  - Debriefing sessions, e.g., regarding difficult cases/situations
  - Referral for outside mental health services
  - Wellness resources (short email blasts, art therapy activities, websites, apps)
  - Compassion fatigue group
  - Training for the team on issues such as de-escalation strategies, diffusing difficult and stressful client situations, animal cruelty/neglect recognition and reporting, and hoarding

- Develop/update:

  - Brochures/handouts (pet loss, quality of life, children and grief, and others).
  - Pet loss resources, such as therapists, support groups, home euthanasia services, pet loss support hotlines, online resources, booklist.
  - Other client resources including, but not limited to, financial, mental health, housing, transportation, and rental assistance.
  - Website.
  - Remembrance ceremony/memorial event.
  - Pet loss support group.
  - Forms, procedures, materials, and scheduling system for outreach program.
  - Protocols for staff to effectively utilize social work support during stressful client situations.
  - Collaborate with local human health/social service agencies to develop/add questions about pets on their patient/client paperwork (Do you have any animals in your household? Do you have any worries or concerns about your pets? What part does your pet play in your family?).

Competency 9: Evaluate with Individuals, Families, Groups, Organizations, and Communities

- Evaluate response to workshops provided to teams and/or clients.
- Evaluation of any new programs (outreach clinic, memorial events, etc.).
- Make recommendations to administrators.

References

Abram, F., Hartung, M., & Wernet, S. (2000). The nonMSW task supervisor, MSW field instructor, and the practicum student: A triad for high quality field education. *Journal of Teaching in Social Work, 20*(1/2), 171–185.

American Pet Products Association. (n.d.). *2019–2020 APPA national pet owners survey*. https://www.americanpetproducts.org/pubs_survey.asp

Bikales, G. (1975). The dog as "significant other". *Social Work, 20*, 150–152.

Cima, G. (2020). Social work expands in veterinary hospitals: Emergency, specialty practices hiring to counsel staff members, clients. *Journal of the American Veterinary Medical Association, 256*(12), 1310–1314. https://www.avma.org/javma-news/2020-06-15/social-work-expands-veterinary-hospitals

Council on Social Work Education. (2015, June 11). *Education policy and accreditation standards*. https://www.cswe.org/getattachment/Accreditation/Accreditation-Process/2015-EPAS/2015EPAS_Web_FINAL.pdf.aspx

Council on Social Work Education. (2021). *Information for students and social workers*. https://www.cswe.org/accreditation/info/student-and-social-worker-information/

Hediger, K., Meisser, A., & Zinsstag, J. (2019). A One Health research framework for animal-assisted interventions. *International Journal of Environmental Research and Public Health, 16*(4), 640.

Hoy-Gerlach, J., Delgado, M., Sloane, H., & Arkow, P. H. (2019). Rediscovering connections between animal welfare and human welfare: Developing master's level social work internship at a humane society. *Journal of Social Work, 19*(2), 216–232. https://doi.org/10.1177/1468017318760775

Miech, E., Rattray, N., Flanagan, M., Damschroder, L., Schmid, A., & Damush, T. (2018). Inside help: An integrative review of champions in healthcare-related implementation. *SAGE Open Medicine, 6*, 1–11.

Larkin, M. (2016). For human needs, some veterinary clinics are turning to a professional: Social workers see a place for themselves in veterinary practice. *Journal of American Veterinary Medical Association, 248*(1), 8–12. https://doi.org/10.2460/javma.248.1.8

Nett, R. J., Witte, T. K., Holzbauer, S. M., Elchos, B. L., Campangnolo, E. R., Musgrave, K. J., … Funk, R. H. (2015). Risk factors for suicide, attitudes toward mental illness, and practice-related stressors among US veterinarians. *Journal of American Veterinary Medical Association, 247*(8), 945–955. https://doi.org/10.2460/javma.247.8.945

Tomasi, S. E., Fechter-Leggett, E. D., Edwards, N. T., Reddish, A. D., Crosby, A. E., & Nett, R. J. (2019). Suicide among veterinarians in the United States from 1979 through 2015. *Journal of the American Veterinary Medical Association, 254*(1), 104–112. https://doi.org/10.2460/javma.254.1.104

University of Tennessee. (2021). *Veterinary social work.* https://vetsocialwork.utk.edu/about-us/

University of Toledo. (2021). *MSW Student Handbook.* https://www.utoledo.edu/hhs/socialwork/gradprogram.html

Chapter 14
Ethical and Legal Issues in Veterinary Social Work Research

Sana Loue

Introduction

Social workers may engage in research in the context of their employment with nonprofit organizations, governmental entities, or academic institutions. Less frequently, they may be involved as independent consultants to research teams or enterprises. Most often, veterinary social workers (VSWs) conducting research will be concerned with human participants. As examples, research might involve a study of various dimensions of the human-animal bond from the perspective both of the human companions of animals and of the social workers who include animals in their practices (Risley-Curtiss, 2010). They might be members of research teams investigating the mental health of veterinary professionals (see Bartram & Baldwin, 2008; Scotney et al., 2015), the effects of pet support services for homeless populations, the relationship between animal abuse and family violence, or best practices for the inclusion of animals in clinical practice (Arkow, 2020). The findings of such research may be critical to advocacy efforts on behalf of clients and for the formulation of policy (Maschi & Youdin, 2012).

The first portion of this chapter considers ethical issues that may arise when social workers are involved in research efforts that focus on the humans involved. The second portion of this chapter examines the ethical issues that may face the social worker when conducting research that is designed to focus on both the humans and the animals involved. In each case, the researchers may be concerned

S. Loue (✉)
Department of Bioethics, Case Western Reserve University School of Medicine, Cleveland, OH, USA
e-mail: Sana.Loue@case.edu

with the relationship between the animals and the humans, but the ethical and legal issues that arise may vary somewhat due to the nature and focus of the research.

Ethical and Legal Issues in Veterinary Social Work Research with Humans

Consider the following hypothetical study. *The research team wishes to understand whether people who own dogs are better able to manage daily levels of stress compared to those who have no pets. They design a study to compare the daily stress levels and stress management strategies of people who currently own dogs versus people who do not currently own dogs. They will assess stress level using a self-report measure to be completed by each participant, as well as daily measures of blood pressure and cortisol levels.*

In this scenario, the focus of the research is on the human beings. Although the researchers are responsible for safeguarding the safety of the humans as research participants, many would likely argue that they are not responsible for the safety of the dogs as research participants because they played no role in whether people did or did not have dogs. Indeed, as Moga notes in her Chap. 7 in this volume, social work codes of ethics fail to acknowledge the role of animals, whether in the clinical or research context. However, depending on the laws pertaining to animal abuse and neglect that exist where the study is being carried out, the researchers may have a legal responsibility to report any animal abuse or neglect that they suspect or witness.

It may come as a surprise to some readers to learn that many ethical and legal obligations involving responsibilities to human research participants that are often associated with biomedical research are arguably relevant to social work research. As the result of several court decisions, social workers conducting research with human participants are likely also obligated to adhere to the norms of international law that pertain to research (*Abdullahi v. Pfizer*, 2009). These laws and norms are embodied in the Nuremberg Code (1946), the Declaration of Helsinki (World Medical Association, 2013), and the International Covenant on Civil and Political Rights (1966)[1]; each of these three international documents expressly requires that a researcher obtain the informed consent of an individual as a prerequisite to his or her participation in research. This requirement is reflected in US federal regulations governing the conduct of human subjects research (45 C.F.R. Part 46, 2018). Depending upon the state in which US-based research is undertaken and the focus

---

[1] The Nuremberg Code was promulgated in 1947 by a military tribunal as part of its final judgment against 15 Nazi physicians who were found guilty of war crimes and crimes against humanity due to their conduct of medical experiments on individuals without their consent (Annas, 1992). The International Covenant on Civil and Political Rights, which is legally binding on the more than 160 nations that have ratified it, guarantees the right to individuals to be free from nonconsensual medical experimentation by any entity.

of the particular research, social work research may also fall within the scope of state laws and/or regulations.

The Nuremberg Code provides the foundation for three basic principles that guide the conduct of research involving human beings: respect for persons, beneficence, and justice. *Respect for persons* encompasses the concept of autonomy and the requirement that research with human beings be conducted only with the informed consent of the individual. How we understand autonomy, however, depends upon our notion of personhood. In the USA, autonomy is often interpreted to refer to individual rights, self-determination, and privacy (De Craemer, 1983). *Beneficence* refers to the researcher's obligation to maximize good to the research participants. This principle is sometime framed as two, the second being *nonmaleficence*, or the obligation to minimize harm to the research participants. The principle of *justice* is frequently interpreted as distributive justice; this refers to the researcher's responsibility to equitably distribute the benefits and burdens of research across groups. The Nuremberg Code specifies that research involving human participants should not be conducted unless the prospective participants have given their voluntary consent, there is no prior reason to believe that death or disabling injury will occur, the researchers are qualified to conduct the research, and the participant may end their participation in the research at any time.

Respect for Persons

Respect for persons refers to both the concept of autonomy and the requirement that special protections in research be provided for vulnerable persons. This principle suggests that (1) individuals and groups may be different in ways that are relevant to their worldview and their response to any variety of situations; (2) the researcher must respect these differences and fashion their research protocols in a way that is sensitive to these varying understandings while still ensuring that fundamental principles of informed consent are observed; and (3) the researcher is responsible for ensuring that individuals with impaired or diminished autonomy who are participating in the research are protected from harm or abuse (Loue, 2017).

Autonomy requires that an individual be able to act "(1) intentionally, (2) with understanding, and (3) without controlling influences" (Faden & Beauchamp, 1986). In order to act with understanding, the individual must have the capacity to do so and must have the information necessary for understanding. Influences on a person's decision-making exist along a continuum, ranging from controlling to non-controlling; beyond a certain point on that continuum, the degree of control becomes so great that a decision cannot be said to be voluntary.

Capacity refers to the ability of an individual to evidence a choice, the ability to understand relevant information, the ability to appreciate a situation and its consequences, and the ability to manipulate information rationally. Although the term is often used interchangeably with "competence," the two concepts are distinct.

Competence is a legal determination relating to an individual's ability to care for him- or herself and/or his or her financial affairs.

Adults are presumed to have the capacity to consent unless there is reason to believe otherwise (Children are by law presumed to lack adequate capacity to consent, although the age at which childhood ends and adulthood begins may differ across states in the USA and across countries). The ability to decide whether or not to participate in research requires that the individual be able to understand basic study information, including the procedures to be performed, the risks associated with participation, the potential benefits to be gained from participation, alternatives to study participation, the difference between research interventions and established therapy, and the individual's ability to refuse to participate without suffering a penalty (Dresser, 2001).

Vulnerable participants are often thought to be individuals with "insufficient power, prowess, intelligence, resources, strength or other needed attributes to protect their own interests through negotiations for informed consent" (Levine, 1988). Vulnerability and capacity may be interrelated; as an example, individuals may have illnesses that affect capacity, such as advanced Alzheimer's dementia and active psychosis. The capacity to provide informed consent may be understood as fluctuating (National Bioethics Advisory Commission, 1998), such as when a participant is experiencing delusions due to mental illness.

The concept of vulnerability has traditionally been used to refer to members of specific groups that share a common characteristic, such as children, prisoners, and pregnant women. However, it is now recognized that vulnerability is inherent in situations, not people (Kipnis, 2001). As an example, a pregnant woman may be vulnerable in a clinical trial to test a new drug for the treatment of depression, but is likely not vulnerable in survey research about the contribution of pet ownership to stress management during pregnancy. Further, although often treated as a binary classification (one is either vulnerable or not), it is open to debate whether vulnerability is better conceptualized as a spectrum of attributes with greater and lesser vulnerability. Vulnerability has also been conceived of as existing in layers, whereby characteristics possessed by an individual can cumulatively add layers of vulnerability, e.g., poverty, race, and illiteracy may combine in a particular research context to compound the vulnerability of an individual beyond that which would result from the existence of only one such characteristic (Luna, 2009).

Relying on the definition of vulnerability above, it appears that many of the populations that might be involved as participants in social work research could be considered vulnerable depending upon the nature of the research and the context in which it is conducted. This may include students; elderly persons; residents of nursing homes; hospitalized patients; people receiving welfare benefits or social assistance and other poor people and the unemployed; some ethnic, racial, and religious minority groups; homeless persons; nomads; refugees or displaced persons; prisoners; patients with incurable diseases; individuals who are politically powerless; members of relatively isolated communities; and individuals with serious, potentially disabling, or life-threatening diseases. Accordingly, it is important for researchers to understand the social, historical, and other contextual realities in which the research participants are living in order to understand whether and the degree to which they may be vulnerable in the proposed research (Kipnis, 2003; Levine et al., 2004).

Understanding and Information   In order to act with understanding, a prospective research participant has been provided with adequate information regarding the nature of the research and its potential implications and consequences to enable him or her to make an informed choice regarding participation. Many of these elements are also included in US federal regulations that apply to all research conducted in institutions that receive federal funding, such as hospitals and institutions that receive Medicare or Medicaid payments, universities that receive federal research grants, and nonprofit clinics and organizations that receive certain forms of government funding.

Ethical guidelines relating to the conduct of social work research reflect the norms embodied by these international documents and federal regulations. Social workers are ethically obligated to ensure that participants in their research are adequately informed and protected. The *Code of Ethics* of the National Association of Social Workers (2021) advises that:

> Social workers engaged in evaluation or research should obtain voluntary and written informed consent from participants, when appropriate, without any implied or actual deprivation or penalty for refusal to participate; without undue inducement to participate; and with due regard for participants' well-being, privacy, and dignity. Informed consent should include information about the nature, extent, and duration of the participation requested and disclosure of the risks and benefits of participation in the research.
>
> (g) When evaluation or research participants are incapable of giving informed consent, social workers should provide an appropriate explanation to the participants, obtain the participants' assent to the extent they are able, and obtain written consent from an appropriate proxy.
>
> (h) Social workers should never design or conduct evaluation or research that does not use consent procedures, such as certain forms of naturalistic observation and archival research, unless rigorous and responsible review of the research has found it to be justified because of its prospective scientific, educational, or applied value and unless equally effective alternative procedures that do not involve waiver of consent are not feasible.
>
> (i) Social workers should inform participants of their right to withdraw from evaluation and research at any time without penalty. (National Association of Social Workers, 2021, par. 5.02(g)–(i))

Even after providing an individual with all of the information that can possibly be provided, a person may misunderstand the purpose of the study because of a misbelief about the underlying purpose of inviting his or her participation. Suppose, for example, that the social worker wishes to evaluate whether individuals who are diagnosed with a chronic illness-associated depression do better with animal-assisted psychotherapy compared to similar individuals who receive cognitive behavioral therapy (CBT). He or she proposes to randomize the agency's clients into two groups, one of which will receive the usual CBT for depression management, and the other of which will receive CBT augmented with animal-assisted therapy. A client may erroneously believe that the social worker truly does know what will work best for the client and is offering this opportunity because it will be of clinical benefit to the client. This misbelief, known as the therapeutic misconception (Appelbaum et al., 1987; Grisso & Appelbaum, 1998), may be difficult to detect when discussing research participation with an ongoing client.

The Nuremberg Code suggests that there must be a balance of the risks and benefits to the prospective research participants that are involved in any specific research undertaking and that provisions be made to reduce the likelihood of or impact of the potential risks. In the context of social work research, these provisions might focus on access to supportive services and protecting participants from unwarranted distress. In almost every research situation involving human participants, there exists a potential risk that confidentiality may be inadvertently breached. The National Association of Social Workers' *Code of Ethics* reflects these principles:

> (j) Social workers should take appropriate steps to ensure that participants in evaluation and research have access to appropriate supportive services.
> (k) Social workers engaged in evaluation or research should protect participants from unwarranted physical or mental distress, harm, danger, or deprivation. (National Association of Social Workers, 2021, par. 5.02(j)–(k))

Voluntariness What constitutes a "controlling influence" varies across cultures. Many Americans think of themselves as independent agents who are free to make decisions without consulting others or considering the consequences to others. However, in some cultures, an individual may view themselves as an "enlarged self," that is, the aggregation and integration of various roles and relationships, each with corresponding responsibilities. Individuals who see themselves this way may want to consult with important others before deciding whether or not to participate in a research study. As long as this consultation by a prospective research participant with others is voluntary, it is entirely consistent with the principle of respect for persons.

Social workers conducting research must also consider the power differential that exists between the researcher and the potential participant. One scholar explained:

> The process of conducting research tends to reinforce the power imbalances of society. Researchers usually turn their gaze downward in the social power hierarchy, studying people who are poorer, less educated, more discriminated against, and in a variety of ways less socially powerful than themselves. (Aronson Fontes, 1998, p. 54)

In some research situations, there may be little likelihood of a power differential. For example, a researcher sends out a survey to everyone living in a specific neighborhood to ascertain how many school-aged children would be interested in participating in an after-school program that involves animals. The power differential may not be an issue because the potential participant can easily ignore the mailed survey. It is a very different situation, however, if a social worker wishes to conduct research using his or her own clients as the research cases or participants. The client might feel that he or she would not receive the same quality of care if they do not agree to be part of a study or that the social worker might prepare a negative report that would later come back to haunt them. Even if the client is no longer receiving services from the social worker, e.g., case management or counseling, he or she might fear that a refusal to participate in the research would lead to a refusal by the social worker to provide future services if the client wished to have them.

Monetary payments are frequently offered to individuals to increase the likelihood that an adequate number of participants will be recruited for a particular study; to overcome "opportunity costs" and increase the recruitment of individuals from underrepresented groups; to reimburse individuals for the costs associated with their participation, such as lost wages, transportation, and child care expenses; and/or to provide participants with fair compensation for their contribution of their time and any associated inconvenience (Grady, 2005). Concerns have been raised as to whether such payments are coercive or represent undue influence, particularly when made to individuals who are economically disadvantaged with lower educational levels that may impede their comprehension and heighten their vulnerability (Denny & Grady, 2007; Grady, 2001; Largent et al., 2012).

Most scholars agree that coercion involves a threat of harm, so that payments to research participants are not coercive because coercion is absent from such interactions (Beauchamp & Childress, 1994; Largent et al., 2012). Modest payments to research participants to compensate them for their contribution are unlikely to induce individuals to ignore potential study risks and agree to participate in proposed research (Faden & Beauchamp, 1986).

In addition to the risks and benefits, individuals must also understand several particular aspects in order to understand that a study involves research:

- That they will be contributing to the development of generalizable knowledge that will be used to help others in the future (research contribution).
- That the investigators will rely on the participants to gather this generalizable knowledge (research relationship).
- The extent to which what the participants do and what happens to them will be altered because of their participation in the particular research (Wendler & Grady, 2008).

Social work researchers can utilize a number of strategies to enhance the communication of these elements. These include:

- Ensuring that the literacy level of the informed consent document is consistent with the prospective participant's reading level.
- Using language and terms in both the written informed consent form and in discussions about the study that non-researchers and nonprofessionals can understand.
- Formatting the informed consent form and process to facilitate understanding, e.g., using a video to explain the study.
- Assessing the prospective participant's understanding about the study by asking him or her questions about the study how it will affect them.
- Providing a stipend in an amount and/or form that is commensurate with what is expected of the participant.
- Allowing the prospective participant adequate time to consult with others regarding their participation prior to deciding whether or not to participate (Flory & Emanuel, 2004).

Beneficence and Nonmaleficence

As indicated previously, this dual principle states that the benefits of the research are to be maximized and the harms are to be minimized. Accordingly, the potential risks of the research must be outweighed by the potential benefits, the research design must be sound, the researcher must be competent to conduct the proposed research, and the welfare of the research participants must be protected. The principle might be unintentionally violated if the social worker does not adequately consider all possible scenarios in designing the research. As an example, the questions asked by a social worker conducting research on moral distress among veterinary personnel may trigger additional distress. In conducting such a study, the social worker should be prepared ahead of time to provide research participants with a listing of mental health support services that they would be able to consult if needed.

Justice

The *Belmont Report* (National Commission for the Protection of Human Subjects of Biomedical and Behavioral Research, 1979, pp. 7–8) noted:

> Justice is relevant to the selection of subjects of research at two levels: the social and the individual. Individual justice in the selection of subjects would require that researchers … not offer potentially beneficial research only to some patients who are in their favor.
>
> Injustice may appear in the selection of subjects, even if individual subjects are selected fairly by investigators and treated fairly in the course of research. This injustice arises from social, racial, sexual, and cultural biases institutionalized in society ….
>
> Although individual institutions or investigators may not be able to resolve a problem that is pervasive in their social setting, they can consider distributive justice in selecting research subjects.

These observations suggest that prior to beginning a research study, the social worker conducting research should consider whether the individuals who are to be burdened by their participation will also benefit from the study findings. As an example, if individuals participate in a study to evaluate the effectiveness of an intervention, will they have access to that intervention following the conclusion of the study?

Legal Obligations Associated with Data

Discussions related to legal obligations associated with data often focus on confidentiality protections, limitations on confidentiality, and data ownership and sharing. (The concept of confidentiality is to be distinguished from privacy, which refers specifically to the person, rather than the data.) Although an extended discussion of these obligations is beyond the scope of this chapter, the following section provides a brief overview of various salient issues.

Confidentiality and Its Limits

Legal Obligations   In general, social workers who conduct research are legally required to maintain the confidentiality of the data that they collect from research participants.

Depending upon the nature and the source of the data collected, the federal Health Insurance Portability and Accountability Act of 1996, known as HIPAA, and related regulations may be the sources of that legal obligation. Every healthcare provider who transmits health information in connection with certain transactions is covered by the law. Even if a social worker is acting in his or her capacity as a researcher, if he or she receives or sends health-related information electronically, that communication is likely to fall within HIPAA's scope. As an example, a social worker conducting research relating to mental health outcomes associated with animal-assisted psychotherapy may wish to obtain copies of the participants' clinical records to compare provider observations with the participants' subjective opinions about their mental health status. A participant might ask the social worker-researcher to transmit copies of their assessment to their healthcare providers. Using electronic technology alone, such as e-mail will not bring the transmission under HIPAA; "the transmission must be in connection with a standard transaction" (United States Department of Health and Human Services, n.d.). It could be argued, however, that the request for or release of such information constitutes a standard transaction.

The HIPAA privacy rule covers "protected health information," which refers to information about an individual's past, present, or future physical or mental health condition and identifies the individual or provides information such that there is a reasonable basis to believe that the individual could be identified (45 C.F.R. § 160.103, 2013). If the individual providing the information is considered to be a covered entity under the law, such as a psychiatrist's office providing a previous mental health assessment, that entity must obtain the individual's written consent to use or disclose the private health information if that disclosure is not for payment, treatment, or healthcare operations or otherwise permitted or protected by the privacy rule (45 C.F.R. § 164.508, 2013). The provisions of HIPAA's privacy rule are quite complex, and social workers conducting research relating to individuals' health status are urged to consult its provisions to ensure that they are in compliance.

Although electronic media such as e-mail, chat rooms, instant messaging, videoconferencing programs, and videoteleconferencing systems are frequently used in the research context to convey information between members of the research team or between participants and members of the research team (Neukrug, 1991; Smith et al., 1998), reliance on these mechanisms may increase risks to confidentiality. A variety of strategies can be utilized in an effort to reduce risks associated with electronic transmissions. These include the use of complex passwords for computers, iPads, and cell phones, screen savers to prevent others from seeing computer screens while they are in use, establishment of a virtual private network (VPN) to further safeguard communications from being accessed over public networks, and encryption software.

The *Code of Ethics* of the National Association of Social Workers addresses the need to maintain individuals' privacy and the confidentiality of their data. The *Code* provides that:

> Social workers should respect clients' right to privacy. Social workers should not solicit private information from clients unless it is essential to providing services or conducting social work evaluation or research. Once private information is shared, standards of confidentiality apply. (National Association of Social Workers, 2021, standard 1.07(a))

Legal Limitations on Confidentiality in Research   There are, however, legal limitations on the ability of a social worker-researcher to assure confidentiality. The now famous 1976 case of *Tarasoff v. Regents of the University of California* established what has become known as a "duty to warn." The case involved a lawsuit by the Tarasoff family against the University of California and a psychologist at the Berkeley campus of the university following the murder of their daughter by a graduate student after she rebuffed his romantic overtures. The would-be suitor had revealed his intent to kill Tatiana during the course of counseling sessions with a psychologist at the school's counseling services. Although the psychologist and several colleagues attempted to have this student involuntarily hospitalized for observation purposes, he was released after a brief observation period and subsequently killed the daughter.

The psychologist claimed that he could not have advised either the family or Tatiana of the threat because to do so would have breached the traditionally protected relationship between the therapist and the patient. The court held otherwise, holding that when a patient "presents a serious danger … to another [person], [the therapist] incurs an obligation to use reasonable care to protect the intended victim against such danger." That obligation could be satisfied by warning the intended victim of the potential danger, by notifying authorities, or by taking "whatever other steps are reasonably necessary under the circumstances" (*Tarasoff v. Regents of the University of California*, 1976, p. 340). The court specifically noted that the therapist-patient privilege was not absolute. Some later court cases in various jurisdictions have followed the reasoning of the *Tarasoff* court (*Davis v. Lhim*, 1983; (*Ewing v. Goldstein*, 2004; *Ewing v. Northridge Hospital Medical Center*, 2004; *McIntosh v. Milano*, 1979). (It should be noted, however, that a duty to warn no longer exists in California, and there is now only a duty to protect due to statutory revisions subsequent to these judicial decisions. See Weinstock et al., 2014 for additional analysis.) Judicial opinions differ, however, on whether the patient/client must make threats about a specific, intended victim to trigger the duty to warn (*Jablonski v. United States*, 1983; *Thompson v. County of Alameda*, 1980).

Depending on the particular state, however, researchers may also be required to report suspected instances of child sexual abuse, child abuse or neglect, elder abuse, or intimate partner violence that may be committed by or perpetrated on a research participant. Whether such an obligation exists often depends on the age and state of residence of the victim, the state's definition of the offense, the recency of the event, and the status of the reporter, that is, whether a researcher who holds a social work license under that state's laws is a mandated reporter, even when acting in the role of a researcher rather than as a provider of social work services. Some states, such as Ohio, now require that under specified circumstances, social workers must report suspected animal abuse or neglect (Ohio Counselor, Social Worker and Marriage and Family Therapist Board, n.d.).

Confidentiality may also be limited due to a subpoena. A subpoena is an order from a court or administrative body to compel the appearance of a witness or the production of specified document or records. This discussion focuses on subpoenas issued to compel the production of records or documents associated with the research.

A subpoena can be issued by a court or administrative body at the state or federal level. The information sought may be believed to be important to the conduct of an investigation, a criminal prosecution, or a civil lawsuit. As an example, a social worker conducting research into the link between animal abuse and family violence might be served with a subpoena demanding his or her research records relating to a particular research participant who has been charged with animal cruelty or child abuse. The issuance of subpoenas against researchers had become increasingly common (Auriti, 2013), and they have been used as a mechanism to obtain data relating to identifiable research participants (e.g., Hayes, 2011). In some cases, social workers conducting research on a sensitive issue, such as mental health or substance use, may be able to obtain a certificate of confidentiality from the National Institutes of Health (NIH), even if the study is not funded by the NIH. Certificates may protect the data from being accessed through a subpoena. Information relating to certificates of confidentiality and the application process may be found at https://grants.nih.gov/policy/humansubjects/coc/what-is.htm.

The legal and ethical obligations to maintain confidentiality extend even beyond the close of a study. Social workers who are engaged in research are required to report the research findings accurately and continue to preserve the confidentiality and privacy of the research participants (National Association of Social Workers, 2021). The identity of the research participants and the safeguarding of their individual data can often be accomplished by aggregating the data from multiple individuals, excluding identifying descriptions of individuals, and conflating multiple accounts or scenarios into one representative account or case study (see Australian Government, 2018).

Research Oversight

The US Regulatory Framework and Compliance

The basic ethical principles governing research have been integrated into federal law through statutes and regulations. Although a researcher's ethical and legal obligations are not always congruent, this legal framework mandates a researcher's

minimum obligations to research participants. In 1991, 15 different federal departments and agencies codified in their regulations the Federal Policy for the Protection
of Human Subjects, known as the "Common Rule." The Common Rule was revised
in 2017 and amended in January 2018; these most recent revisions became effective
on January 21, 2019. Twenty different federal agencies are either signatories to the
revised Common Rule or have indicated their intent to become an official signatory.
These include many agencies to which social worker-researchers may apply for
funds to support their research, such as the Agency for International Development,
the Department of Defense, the Department of Veterans Affairs, the Department of
Health and Human Services, and the National Science Foundation (United States
Department of Health and Human Services, Office for Human Research
Protections, 2016).

The revised Common Rule now specifies that the information provided to each
participant must be such that a reasonable person would want in order to decide
whether or not to participate. Portions that are relevant in the context of most veterinary social work research are:

1. A statement that the study involves research, an explanation of the purposes of
   the research and the expected duration of the subject's participation, a description of the procedures to be followed, and identification of any procedures that
   are experimental
2. A description of any reasonably foreseeable risks or discomforts to the subject
3. A description of any benefits to the subject or to others that may reasonably be
   expected from the research
4. A disclosure of appropriate alternative procedures or courses of treatment, if any,
   that might be advantageous to the subject
5. A statement describing the extent, if any, to which confidentiality of records
   identifying the subject will be maintained
6. For research involving more than minimal risk, an explanation as to whether any
   compensation and an explanation as to whether any medical treatments are available if injury occurs and, if so, what they consist of, or where further information
   may be obtained
7. An explanation of whom to contact for answers to pertinent questions about the
   research and research subjects' rights, and whom to contact in the event of a
   research-related injury to the subject
8. A statement that participation is voluntary, refusal to participate will involve no
   penalty or loss of benefits to which the subject is otherwise entitled, and the
   subject may discontinue participation at any time without penalty or loss of benefits to which the subject is otherwise entitled
9. One of the following statements about any research that involves the collection
   of identifiable private information or identifiable biospecimens:

   (i) A statement that identifiers might be removed from the identifiable private
       information or identifiable biospecimens and that, after such removal, the
       information or biospecimens could be used for future research studies or

distributed to another investigator for future research studies without additional informed consent from the subject or the legally authorized representative, if this might be a possibility

(ii) A statement that the subject's information or biospecimens collected as part of the research, even if identifiers are removed, will not be used or distributed for future research studies (46 C.F.R. § 46.116, 2018)

Additional information may be required depending upon the nature of the study.

Monitoring Mechanisms

One of the primary concerns in conducting research is that of participant safety. As noted earlier, researchers are ethically required to make efforts to maximize benefit and to avoid all unnecessary harm. Accordingly, efforts must be made to oversee the study and assure participant safety during the course of the research. These concerns are reflected in federal policy.

Institutional review boards (IRBs) are administrative bodies that are charged with the responsibility of following ethical standards for the conduct of studies and ensuring that the identity, privacy, safety, and health of the research participants are protected. Academic institutions and hospitals that engage in research and receive federal funds generally have an IRB. Some nonprofit entities and local departments of health may contract with a university-based IRB to review their research protocols. Alternatively, in some cases, the researcher will wish to utilize an independent IRB for the review of their protocol.

IRB review of studies involving human participants is required by federal regulations of "all research involving human subjects conducted, supported, or otherwise subject to regulation by any Federal department or agency that takes appropriate administrative action to make the policy applicable to such research" (45 C.F.R. § 46.101). Every IRB must have at least five members with varying disciplinary backgrounds in order to ensure that its review of research protocols will encompass the institutional, legal, scientific, and social implications of the proposed research and will be complete and adequate (45 C.F.R. § 46.107).

In some situations, the funding entity or an IRB will require that the researcher also have an independent data safety monitoring board (DSMB) or an independent safety monitor (National Institute of Mental Health, 2015a). This is often required in clinical trials, but is less common in the context of behavioral studies. An independent safety monitor (ISM) is an independent physician or other expert who is engaged to provide independent monitoring of a clinical trial (National Institute of Mental Health, 2015b). The ISM must not have any conflict of interest with either the study to be monitored or any member of the study team in order to ensure that he or she will maintain the objectivity necessary to ensure the safety of the trial participants and the integrity of the data. The ISM can be affiliated with the researcher's institution or the study site, but he or she cannot be a collaborator, mentor, mentee, supervisor, supervisee, co-author, or member of the investigator's department during the preceding 3 years.

A DSMB consists of individuals who are considered to be experts in their respective fields and who are independent of the study to be monitored (National Institute of Mental Health, 2015b). NIMH requires that a board have at least three members, who must include at least one content expert and one biostatistician. Additional members may include a bioethicist, pharmacologist, clinical trials expert, patient advocate, or community representative (National Institute on Drug Abuse, 2018). Members must be free of any professional or financial conflict of interests in order to assure objectivity. A member may be affiliated with the same institution as the investigator, but may not be a collaborator, co-author, supervisor, mentor, mentee, subordinate of the investigator, or member of the investigator's institutional department during the previous 3 years (National Institute of Mental Health, 2015b). The DSMB meets at predetermined intervals, such as semiannually or quarterly, but must in all cases meet at least once a year. They usually first meet in an open session that may include the investigators, and the program officers associated with the funding source. Unlike the IRB, DSMB members may have access to the study data if required to evaluate safety concerns (Loue, 2021).

Ethical and Legal Obligations in Research with Animal Subjects

Consider the following hypothetical study. Like the hypothetical study presented at the beginning of this chapter, the researchers wish to test their hypothesis that individuals who own dogs are better able to manage stress and have a broader range of stress management strategies. In order to do so, *they recruit individuals to the study who do not currently own dogs. They then randomize the individuals into two groups and provide dogs to people in one of the groups, but not the other. The researchers follow the study participants for a predesignated period of time, periodically assessing their levels of stress.*

In this scenario, many might agree that the researchers are ethically responsible not only for the safety of the human participants as research subjects but also for the safety and well-being of the dogs, because they provided them to the humans as a part of this experiment. In this case, their ethical and legal obligations to the dogs extend beyond the obligations that might be imposed for the reporting of animal abuse and neglect.

However, social work codes of ethics are silent with respect to the ethical obligations owed to animals in the context of research. Although animals have been used in research ever since the third century B.C. (Straight, 1962), discussion relating to ethical issues in the context of social work research has been relatively rare until recently. Views relating to the use of animals in research differ greatly across cultures, societies, and religion. (See Loue's Chap. 16, this volume, focusing on veterinary social work across diverse cultures. See also Loue, 2017). Some argue that humans are to be concerned for animals' welfare not because of a sensitivity to the animal, but rather because of the effect that acting cruelly would have on the human doing so (Francione, 2000; Gaffney, 1986). Others suggest that humans should be concerned with the animal itself (Kalechofsy, 1992), while still others object to the use of animals in any research (Regan, 1983, 1997; Singer, 1980). Too much of this discourse has focused attention on the use of animals for biomedical research, including laboratory-based research, and has not paid significant attention to researchers' reliance on animals in environments outside of laboratories.

Social workers who conduct their research in the context of their employment with an academic institution, a hospital, a nonprofit agency that receives specified federal funding, or a governmental entity are required to comply with federal regulations that set forth minimum standards for the care of the animals involved in the research. However, a large proportion of these requirements apply specifically to the use of animals in laboratory-based research.

Consider again the hypothetical study introduced at the beginning of this section. If that study were to occur at an academic institution or at a nonprofit organization or a hospital that receives specified types of federal funding, the researcher would be required to have his or her study protocol reviewed and approved by an institutional animal care and use committee (IACUC) prior to initiating the research. Specific requirements for the composition and function of the IACUC have been established by federal regulations. IACUCs must have a minimum of three members, one of whom is a veterinarian not involved in the proposed research. In general, the IACUC is concerned with the welfare of the animals in the research, including the extent to which pain, distress, and discomfort are minimized, the appropriateness of the animals' living conditions, the availability of needed veterinary care during the course of the research, and the qualifications of the individuals conducting the research (Health Research Extension Act of 1985; 9 C.F.R. § 2.31, 1998). Because the researchers conducting this hypothetical study have provided the human participants with the dogs as part of the study protocol, this study would likely be monitored by both an IRB, with its focus on the welfare of the human participants, and an IACUC, with its focus on the animals.

Data Ownership, Storage, and Sharing

Data ownership refers to the legal right to possess the data and to retain the data following completion of a particular study (Clinical Tools, Inc., 2006). Data sharing concerns the dissemination of the data to other researchers, institutions, and the public. "Data" encompasses both observable details, such as someone's sex, and the sources of and processes through which those data were collected, such as questionnaires and interviews. Examples of issues related to the ownership and/or sharing of collected data include disputes relating to publication from the collected data; concerns of an individual or community relating to the potential consequences of the data use, sharing, or publication; and the archiving of data for future unspecified research use by unspecified persons. Issues of ownership are often layered and complex, as illustrated by the following example.

Assume that a social worker-researcher conducts interviews with divorced parents to explore the challenges associated with co-parenting and strategies to address their child's openly defiant behaviors. According to copyright law, the parents own the words that they use in their interviews because they are the ones who initially uttered them. In contrast, the recording of those words, whether by video or computer or on paper, is generally owned by the entity in which the social worker-researcher is employed, such as a nonprofit organization, a governmental agency, or an academic institution. The researcher is, in essence, granted "stewardship" over the data and may use the data in a manner that is consistent with the representations and assurances under which the data were collected from the interviewees, e.g., presentation at conferences and publications (Clinical Tools, Inc., 2006). In many cases, the organization or institution will allow the social worker-researcher to take a copy of the data with them if they were to change employers, but would likely also require that a copy of the data or the original dataset be left with the organization.

In some cases, the researcher may have an obligation to share their final data with other researchers. As an example, the National Institutes of Health may require that recipients of its funding make their final data available to other researchers (National Institutes of Health, 2003a).

Data archives have become an important source of data due to a greater emphasis on cross-disciplinary collaboration to promote better understanding and conserve scarce research resources (Parry & Mauthner, 2004). Many data archives consist of quantitative data that have been at least partially de-identified or anonymized in order to maintain research participants' confidentiality, such as their names, specific residence, and telephone number (Corti, 2000).[2] Researchers may be required to execute a data use agreement, also known as a data sharing agreement, licensing agreement, and data distribution agreement, to access such data. A data use agreement generally specifies the intended uses of the data and a finite period of time during which the data may be used (National Institutes of Health, 2003b). In some cases, archived quantitative data may be available for public use, such as the Center for Medicare and Medicaid Services data at http://hrsonline.isr.umich.edu/rda/ user-docs/cmsdua.pdf. Examples of international data archives relevant to social work

---

[2] In some cases, individuals' identities may be deductively disclosed, such as in the case of small geographic areas, specific small populations, and linked databases (National Institutes of Health, 2003b). As an example, a social worker investigating community poverty levels might wish to link information from several databases to better understand not only whether poverty exists, but its implications for access to needed services. Although likely not relevant to most social work research, identification of specific individuals is theoretically possible in the context of genetic research that utilizes archived tissue samples, since DNA information is specific to an individual.

research include the South African Data Archive (http://sada.nrf.ac.za/), which includes social work data; the Centre for International Statistics at the Canadian Council on Social Development (http://www.ccsd.ca/), which includes data on poverty, welfare, and income; and the Australian Social Science Data Archives (http://www.ccsd.ca/), which houses data relating to social, political, and economic affairs, as well as data from opinion polls. Access to international data archives often requires that the investigator agree to the "responsible use" of the data and refrain from the intentional disclosure of individuals' identity (see Inter-University Consortium for Political and Social Research, n.d.; South African Data Archive, n.d.).

The sharing and archiving of qualitative data present unique issues. Qualitative data most frequently includes details related to the specific community and inclusion of field notes. Removal of identifying data to ensure the anonymity of the study participants would threaten the integrity of the remaining data, potentially making it unusable (Mauthner et al., 2000; Parry & Mauthner, 2004), but inclusion of such information could lead to the identification of individual participants and/or their community. The falsification of some data has been used as a strategy to protect the identity and confidentiality of participants, but this approach raises concerns about the integrity of the data (Parry et al., 1997).

Authorship and Publication

Legal and ethical issues extend even after the completion of the study. The author of manuscripts originating from the research has an intellectual property interest in that work (United States Copyright Office, 2012. See also United States Copyright Office, 2016). In general, individuals who have made a significant intellectual contribution to the research should be included as co-authors. Others who assisted with the research, such as an assistant for the transcription of recorded interviews or for data entry, can be thanked in an acknowledgment section (Wager & Kleinert, 2010; International Committee of Medical Journal Editors, 2014; National Association of Social Workers, 2008). Best practice suggests that a researcher should obtain the permission of individuals to be acknowledged in a publication, rather than noting their contribution without their input.

A researcher's organization and/or funding source may require that the researcher maintain the data underlying publication(s) for a specific period of time; that period of time often depends upon the requirements of the funding entity, the policies of the researcher's employer, and the intended uses of the data. Retention of the data allows the same or other researchers to reanalyze the data to verify or refute the original findings, to conduct alternate analyses to refine the study results, and to conduct analyses to assess the robustness of the data in light of varying assumptions (Fienberg et al., 1985).

References

Annas, G. J. (1992). The Nuremberg Code in U.S. courts: Ethics versus expediency. In G. J. Annas & M. A. Grodin (Eds.), *The Nazi doctors and the Nuremberg Code: Human rights in human experimentation* (pp. 201–222). Oxford University Press.

Appelbaum, P., Roth, L., Lidz, C., & Bensen, P. W. W. (1987). False hopes and best data: Consent to research and the therapeutic misconception. *Hastings Center Report, 2,* 20–24.

Arkow, P. (2020). Human-animal relationships and social work: Opportunities beyond the veterinary environment. *Child and Adolescent Social Work Journal, 37,* 573–288.

Aronson Fontes, L. (1998). Ethics in family violence research: Cross-cultural issues. *Family Relations, 47*(1), 53–61.

Auriti, E. (2013). Who can obtain access to research data? Protecting research data against compelled disclosure. *NACUA Notes, 11*(7). National Association of College and University Attorneys. https://www.calstate.edu/gc/documents/NACUANOTES-WhoCanObtainAccess-to-Research-ProtectingData.pdf. Accessed 19 Dec 2016.

Australian Government. (2018). Open data toolkit. Available https://toolkit.data.gov.au/Confidentiality_How_to_confidentialise_data_the_basic_principles.html. Accessed 30 Jul 2022.

Bartram, D. J., & Baldwin, D. S. (2008). Veterinary surgeons and suicide: Influences, opportunities and research directions. *Veterinary Record, 162,* 36–40.

Beauchamp, T., & Childress, J. (1994). *Principles of biomedical ethics.* Oxford University Press.

Clinical Tools, Inc. (2006). *Guidelines for responsible data management in scientific research.* Office of Research Integrity, United States Department of Health and Human Services. https://ori.hhs.gov/education/products/clinicaltools/data.pdf. Accessed 15 Mar 2017.

Corti, L. (2000). Progress and problems of preserving and providing access to qualitative data for social research: The international picture of an emerging culture. *Forum: Qualitative Social Research, 1*(3). http://www.qualitative-research.net/index.php/fqs/article/view/1019. Accessed 15 Mar 2017.

De Craemer, W. (1983). A cross-cultural perspective on personhood. *Milbank Memorial Fund Quarterly: Health and Society, 61*(1), 19–34.

Denny, C. C., & Grady, C. (2007). Clinical research with economically disadvantaged populations. *Journal of Medical Ethics, 33,* 382–385.

Dresser, R. (2001). Advance directives in dementia research: Promoting autonomy and protecting subjects. *IRB: Ethics & Human Research, 23*(1), 1–6.

Faden, R. R., & Beauchamp, T. L. (1986). *A history and theory of informed consent.* Oxford University Press.

Fienberg, S. E., Martin, M. E., & Straf, M. L. (1985). *Sharing research data.* National Academy Press.

Flory, J., & Emanuel, E. (2004). Interventions to improve research participants' understanding of informed consent for research: A systematic review. *Journal of the American Medical Association, 292*(13), 1593–1601.

Francione, G. L. (2000). *Introduction to animal rights: Your child or the dog?* Temple University Press.

Gaffney, J. (1986). The relevance of human experimentation to Roman catholic ethical methodology. In T. Regan (Ed.), *Animal sacrifices* (pp. 149–170). Temple University Press.

Grady, C. (2001). Money for research participation: Does it jeopardize informed consent? *American Journal of Bioethics, 1*(2), 40–44.

Grady, C. (2005). Payment of clinical research subjects. *Journal of Clinical Investigation, 115*(7), 1681–1687.

Grisso, T., & Appelbaum, P. (1998). *Assessing competence to consent to treatment: A guide for physicians and other health professionals.* Oxford University Press.

Hayes, C. (2011, September 2). *IRA researchers at Boston College file suit against US govt.* Irish Central. Available at: http://www.irishcentral.com/news/others-from-boston-college-project-file-separate-suit-to-suppress-ira-interviews-129168208-237409721.html. Accessed 19 June 2014.

International Committee of Medical Journal Editors. (2014). *Defining the role of authors and contributors.* http://www.icmje.org/recommendations/browse/roles-and-responsibilities/defining-the-role-of-authors-and-contributors.html. Accessed 19 June 2014.

Inter-University Consortium for Political and Social Research. (n.d.). https://www.icpsr.umich.edu/icpsrweb/content/datamanagement/confidentiality/index.html. Accessed 15 Mar 2017.

Kalechofsy, R. (1992). Jewish law and tradition on animal rights: A usable paradigm for the animal rights movement. In R. Kalechofsy (Ed.), *Judaism and animal rights: Classical and contemporary responses* (pp. 46–55). Micah Publications, Inc.

Kipnis, K. (2001, March). Vulnerability in research subjects: A bioethical taxonomy. In *Ethical and policy issues in research involving human participants. Vol. II: Commissioned papers and staff analysis* (pp. G-1–G-13). National Bioethics Advisory Commission.

Kipnis, K. (2003). Seven vulnerabilities in the pediatric research subject. *Theoretical Medicine, 24*, 107–120.

Largent, E. A., Grady, C., Miller, F. G., & Wertheimer, A. (2012). Money, coercion, and undue inducement: A survey of attitudes about payments to research participants. *IRB, 34*(1), 1–8.

Levine, R. J. (1988). *Ethics and regulation of clinical research.* Yale University Press.

Levine, C., Faden, R., Grady, C., Hammerschmidt, D., Eckenwiler, L., Sugarman, J., & Consortium to Examine Clinical Research Ethics. (2004). The limitations of "vulnerability" as a protection for human research participants. *American Journal of Bioethics, 4*(3), 44–49.

Loue, S. (2017). *Handbook of religion and spirituality in social work practice and research.* Springer Science+Business.

Loue, S. (2018). Legal issues in social work research. In S. Loue (Ed.), *Legal issues in social work practice and research* (pp. 81–101). Springer. https://doi.org/10.1007/978-3-319-77414-5_5

Loue, S. (2021). Ethical considerations in global mental health research. In A. R. Dyer, B. A. Kohrt, & P. J. Candilis (Eds.), *Global mental health ethics.* Springer.

Luna, F. (2009). Elucidating the concept of vulnerability: Layers not labels. *International Journal of Feminist Approaches to Bioethics, 2*(1), 121–139.

Maschi, T., & Youdin, R. (2012). *Social worker as researcher: Integrating research with advocacy.* Pearson Education, Inc.

Mauthner, N. S., Maclean, C., & McKee, L. (2000). "My dad hangs out of helicopter doors and takes pictures of oil platforms": Children's accounts of parental work in the oil and gas industry. *Community, Work, and Family, 3*, 133–162.

McIntosh v. Milano. (1979). 168 N.J. Super. 466.

National Association of Social Workers. (2021). *Code of ethics.* https://www.socialworkers.org/About/Ethics/Code-of-Ethics/Code-of-Ethics-English#standards. Accessed 30 Jul 2022.

National Bioethics Advisory Commission. (1998). *Research involving persons with mental disorders that may affect decisionmaking capacity. Vol. 1: Report and recommendations of the National Bioethics Advisory Commission.* U.S. Government Printing Office.

National Commission for the Protection of Human Subjects of Biomedical and Behavioral Research. (1979). *The Belmont Report: Ethical principles and guidelines for the protection of human subjects of research.* United States Department of Health, Education, and Welfare [DHEW Pub. No. OS 78-0012].

National Institute of Mental Health. (2015a, April 6). *Data safety monitoring plan writing guidance: Guidance for developing a data and safety monitoring plan for clinical trials sponsored by NIMH.* Available at https://www.nimh.nih.gov/funding/clinical-research/data-and-safety-monitoring-plan-writing-guidance.shtml. Accessed 24 Feb 2020.

National Institute of Mental Health. (2015b, April 24). *Policy governing independent safety monitors and independent data and safety monitoring boards.* Available at https://www.nimh.nih.gov/funding/clinical-research/policy-governing-independent-safety-monitors-and-independent-data-and-safety-monitoring-boards.shtml. Accessed 24 Feb 2020.

National Institute on Drug Abuse. (2018, October). *Guidelines for establishing and operating a data and safety monitoring board*. Available at https://www.drugabuse.gov/research/clinical-research/guidelines-establishing-data-safety-monitoring. Accessed 24 Feb 2020.

National Institutes of Health. (2003a, 26 February). *Final NIH statement on sharing research data [NOT-OD-03-032]*. https://grants.nih.gov/grants/guide/notice-files/NOT-OD-03-032.html. Accessed 15 Mar 2017.

National Institutes of Health. (2003b, March 5). *NIH data sharing policy and implementation guidance*. https://grants.nih.gov/grants/policy/data_sharing/data_sharing_guidance.htm#imp. Accessed 15 Mar 2017.

Neukrug, E. S. (1991). Computer-assisted live supervision in counselor skills training. *Counselor Education and Supervision, 31*, 132–138.

Nuremberg Code. (1946). Lebacqz, K., & Levine, R. J. (1982). Informed consent in human research: Ethical and legal aspects. In W. T. Reich (Ed.). *Encyclopedia of bioethics* (p. 757). The Free Press.

Ohio Counselor, Social Worker and Marriage and Family Therapist Board. (n.d.). *New mandated reporting requirement—Animal abuse*. https://cswmft.ohio.gov/wps/portal/gov/cswmft/for-professionals/resources-for professionals/Guidance_Animal_Abuse_Reporting_HB33. Accessed 21 Aug 2021.

Parry, O., & Mauthner, N. S. (2004). Whose data are they anyway? Practical, legal and ethical issues in archiving qualitative research data. *Sociology, 38*(1), 139–152.

Parry, O., Atkinson, P., & Delamont, S. (1997). The structure of PhD research. *Sociology, 31*, 121–129.

Regan, T. (1983). *The case for animal rights*. University of California Press.

Regan, T. (1997). The rights of humans and other animals. *Ethics & Behavior, 7*(2), 103–111.

Risley-Curtiss, C. (2010). Social work practitioners and the human-companion animal bond: A national study. *Social Work, 55*(1), 38–46.

Scotney, R. L., McLaughlin, D., & Keates, H. L. (2015). A systematic review of the effects of euthanasia and occupational stress in personnel working with animals in animal shelters, veterinary clinics, and biomedical research facilities. *Journal of the American Veterinary Medical Association, 247*(10), 1121–1130.

Singer, P. (1980). Animals and the value of life. In T. L. Beauchamp & T. Regan (Eds.), *Matters of life and death: New introductory essays in moral philosophy*. Temple University Press.

Smith, R. C., Mead, D. E., & Kinsella, J. A. (1998). Direct supervision: Adding computer-assisted feedback and data capture to live supervision. *Journal of Marital and Family Therapy, 24*, 113–125.

South African Data Archive. (n.d.). http://sada.nrf.ac.za/icpsr.html. Accessed 15 Mar 2017.

Straight, W. (1962). Man's debt to laboratory animals. *Miami University Medical School Bulletin, 16*, 106.

United States Copyright Office. (2012). *Copyright basics [Circular 1]*. Author. https://www.copyright.gov/circs/circ01.pdf. Accessed 07 May 2017.

United States Copyright Office. (2016). *Copyright registration of books, manuscripts, and speeches [FL-109]*. https://www.copyright.gov/fls/fl109.pdf. Accessed 06 May 2017.

United States Department of Health and Human Services. (n.d.). *Summary of the HIPAA privacy rule*. http://www.hhs.gov/hipaa/for-professionals/privacy/laws-regulations/index.html. Accessed 23 Mar 2017.

United States Department of Health and Human Services, Office for Human Research Protections. (2016). *Federal policy for the protection of human subjects ('Common Rule')*. https://www.hhs.gov/ohrp/regulations-and-policy/regulations/common-rule/index.html. Accessed 17 Feb 2020.

Wager, E., & Kleinert, S. (2010, July 22–24). *Responsible research publication: International standards for authors*. A position statement developed at the Second World Conference in Research Integrity, Singapore. http://publicationethics.org/files/International%20standards_authors_for%20website_11_Nov_2011.pdf. Accessed 19 June 2014.

Weinstock, R., Bonnici, D., Seroussi, A., & Leong, G. S. (2014). No duty to warn in California: Now unambiguously solely a duty to protect. *Journal of the American Academy of Psychiatry and the Law, 42*(1), 101–108.

Wendler, D., & Grady, C. (2008). What should research participants understand to understand they are participants in research? *Bioethics, 22*(4), 203–208.

World Medical Association. (2013). *Helsinki Declaration—Ethical principles for biomedical research involving human subjects.* http://www.wma.net/en/30publications/10policies/b3/index.html. Accessed 14 Mar 2017.

Legal References

Cases

Abdullahi v. Pfizer, 562 F.3d 163 (2d Cir. 2009).

Davis v. Lhim, 124 Mich. App. 291 (1983), *aff'd on rem* 147 Mich. App. 8 (1985), *rev'd on* grounds of government immunity in *Canon v. Thumudo*, 430 Mich. 326 (1988).

Ewing v. Goldstein, 120 Cal. App. 4th 807 (2004).

Ewing v. Northridge Hospital Medical Center, 120 Cal. App. 4th 1289 (2004).

Jablonski v. United States, 712 F.2d 391 (9th Cir. 1983).

Tarasoff v. Regents of the University of California, 17 Cal. 3d 425 (1976).

Thompson v. County of Alameda, 27 Cal. 3d 741 (1980).

Statutes

Health Insurance Portability and Accountability Act of 1996. Pub. L. 104–191.

Health Research Extension Act of 1985, Pub. L. No. 99–158.

U.S. Regulations

9 C.F.R. § 2.31 (1998).

45 C.F.R. Part 46 (2009).

45 C.F.R. § 46.101.

45 C.F.R. § 46.107.

45 C.F.R. § 160.103 (2013).

45 C.F.R. § 164.508 (2013).

46 C.F. 46.116 R. § (2018).

Other

International Covenant on Civil and Political Rights, December 19, 1966, 999 U.N.T.S. 171.

Part V
Looking to the Future

Chapter 15
The Current State of Research in Veterinary Social Work

Maya Gupta

Introduction

Why should the veterinary social worker be interested in the foundation of research underlying this field? It is the position of this author that whether focused at the micro, mezzo, or macro level, the veterinary social work (VSW) practitioner has much to take from—and give to—research. For clinicians, research provides a knowledge base to guide the formulation of presenting problems and the selection and implementation of evidence-based approaches while pointing to new directions in advancing interventions toward increased efficacy and effectiveness. In turn, clinicians' experiences in practice inform new research questions aimed at these same goals. On the programmatic and policy fronts, decisions about allocation of resources can and should be informed by data. Reciprocally, applied research and program evaluation to address the question "OK, we tried it—so did it work?" is vital to accountability and iteration, ensuring maximum impact relative to effort.

Therefore, reinforcing the girders of this two-way bridge between science and practice stands to bolster the VSW field across its span. While not every veterinary social worker need be directly involved in doing research hands-on, it adds value both to one's own practice and to the field as a whole to serve as an informed consumer of research: able to critically analyze its strengths, limitations, and practical implications, and actively participating in the conversation about its future development. It is in this spirit in which this chapter sets forth.

Research at the intersection of humans and animals has accelerated and compounded impressively in recent years following a long, yet intermittent, period of scholarship across various disciplines. This chapter cannot do justice to the full scope of research in each of the four domains of VSW, but will provide the reader

M. Gupta (✉)
American Society for the Prevention of Cruelty to Animals, New York, NY, USA
e-mail: maya.gupta@aspca.org

© The Author(s), under exclusive license to Springer Nature Switzerland AG 2022
S. Loue, P. Linden (eds.), *The Comprehensive Guide to Interdisciplinary Veterinary Social Work*, https://doi.org/10.1007/978-3-031-10330-8_15

new to these topics (or new to the research aspect of these topics) with an overview of current knowledge and recent developments in the literature. In keeping with this goal, systematic reviews will be prioritized where available. This approach to synthesizing research also conveys the benefits of examining the methodological quality of included studies, peer review of the methodology and conclusions of the review itself, and (in the case of meta-analysis) amalgamating heterogeneous findings into overall estimates of effect size.

Animal-Assisted Interventions

Of the four domains of VSW, the largest literature base by far is in the area of animal-assisted interventions (hereafter AAI). The increase of funding for research in this area in recent years, for example, through the Human-Animal Bond Research Institute (HABRI) and the public-private partnership between Mars/Waltham and the Eunice Kennedy Shriver National Institute of Child Health and Human Development, has doubtless played a role in attracting the attention of researchers; interest from the field also builds the case for funder interest in a topic. Due to the volume of literature in this area and a resulting proliferation of systematic reviews, in some cases, only more recent reviews (where several exist on a given subtopic) are covered here.

Autism

A review by Hoagwood et al. (2017) included nine studies of AAT for youth with autism, finding support for the intervention in five studies and partial support in an additional two studies. However, in a review focused on equine therapies, Srinivasan et al. (2018) found support primarily for an effect of the interventions on behavior skills, and to a lesser extent on social communication skills; there was limited evidence for impact on other skills. A more recent meta-analysis across all forms of AAT for autism (Dimolareva & Dunn, 2020) identified small effect sizes of AAIs on social interaction, communication, and overall autism symptoms, concluding that there may be little gain beyond active control conditions (comparison groups in experimental studies in which participants engage in a task of some type to separate the effect of the intervention from the effect of simply "doing something").

Given the high prevalence of interest in autism in the AAT research and clinical domains, and the completion of a number of systematic reviews on this topic, it is noteworthy that there are not clearer takeaways from the research thus far. It is also noteworthy that, to date, only one study to this author's knowledge has examined AAT for adults with autism, providing some preliminary evidence of utility (Wijker et al., 2020).

Older Adults

A review by Gee and Mueller (2019) across a range of target outcomes of AAI for older adults (including physical health, depression, anxiety/agitation, and loneliness/social functioning) identified a number of promising results, but results overall were mixed and the rigor of the included studies varied widely. More recently, Chang et al. (2020) reviewed 47 studies (of which 21 were randomized controlled trials), the majority involving dogs and the second highest number involving horses. Meta-analysis across 14 of these studies identified a significant effect of AAT on depression in older adults, but meta-analyses could not be completed for other outcomes due to heterogeneity of the studies reviewed.

Among several systematic reviews focused on dementia, two recent papers (Klimova et al., 2019; Yakimicki et al., 2019) identified positive effects of AAI on behavior (both reviews), psychological symptoms (Klimova), and overall quality of life (Yakimicki). However, again focusing on dementia but including only randomized controlled trials, Lai et al. (2019) found evidence only for reduction of depressive symptoms.

It is important to note that older adults are not a homogeneous population; as seen here, AAIs have been targeted to a variety of symptoms with a variety of individuals and settings. Further, AAIs themselves vary, as do the animals involved. Some variability in the literature is therefore to be expected for this reason alone; however, further research should continue to elucidate specific interventions, populations, settings, and other variables associated with differing outcomes. As with all syntheses of literature, inclusion/exclusion criteria for which studies are reviewed (e.g., whether only randomized controlled trials are included; whether unpublished theses and dissertations are included) can also play a considerable role in findings.

Trauma

Hoagwood et al. (2017) found that the use of AAT for childhood trauma demonstrated positive effects across the three studies reviewed, though there was no random assignment to treatment condition and no measure of effect size was calculated by the reviewers. A previous review by O'Haire et al. (2015) across both childhood trauma and veterans with post-traumatic stress disorder (PTSD) found some evidence for reduction of depression (6/10 studies), PTSD symptoms (5/10), and anxiety (4/10); however, these effects tended to be short-lived. Focusing solely on equine interventions for PTSD, Boss et al. (2019) found mixed evidence among nine studies.

Other Outcomes

Applications of AAI to a number of other populations and symptoms have begun accumulating enough literature to conduct systematic reviews:

- Across studies using AAI with dogs and incarcerated individuals, Villafaina-Domínguez et al. (2020) identified promising findings, but noted that only 3 of the 20 studies were RCTs.
- Cotoc et al. (2019) reviewed five studies of the use of AAIs with pediatric oncology patients, demonstrating promise for both psychological and physical symptoms and for stress/anxiety reduction in individuals associated with the patients. However, methodological weaknesses in the included studies and heterogeneity in the AAI approaches reviewed limited the strength and generalizability of these conclusions.
- A review of seven studies of animal-assisted therapy for pain in children concluded that this treatment shows some promise in pain reduction, but that additional research is needed (Zhang et al., 2020).
- A review of seven RCTs was inconclusive as to the effects of AAT on schizophrenia (Hawkins et al., 2019a).
- A review of AAI in classroom settings demonstrated promise, albeit with similar caveats about heterogeneity (Brelsford et al., 2017).
- A review of AAI in psychosocial outcomes for individuals (mostly children and adolescents) with intellectual disabilities indicated support for the interventions, but 8/10 of the studies were rated weak in quality and the remaining 2 of moderate quality (Maber-Aleksandrowicz et al., 2016).

Future Directions

Though only in mid-career at present, this author has been in the field long enough to remember dire proclamations of the lack of rigor in AAI research—often coupled with prognostications that little would change because of the lack of funding for larger-scale data collection and more sophisticated research designs. In less than two decades, the narrative has changed considerably in many areas of AAI, and the field is to be commended for its advancements even as further work is necessary to build upon this base.

However, researchers should bear in mind that demonstrating success in tightly controlled studies, no matter how high in quality, is only one step in identifying and establishing empirically supported treatments. The translation from demonstrating experimental efficacy to documenting real-life effectiveness in programmatic settings—including such factors as dissemination, replicability and implementation fidelity, cost, patient satisfaction and adherence, and maintenance of treatment gains across time—requires additional effort and a tolerance for the "messiness" of applied research. Simultaneously, to close the research-to-practice gap, AAI practitioners must be willing to adopt an evidence-based approach to their intervention approaches, taking cues from the research to guide their practice efforts and (where practicable) participating in effectiveness research themselves.

Further, even when AAI is demonstrated to be both efficacious and effective, its impact must be weighed against that of current "treatment as usual" and not simply against a no-treatment group. Kazdin (2010) explains that this experimental condition controls for potential effects of simply receiving any form of treatment at all, such as expectancy effects. In the opinion of this author, there is also a compelling pragmatic and ethical rationale beyond the research rationale: the principle that healthcare providers should offer the most effective treatment available. If AAI is superior to no treatment, yet inferior to another form of treatment, what is the basis for providing AAI instead of the other treatment? In the same spirit, researchers should consider whether AAI offers clinically meaningful enhancement to gains made via treatment as usual and, if so, whether it may be worth the additive investment.

Fuller reviews of future directions in AAI research are available in Fine et al. (2019), Kazdin (2010), and Serpell et al. (2017), but several themes prominent in those papers are worthy of reiteration here: (1) the importance of basing outcomes research on theoretical frameworks of AAI's mechanisms of action, including explicitly testing connections among the interventions, mechanisms of action, and outcomes, and (2) closer examination of the welfare of animals involved in AAI. Glenk (2017) reviewed studies assessing physiological, behavioral, and perceptual indicators of therapy dog welfare, finding some evidence of stress markers during AAIs but concluding that there is currently no basis for acute concern based on available literature. However, Glenk noted that the limitations and variability of this literature preclude a comprehensive overview of how AAI relates to the welfare of therapy dogs, including assessment of longer-term effects and measurement of both negative and positive welfare indicators. Studies of other species involved in AAI, including those in whom signs of stress may be less readily recognized, are urgently needed.

Central to AAI's broad appeal is the idea of a win-win: using the human-animal bond for good, and affording AAI practitioners the joy of working with animals while bringing benefit to others. In the spirit of ensuring a win-win (or at least a "win-no lose") for all parties, it is time for knowledge about the animal side of these human-animal interactions to catch up with knowledge about the human side. Accordingly, assessment of animal welfare should become a standard component of all AAI research, even when human outcomes are the primary variables of interest.

Animal-Related Grief and Bereavement

Research on animal-related grief and bereavement draws heavily from both the theory and science of adjustment to human death. Coverage of the full spectrum of human loss is beyond the scope of this chapter, but the reader is referred to Bui (2018) for a review.

The majority of research attention on this topic has been directed toward pet loss, as opposed to other situations in which humans may grieve animals. Where applicable, studies that address grief and bereavement in relation to different types of human-animal relationships will be noted.

Effects of Animal-Related Bereavement

A primary swath of the animal-related grief and bereavement literature focuses on its effects on animal owners/guardians, which may range from normative sadness, anger, and disbelief to severe disturbances of functioning. Perhaps due to human tendencies to anthropomorphize animal companions (Behler et al., n.d.), several studies suggest that these effects may resemble grief in relation to the loss of a human, though potentially with somewhat less severity on average (Eckerd et al., 2016). Disenfranchised or un- or underacknowledged grief (Doka, 1999) may also be prominent in human-animal relationships (Packman et al., 2014; Spain et al., 2019), perhaps more so than in human-human relationships due to societal perceptions that "it's just an animal." As a result, there may be fewer socially sanctioned opportunities to mourn. Qualitative research (e.g., Bussolari et al., 2019; McKinney, 2019; Packman et al., 2014, 2017; Reisbig et al., 2017) has been helpful in understanding the human experience of animal loss. Kemp et al. (2016) completed a systematic review of qualitative studies, including a small number of studies involving other species (birds, fish, hamsters, rabbits, and horses). They found that animal-related grief was individualized, though such factors as social expectations, life stage, personal events, disenfranchised grief, and social support were relevant to the grief experience.

The construct of complicated grief (Shear et al., 2011) and the diagnoses of Prolonged Grief Disorder in ICD11 (World Health Organization, 2019) and Persistent Complex Bereavement Disorder in DSM-5 (American Psychiatric Association, 2013) illustrate efforts to codify a form of grief beyond normal adjustment. Though research continues into nosological similarities and differences among these terms, and researchers contributing to this work have typically paid scant attention to animal-related grief, there is recent preliminary evidence that the DSM-V construct of PCBD is valid for pet loss also (Lee, 2020) and that complicated grief can be present in pet loss study samples (Adrian & Stitt, 2017). Interestingly, as highlighted by Schroeder (2019), Adrian and Stitt's survey sample contained four horse owners, all of whom had high PTSD symptom scores.

Risk and Resilience

Consistent with the literature on human loss, the degree of closeness or attachment to the animal appears to be associated with the degree of grief experienced (Barnard-Nguyen et al., 2016; Eckerd et al., 2016). On the other hand, a growing body of research indicates that continuing bonds (Klass et al., 2014)—efforts to remain connected to the deceased person or pet while creating a new type of relationship with the deceased—may be associated with both distress and comfort in relation to pet loss (e.g., Habarth et al., 2017; Packman et al., 2017). Habarth et al. observed associations between attachment, grief, and the variety of ways in which continuing bonds were expressed, along with relationships between attachment and post-traumatic growth in predicting the degree of comfort derived from these continuing bonds. They suggest that meaning-making ability may influence the relationship between continuing bonds and adaptive vs. maladaptive effects. Bussolari et al. (2018) identified self-compassion as a potentially important contributor to willingness to engage in continuing bonds.

The role of emotion regulation in overall psychological functioning is also prominent in grief studies. A recent systematic review (Eisma & Stroebe, 2020) highlighted the role of emotion regulation in complicated grief, identifying experiential avoidance and rumination as being particularly associated with persistence of complicated grief. Broadly consistent with this finding although not expressly focused on complicated grief, a small study by Green et al. (2018) found that emotion regulation skills were associated with degree of symptoms following the death of a pet. Adaptive skills such as reappraisal, refocusing, and perspective-taking were associated with positive affect and less grief, anger, trauma, and guilt, while the opposite was broadly true of maladaptive emotion regulation strategies such as catastrophizing, rumination, and blaming. Thus, emotion regulation appears to be both a risk (when maladaptive strategies are employed) and a resilience factor (adaptive skills) in pet-related grief.

The base of scholarship on grief is understandably broad and complex. In continuing to elucidate the factors responsible for risk and resilience in animal-related grief and bereavement, it seems important to tie together pockets of research on this topic to better understand interconnections among attachment, continuing bonds, emotion regulation, and other key variables in predicting grief adjustment.

Tailoring Services in the VSW Practice Setting

Given the above research, how can veterinary social workers and animal care professionals identify who is most at risk for severe or disordered grief so they can direct measures appropriately? Are those at greatest risk typically the same individuals who choose to avail themselves of VSW resources in, say, a veterinary clinic setting? Are services provided at or near the time of the animal's death effective in preventing the development of grief disorders? These and other next-level research questions in the applied setting are essential to inform more effective service delivery.

An early study seeking to identify predictors of owner response to the death of their pets (Adams et al., 2000) found that human-related variables were more strongly associated with grief response than pet-related variables. Human-related variables included attachment, attitudes toward pet death and euthanasia, and the support owners received from the veterinarian. However, a more recent study similarly seeking to identify risk factors for developing severe grief among veterinary practice clients—this time focusing on euthanasia—provided evidence that in addition to attachment, the circumstances surrounding the loss of the animal may also be associated with the grief response (Barnard-Nguyen et al., 2016). Cancer diagnosis was inversely associated with anger and guilt, whereas sudden loss was associated with increased anger. A recent systematic review of the human-human grief literature (Djelantik et al., 2020) indicated that the prevalence of Prolonged Grief Disorder may be as high as 49 percent for unnatural losses such as accidents. In light of these findings, it may be fruitful to conduct further exploration into potentially unique consequences of unexpected animal deaths for owners' well-being. These cases may also have special bearing in situations where animal cruelty takes place, including as a component of human violence, for which reason owners' grief reactions to violent death may also be an important topic of further study.

Several other circumstances that may be uniquely associated with the grief experience and/or warrant tailored approaches to intervention bear mention here:

- Behavioral euthanasia has received scant research attention. However, forthcoming qualitative research by M.K. Workman (personal communication, January 21, 2021) suggests that disenfranchised grief is a key theme among individuals who euthanized animals for behavioral reasons, and that it may be shaped by "double disenfranchisement" insofar as (1) the fact that the animal posed a safety risk makes expressions of grief even less acceptable, as does (2) the fact that the individual made the choice to end the animal's life. Workman also identifies a guilt-relief cycle as one of the most common themes in her data: "The guilt for making the decision is often followed by relief of not having to live in a state of hypervigilance and chronic stress followed by guilt about feeling relief when they chose to take a life." Guilt further emerged about stress experienced by other animals in the household who were affected by the animal prior to euthanasia.
- Whereas the preponderance of research and clinical interest has focused on grief following the loss of the animal, anticipatory grief appears to be a prominent theme for some animal owners contemplating the eventual or impending loss and may have particular relevance to euthanasia (Laing & Maylea, 2018). Anticipatory grief may therefore also merit further study in palliative care for animals.
- Other types of animal losses that may produce grief are worthy of further examination in VSW research and practice. Davies and James (2018) investigated equestrians' responses to the experience of injury to their horses, observing that time investment in the horse, length of ownership, and projected length of rehabilitation from the injury were associated with the degree of distress experienced. Relationships with animals may also end through relinquishment/rehoming or through the animal becoming lost. In such circumstances, it may not be known whether the animal is still alive. One study found no difference between the severity of grief between those whose loss was ambiguous in this way and

those who knew the animal had died; however, the small sample size in the ambiguous-loss group likely underpowered the study (Green et al., 2018).

How can practice settings make use of these findings, and what else remains to be known in order to guide practice? In a recent survey of individuals following euthanasia of a pet, the most commonly reported form of mourning was in private (75%), although a majority (58%) also sought support from family or friends (Park & Royal, 2020). Fewer than 1 percent had participated in support groups. Understanding what factors influence willingness to engage in supportive services and whether any of these factors can be modified (e.g., through client communication, marketing of services, or service structure) could assist VSW professionals in reaching more individuals. (However, as previously stated, given resource constraints and the desire for services to have maximum impact, it is also important to better understand which individuals cope effectively with animal bereavement without additional services, and which individuals tend to seek services without benefiting substantially from them.) In addition to direct support for grief, recent research has also explored veterinary clients' expectations and concerns regarding end-of-life decision-making and after-death body care, offering insight into how veterinary practices can better structure these services (Cooney et al., 2020).

In the practice setting, evidence also indicates that VSW professionals should not solely focus attention on animal owners. The role of animal death in compassion fatigue among veterinarians, animal shelter workers, and other animal care professionals is addressed in the next section of this chapter. Nevertheless, it is worthy of mention here that a small Australian survey expressly tying end-of-life issues to veterinary well-being found that 88 percent of respondents had themselves experienced grief related to the death of an animal in practice, and 40 percent reported effects on their mental and/or physical health from both this and the experience of their clients' grief (Dow et al., 2019). Additionally, over one-half of these veterinarians felt unprepared by their veterinary school curricula to deal with grieving owners. While survey research indicates that the majority of veterinary schools in the USA and UK expose students to end-of-life issues, an average of only 7 h are devoted to these topics in US curricula compared with 21 in the UK (Dickinson, 2019). Littlewood et al. (2020) reported on grief management training in Australasian veterinary schools, concluding that stronger and well-rounded content is needed to facilitate better response by veterinarians both to their own grief and to that of clients.

Interventions

In a systematic review of psychological interventions for grief, Johannsen et al. (2019) identified a statistically significant but small effect (effect size = 0.45 at post-intervention and 0.41 at follow-up; for an overview of effect size in relation to clinical relevance vs. statistical significance, see Ferguson, 2009). Factors associated with stronger effects included individual (as opposed to group) intervention formats and bereavement occurrence 6 or more months earlier, consistent with the ICD-11 criteria for Persistent Grief Disorder. Notably, this review explicitly excluded pet bereavement. Stringent outcome research (e.g., randomized controlled trials) investigating the efficacy of various interventions for animal-related grief would add heft to VSW practice in this area and would likely illustrate pathways for refining existing approaches.

For a thorough treatment of the topic of animal-related grief and bereavement from the vantage point of the practitioner, including a deeper exploration of relevant research, see the recent edited volume by Kogan and Erdman (2020).

Future Directions

In considering what avenues of further research are worthy of greatest emphasis, it is important to begin by considering the goals of the science. Viewed through the lens of VSW—whether at a micro, mezzo, or macro level—it seems that the natural output of research on this topic should be to aid in addressing the human needs that arise from animal-related grief and bereavement. Working backward from this endpoint, we can see the value of research that illuminates who is most in need, under what circumstances, and what interventions are most effective. A further layer of nuance atop these basic questions includes how to best identify and reach those in need; considerations surrounding treatment timing, duration, and intensity (dose-response); practitioner characteristics and/or behavior associated with effect; and any possible interactions between the above variables and client variables. In this way, we move from the basic question, "Does it work?" (for an individual intervention) to, "What works best?" (comparing interventions) to, "What works *for whom?*" For an excellent discussion of these considerations in psychotherapy research, see the work bearing this title by Roth and Fonagy (2005).

Further, as with all the domains of VSW, it seems important that research attempt to further elucidate the complexity and heterogeneity of human-animal relationships in relation to the topic of interest. While the loss of a dog or cat may be the most commonly encountered situation for a VSW practitioner in a small animal veterinary clinic setting, we would be remiss to proceed as though animal-related grief and bereavement were limited to this scenario. In addition to learning more about grief and bereavement in human relationships with other species, including non-companion animals, we should give greater consideration to differences in the relationships between humans and their pets and to learning which factors may be most salient in predicting response to grief (and to interventions). A further topic of interest might be the degree of association thereof between animal-related grief/ bereavement and interpersonal grief/bereavement within the same individuals, inasmuch as this insight could guide therapeutic practice and further legitimize animal-related grief/bereavement within the context of the study of human grief.

Compassion Fatigue and Management

Drawing on three decades of scholarship in the human healthcare field since first described there by Joinson (1992), research on compassion fatigue (CF) and its management in human-animal interactions has also increased in recent years, though not with the same gusto as research on AAI. This section of the chapter covers current research on CF and related concepts in veterinary, animal welfare organization, and laboratory animal settings. Whereas the latter may be less directly relevant to the majority of veterinary social workers, this area nonetheless bears mention in consideration of the robustness of research and the degree of thematic overlap with more "traditional" VSW practice settings. A thorough review of the constructs of CF, secondary traumatic stress, moral stress/distress/injury, and burnout—including debates about the conceptual and empirical differences and interconnections among these terms—is beyond the remit of this chapter. Generally, the construct(s) examined by a specific study will be noted.

Veterinary Practice

Owing to increased recognition of challenges to mental health and well-being among veterinarians (see, e.g., Tomasi et al., 2019), the topic of CF has received considerable attention in veterinary medicine. In a sample of Canadian veterinarians as compared with the general population, Perret et al. (2020) found increased rates of CF, as well as burnout, anxiety and depression, and lower resilience. A study focused on moral distress (Moses et al., 2018) concluded that a majority of North American veterinarians experienced aspects of moral distress, e.g., distress due to requests to provide care they saw as futile, or due to refusals of care they saw as appropriate. Among Italian veterinarians, Musetti et al. (2020) identified exposure to animal suffering, as well as person-level and other job-level variables, as a factor in professional quality of life. McArthur et al. (2017) observed low compassion satisfaction and high secondary traumatic stress and burnout among Australian veterinary students, identifying psychological factors associated with each: personal distress, coping strategies, and mindfulness were each associated with more than one of these components. Communication styles also appear to be associated with CF among veterinary students, particularly those styles characterized by emotionality, impression manipulation, and aggression (Hess-Holden et al., 2019).

A growing body of research considers CF among other members of the veterinary team, particularly veterinary nurses/technicians. In a mixed-methods study including both veterinarians and technicians, barriers to care and experiencing the grief of clients were associated with CF, while patient/client relationships and feelings of making a difference for animals were associated with compassion satisfaction (Polachek & Wallace, 2018). Recent research by Harvey and Cameron (2020) and by Kogan et al. (2020) observed high rates of burnout among nurses/

technicians, supporting the same finding by Smith (2016), who also observed high rates of secondary traumatic stress (STS) in this population. Given the different roles of veterinarians and nurses/technicians within the practice setting, future research should compare these populations to assess for differences in proximal and distal drivers of CF and related constructs, along with the trajectories of these constructs across the respective careers of veterinarians and nurses/technicians.

Animal Welfare Organizations

Comparatively less scholarly attention has focused on professional quality of life among individuals in other animal care settings, such as animal shelters and rescues. A recent study of 153 animal shelter workers by Andrukonis and Protopopova (2020) identified increased moral injury and secondary traumatic stress associated with involvement in euthanasia. Perhaps surprisingly, both moral injury and secondary traumatic stress were higher in shelters with higher live release rates, as was burnout; on the other hand, compassion satisfaction was higher in these shelters. In a different paper, the same research group (Andrukonis et al., 2020) found that degree of exposure to animals in euthanasia settings (though not the act of euthanasia itself) was associated with burnout and secondary traumatic stress. Baran et al. (2009) classified coping strategies by shelter employees directly involved in euthanasia into eight categories, concluding that performing euthanasia served as a key stressor for these individuals.

Using a qualitative approach, Cavallaro (2016) found that personal histories, the social construction of CF, and the perception of caregiving for animals as "dirty work" are relevant to shelter workers' experience of CF. Another qualitative analysis by Levitt and Gezinski (2020) identified four themes that appeared to underlie resilience in shelter workers: intrinsic motivations, purpose, social supports, and coping strategies.

As in veterinary practice settings, it is possible that different roles within animal welfare organizations (beyond euthanasia involvement) may be associated with different experiences of CF. Some preliminary evidence of this nature was identified by Dunn et al. (2019), who found that support and frontline staff (animal caretakers and especially animal cruelty investigators) at a Canadian animal welfare organization tended to have poorer well-being compared to other staff. An ethnography by Young and Thompson (2020) posited a theoretical model in which lack of support for community cat efforts functions alongside CF and other factors to produce poor outcomes among caregivers of community cats.

Future research may be beneficial in understanding CF among other types of both paid and volunteer roles in animal welfare with respect to volunteer retention, organizational climate, and the welfare of animals in an organization's care. Roles in animal caretaking that may fall outside of the purview of an animal welfare organization, e.g., community cat caretakers and individuals who find/assist strays, should also be further explored using the lens of CF, with an eye to gaining insights into the development and retention of community engagement in the well-being of animals.

Comparisons Across Settings

In a systematic review of studies that included animal shelter, veterinary, and biomedical animal research settings, Scotney et al. (2015) found overall high rates of work-related stress, though heterogeneity in both nosology and methodology precluded clear identification of causes and outcomes. A subsequent survey by the same group (Scotney et al., 2019) again looked across various animal-related roles, though most respondents were veterinarians or veterinary nurses/technicians. Approximately one-fifth to one-fourth of respondents had elevated scores on measures of compassion satisfaction, burnout, and secondary traumatic stress, though it is important to note that this also means that the majority did not. In a large survey of animal care workers across settings by Hill et al. (2019), generally high levels of CF across roles were best predicted by involvement with animal cruelty cases and by stress from involvement in euthanasia. This finding regarding euthanasia aligns with the systematic review by Scotney et al. (2015), where higher rates of work-related stress were reported by those working directly with euthanasia. Similar to findings from studies focusing only on animal shelter settings, two factors that appear to emerge consistently across this literature are the degree of exposure to euthanasia and the individual experience of euthanasia.

Nevertheless, a unidimensional focus on euthanasia may obscure other important factors that, unless addressed, may perpetuate CF in animal care settings even if all euthanasia were to cease immediately. Secondary traumatic stress, as a presumed component of CF, may be caused by exposure to other distressing experiences involving animals, such as animal cruelty as noted above, or concern about the quality of life of sheltered animals. Additionally, burnout could possibly maintain CF even if all sources of secondary traumatic stress were removed. In a sample comprising both paid and volunteer animal care workers across settings, Monaghan et al. (2020) determined that higher levels of job demands, but not paid versus volunteer status, were associated with greater compassion fatigue. Further research to identify not only the greatest factors in CF but also the potential interplay of different factors is sorely needed, as is research that pinpoints which of these factors may be most malleable and whether there are combinations of factors that must be altered together in order to produce change.

Interventions

In the spirit of producing this change, some, but still quite limited, research on interventions for CF in animal care professionals has emerged. A systematic review (Rohlf, 2018) identified only four studies. Some evidence of reduction in symptoms among program participants was noted, but methodological heterogeneity and limitations, e.g., lack of control groups, lack of random assignment when a control group was used, and lack of follow-up in three of the four studies, precluded stronger conclusions. Rohlf recommended that the animal care field borrow from the substantially larger literature on interventions for compassion fatigue in human healthcare. A recent systematic review from human health (Conversano et al., 2020) found that mindfulness training was the most common modality in outcome studies of compassion fatigue interventions, but did not generally improve compassion fatigue, although an impact was demonstrated for other variables such as self-compassion and compassion satisfaction.

Future Directions

The considerable energy directed at discussing CF in both human- and animal-serving settings must be more productively channeled into identifying and implementing effective interventions. As with AAI and animal-related grief, providing interventions without evidence of impact is a misuse of organizational resources (at the opportunity cost of where those resources could be better directed) and raises ethical questions. Further, an apparent focus on intervention after CF has already developed may obscure other important avenues for impact, such as primary and secondary prevention. In addition, as noted by Cavallaro (2016) and alluded to by Young and Thompson (2020), the responsibility for addressing CF may be shared by the individual, the organization/ setting in which the individual works, and society. An excessive focus on altering CF at the individual level is out of keeping with the person-in-context model central to VSW and may ignore more potent avenues for change, such as transforming culture within organizations or even within professions.

In this vein, future research should examine the impact, or lack thereof, of changes that are already happening within animal-related fields. As shifts occur in veterinary demographics, practice models, approaches to care, and both the selection and training of veterinary students, is the prevalence, presentation, and course of CF also shifting? If so, can more deliberate changes be made to drive this shift for the better? Are VSW resources that have been incorporated into academic and other veterinary settings having an effect on CF—and if not, is it something to do with the approaches themselves, the way they are implemented, or some other factor(s) that interfere with or outweigh their effect? In animal shelters, live release rates are generally increasing in the USA (Rowan & Kartal, 2018), but shelter populations anecdotally are shifting to include greater proportions of animals (especially dogs) with medical and behavioral issues. Simultaneously, there is increasing enthusiasm for supporting animals in communities in lieu of bringing them into shelters. As these trends change in animal sheltering, how might CF (and response to CF) morph also? This area is ripe for further study.

Links Between Animal and Human Maltreatment

Of all the areas of VSW, perhaps none has captured attention outside the field as much as the idea of connections or "links" between animal cruelty and interpersonal violence, or more broadly links between animal cruelty and criminal or otherwise deviant acts. Research has played a direct role in driving both public and professional awareness of this issue. Unfortunately, the magnitude of interest in this topic risks allowing the response to outpace the science on which it should be based. This final section of the chapter covers what is known at present alongside what remains to be known. Additional discussion of these links may be found in the Chap. 4 by Susan Hatters Friedman and colleagues in this volume.

Youth-Perpetrated Animal Cruelty

Central to debate in the underlying theories of "the link" has been the contrast between the so-named graduation/progression hypothesis (animal cruelty preceding interpersonal violence) and the deviance generalization hypothesis (animal cruelty occurring in association with other criminal and socially deviant acts, without implication of temporal sequencing). In a systematic review of 32 studies examining associations between animal cruelty and violence among children and adolescents, Longobardi and Badenes-Ribera (2019) found some support for both hypotheses, with those findings fitting the graduation hypothesis generally involving recurrent, as opposed to isolated, acts of animal cruelty. Forms of violence and deviance addressed in the reviewed studies included bullying and criminal acts; among offenses, there was a stronger association between animal cruelty and more serious offending. Several studies demonstrated no association, and the methodological rigor and definitions of animal cruelty used by the reviewed studies varied widely. It should also be noted that the majority of studies included in the review were based on samples of incarcerated individuals, who may not be representative of the overall population. This caveat is also applicable to studies based on clinical samples, such as inpatient psychiatric populations or individuals receiving treatment for mental/behavioral disorders. In a further examination of associations between animal cruelty and other acts among youth involved with the juvenile justice system, Walters (2019) found that animal cruelty and bullying were associated with future delinquency, particularly via the mediation path of moral disengagement.

Animal cruelty perpetrated by youths may also be associated with their own experience of adverse events. Among a group of 81,000 juvenile offenders, Bright et al. (2018) identified 466 individuals who reported harming animals. Compared with those who did not report cruelty, these juveniles were more likely to have had adverse experiences beyond family violence and to have had more than four adverse experiences. Exposure to animal cruelty was not assessed among adverse experiences, as Boat (2014) has suggested it should be. The animal cruelty group was also younger at first arrest, and more likely to be male and White compared with the remaining juveniles. Among a sample of children exposed to intimate partner violence (IPV), lower cognitive empathy and callous/unemotional traits predicted engaging in animal cruelty (Hartman et al., 2019). A qualitative analysis based on a subset of participants in this study identified several themes: witnessing harm to animals by others in the home, co-perpetrating cruelty with other family members, minimizing or normalizing cruelty, believing that animals made humanlike decisions for which punishment was due, punishing pets from anger or annoyance, and curiosity (McDonald et al., 2018). Taken together, these findings indicate needs for assessment and potential opportunities for both prevention and intervention.

The most attention-grabbing narratives about cruelty in relation to other violence involve graphic acts toward animals in childhood/adolescence by serial killers and school-age school shooters. The data are often overstated (as in the frequent casual remark that every serial killer and school shooter has a history of torturing animals) or their implications misconstrued (as in the inference that if a number of serial killers and school shooters had histories of harming animals, a child who harms animals is unquestionably at high risk of committing these acts). It is refreshing that the low base rates of serial killers and mass murderers among the general population limit the ability to analyze large-scale data on this topic. Nevertheless, Arluke and Madfis (2014) studied school shooters in an attempt to identify common features of the animal cruelty perpetrated by these individuals, beyond the simple presence or absence of cruelty. They concluded that up-close-and-personal acts of violence toward socially valued species (e.g., companion animals) were most typical of the 10 (of 23) school shooters who had engaged in animal cruelty, but they also noted cases in which individuals had demonstrated kindness and concern for animals, including one individual who had also abused animals.

Adding similar complexity to the picture, the "Macdonald triad" of co-occurring animal cruelty, fire setting, and enuresis (Macdonald, 1963) continues to be viewed as uniformly indicative of violence risk, yet demonstrates inconclusive research support. In a review, Parfitt and Alleyne (2020) concluded that while individual "triad" behaviors might be associated with future violence, the extreme rarity of co-occurrence of all three behaviors provided little support for the existence of a true triad. Other studies have failed to find a role for enuresis in predicting aggression, identifying animal cruelty and fire setting as relatively more useful predictors of aggressive behavior. Joubert et al. (2021) studied 254 rapists in a forensic mental health setting, finding that overlapping animal cruelty and fire setting were associated with antisocial/aggressive traits. Similarly, Baglivio et al. (2017) examined animal cruelty and fire setting in nearly 300,000 juvenile offenders, finding a rare but statistically significant co-occurrence of the two factors. Males and sexual abuse victims were more likely to display both behaviors.

Adult-Perpetrated Animal Cruelty

Animal cruelty among adults has also been the subject of study in association with other acts, albeit with less intensity than youth-perpetrated violence. In a single systematic review identified to date (Alleyne & Parfitt, 2019), researchers identified 23 studies involving adult perpetrators or individuals with abuse-supportive attitudes. They found little support for the graduation hypothesis insofar as animal cruelty both preceded and followed other acts and was associated with both violent and nonviolent offending. The majority of reviewed studies focused on animal cruelty in the context of IPV, identifying the maltreatment of animals as a form of coercive control (discussed later in this section).

Additional support for the generalized deviance hypothesis arose from analyses of 259 animal cruelty cases by the FBI's Behavioral Analysis Unit (Hoffer et al., 2018), which indicated that 73 percent had committed other crimes whether prior to, concurrently with, and after the animal cruelty incident. Sixty percent of the individuals had committed crimes involving interpersonal violence. Similarly, a classic study at the Massachusetts Society for the Prevention of Cruelty to Animals (Arluke et al., 1999) found that other offenses committed by animal cruelty offenders were no more likely to follow than to precede the animal cruelty. Further, animal cruelty offenders compared to nonoffenders were more likely to commit not only violent crimes but also other crimes. Both of these findings failed to provide support for the graduation hypothesis.

A second substantial body of research in this area of VSW focuses on animal cruelty in association with IPV, child maltreatment, and, to a far lesser extent, elder abuse. Following early work indicating overlaps in the rosters of animal protection and child protection agencies (DeViney et al., 1983), research attention has been directed to the role and sequelae of children's exposure to animal cruelty in the context of violence in the family, including both direct child maltreatment and witnessing other family violence. McDonald et al.'s (2015) interview-based study of IPV-exposed children regarding their exposure to animal cruelty and threats thereof yielded a prominent theme: cruelty was used to coerce and control their mothers. Secondary themes included the use of animal cruelty to discipline pets, siblings' perpetration of cruelty, and attempts by the children to protect their pets. In examining potential sequelae, a pair of recent studies examined youth exposure to animal cruelty as a moderator of associations between IPV exposure and internalizing and externalizing symptoms, respectively (Hawkins et al., 2019b; Matijczak et al., 2020), finding that cruelty exposure moderated the relationship between IPV exposure and internalizing (anxiety and depression) symptoms but not externalizing symptoms.

Research on animal cruelty in the context of IPV, apart from children's experiences, has largely focused on batterer threats/harm to pets or other valued animals as self-reported by (mostly female) victims staying at domestic violence shelters. Some efforts to compare these samples with community controls indicate substantially higher rates of animal cruelty experienced by IPV victims (Ascione et al., 2007). In an epidemiological study across 11 metropolitan areas of the USA, Walton-Moss et al. (2005) found that a history of animal cruelty was one of five primary predictors of engaging in IPV.

More recently, attention has turned to the function of animal cruelty within IPV, commonly identifying the cruelty as part of a pattern of coercive control exerted by the perpetrator over human family members, as noted in the previously described systematic review by Alleyne and Parfitt (2019) and in Collins et al. (2018). However, recent work by Fitzgerald et al. (2019) indicated that this mechanism was clearer for pet-directed threats, emotional abuse, and neglect than for physical animal abuse, at least from the victim's perspective. Several studies suggest that victims of IPV whose partners also harm pets may engage in more frequent and/or severe IPV, potentially rendering animal cruelty an identifier of increased human risk (Barrett et al., 2020; Campbell et al., 2018). Surveys of Canadian domestic violence shelters revealed a general awareness of animal cruelty occurring within IPV, but inconsistent use of questions about animals on shelter crisis lines, in risk assessments, and at intake (Stevenson et al., 2018). Shelter-based research on animal cruelty in the IPV context is limited in that it does not yield any information about those victims who do not enter shelters, yet who may still need assistance in securing safety for themselves, their children, and their animals.

At the opposite end of the lifespan from the intense focus on both victimization and perpetration by children, elder abuse has received scant attention in the literature although anecdotal accounts of threats or harm to elders' animals as a means of control or retaliation, similar to IPV, are common. Peak et al. (2012) found that only 1 of 41 states responding to a survey codified questions about animal concerns in relation to elder abuse in its screening protocols. Further work is urgently needed in this area, not only to establish rates of animal cruelty within elder abuse, but to illuminate pathways for prevention and response.

Future Directions

Patterson-Kane and Piper (2009) catalogued in a review the methodological limitations in this body of research: the wide range of operational definitions of animal "cruelty" and the related term "abuse," variations in approaches to and measures of behavior, and reliance in research on specialized samples, such as psychiatric and/ or incarcerated samples, from which findings may not be generalizable to the overall population. In addition, the current author observes that small sample sizes remain common in "link" research, likely due to difficulties in identifying and accessing large groups of offenders or victims. Additionally, references to these studies in both professional and public discourse frequently extrapolate sample proportions directly to population prevalence rates without the use of confidence intervals, weighted estimates, or other appropriate statistical tools.

As one example, in a foundational study by Ascione (1998), 20 of 28 pet-owning women (71%) at a single domestic violence shelter reported threats or harm to the pet by the perpetrator. Despite a note within the manuscript from the study's author advising caution about generalizing the findings, this proportion—among the highest reported in early research—is repeatedly referenced in websites, presentations, and factsheets as an established national rate: "71% of pet owners entering domestic violence shelters report that their batterer had threatened, injured, or killed family pets" (National Coalition Against Domestic Violence, n.d.).

Overall, despite these limitations, the landscape of available research indicates some support for associations between animal cruelty and other violence/

deviance—more strongly in some areas than others, and with certain factors (e.g., recurrence of cruelty) emerging as more relevant to these associations rather than an outright 1:1 relationship between all cruelty and all other deviant acts. Scholarship that continues to illuminate the nuances of "the link" is important in order to refine our understanding, which will serve as the basis for future programmatic and policy decisions.

In examining animal cruelty in association with other violence/deviance, particularly when identifying implications for decision-making at either the individual or systemic level, it is vital to consider the difference between the statistical and clinical uses of the term "predictor." Identifying a variable (such as animal cruelty) as a statistically significant predictor (explanatory) variable in a regression model does not automatically imply a longitudinal relationship. Further, simply because a variable is statistically significant does not make it clinically meaningful, particularly with large samples where even small associations are likely to yield small p-values in hypothesis testing. Predicting human behavior is notoriously difficult. If we could accurately predict exactly who would commit these acts, there would be no violence or crime because we could take appropriate measures with each individual at risk.

As an example, if a model using animal cruelty in which both the overall model and the cruelty predictor are statistically significant explains 10 percent of the variance in interpersonal violence, what of the factors that account for the remaining 90 percent? In an actuarial sense, it is difficult to target interventions in this way. Animal cruelty may be an interesting and statistically significant predictor, but this alone does not make it the most accurate or useful predictor. Further, statistical models such as these do not provide evidence of causation—meaning that even if animal cruelty were directly targeted for intervention, it could be the wrong target if some other variable (say, genetic predisposition or environmental factors) was causally responsible for both the animal cruelty and the interpersonal violence.

Returning to the question of the graduation hypothesis versus the generalized deviance hypothesis, it is the opinion of this author that taken together across the research on youth- and adult-perpetrated animal cruelty, the greater volume of evidence in both quantity and quality appears to be on the side of generalized deviance. However, both animal cruelty and other deviant/violent acts are heterogeneous behaviors with diverse phenotypes and motivations. It is possible, or even likely, that the answer to the debate is that both hypotheses are true, but for different individuals. It may also be the case that some individuals are characterized by both progression and generalized deviance. Further research, especially using longitudinal designs, can aim to identify these pathways.

A vital area for further research is the impact of programs and policies based on this topic. Do interdisciplinary cross-reporting, the inclusion of animals in domestic violence protective orders, building animal housing facilities at domestic violence shelters, and animal abuser registries—all predicated on the concept of interconnected forms of abuse—actually increase the safety and well-being of people and animals in measurable ways? Other than the references included in the position statement on animal abuser registries by the ASPCA (American Society for the Prevention of Cruelty to Animals, 2021), to which this author contributed, there appear to be scant if any data on any aspects of this topic. This suggests that substantial legislative and advocacy energy are being expended on purported solutions that unbeknownst to their well-intentioned creators and implementers may do little to benefit the intended recipients, or may even cause harm.

A concluding note on this topic: the concept of a "link" has been instrumental in driving attention to animal cruelty among those who might not otherwise have considered it worthy of such attention, and the idea of using understanding of "links" to benefit both animals and humans is seductive (in the same way as AAI utilizes the human-animal relationship). However, it is important to bear in mind that animal cruelty is itself a crime in all 50 US states and involves victims deserving of recognition and assistance, regardless of whether human victims are also involved. In the opinion of this author, treating animal cruelty only as a marker for the "true crime" of human-directed criminality is a disservice to animals and society, incompatible with the spirit upon which VSW is founded.

Conclusion

Whereas suggestions for future research directions have been provided alongside each of the four VSW topic areas reviewed in this chapter, two summary statements bear mention as they apply to all areas of research within the VSW umbrella.

First, even though they have been covered separately here, it would be a mistake to treat the four domains of VSW as independent topics. AAI potentially takes on new angles when delivered for (or by) those experiencing CF or animal-related grief/bereavement, or those who have experienced or perpetrated animal cruelty and/or other aggressive acts. Loss or other harm to animals experienced by victims of family violence in a deliberate attempt to inflict emotional harm can bring additional dimensions to grief. Secondary traumatic stress may contribute to CF in practitioners who work with individuals experiencing animal-related grief/bereavement. While VSW practitioners naturally tend to orient their passion and practice to one topic area more than others, focusing on one area of VSW in isolation risks creating blinders that are inimical to the interconnectedness of social work. Viewing VSW as an effort to promote healthier human-animal relationships through multiple channels, and at all points along a continuum, can be helpful in reminding VSW professionals to keep their eyes open for opportunities to "connect dots" across topics.

Second, as research in these topics continues to proliferate, it is incumbent upon the field as a whole to take steps to prevent and address publication bias. Among the systematic reviews examined for this chapter, only a handful included explicit attention to publication bias either via study selection methods or via calculation of bias in selected studies (funnel plots, Egger's test, etc.). The inherent appeal of the narratives that animals are always good for people, that losing an animal or experiencing animal suffering is always devastating, and that people who harm animals must be depraved and dangerous is a siren song that must be carefully filtered through the decoder of data. When results fail to support hypotheses tied to strongly held implicit beliefs by researchers, reviewers, or funders, either deliberate or inadvertent suppression of null or contradictory findings can distort the dissemination of science. As an example, a research funding solicitation titled "Addressing Evidence-Based Health *Benefits* of Human-Animal Interaction" (my emphasis) currently appears on a website whose cover statement explains that the funder "believes in the powerful relationship between animals and people and the impact of this relationship on the health of individuals, families, and communities" and includes a substantial section dedicated to "the pet effect" (Human-Animal Bond Research Institute, 2021). Presupposing a powerful, impactful relationship makes a worthy and largely well-grounded hypothesis for an approach to most topics in VSW, but when treated as a foregone conclusion instead of a hypothesis, it has the potential to exert undue influence on the scientific process.

It is this author's hope that readers who have persisted to the end of this chapter are not solely those with preexisting interests in research. Echoing the sentiment expressed in the Chap. 1, the entire field of VSW stands to gain from a deeper integration of research and practice. In outlining both available knowledge and gaps therein, this review and analysis of research in the four major domains of VSW seeks to strengthen both scholarly and applied approaches to this growing field, enriching both this growing field and the lives of the humans and animals it touches.

References

Adams, C. L., Bonnett, B. N., & Meek, A. H. (2000). Predictors of owner response to companion animal death in 177 clients from 14 practices in Ontario. *Journal of the American Veterinary Medical Association, 217*(9), 1303–1309. https://doi.org/10.2460/javma.2000.217.1303

Adrian, J. A. L., & Stitt, A. (2017). Pet loss, complicated grief, and post-traumatic stress disorder in Hawaii. *Anthrozoös, 30*(1), 123–133. https://doi.org/10.1080/08927936.2017.1270598

Alleyne, E., & Parfitt, C. (2019). Adult-perpetrated animal abuse: A systematic literature review. Adult-perpetrated animal abuse: A systematic literature review. *Trauma, Violence, and Abuse, 20*(3), 344–357. https://doi.org/10.1177/1524838017708785

American Psychiatric Association. (2013). *Diagnostic and statistical manual of mental disorders* (5th ed.). Author.

American Society for the Prevention of Cruelty to Animals. (2021). *Position statement on animal abuser registries*. https://www.aspca.org/about-us/aspca-policy-and-position-statements/position-statement-animal-abuser-registries

Andrukonis, A., & Protopopova, A. (2020). Occupational health of animal shelter employees by live release rate, shelter type, and euthanasia-related decision. Type. *Anthrozoos*. https://doi.org/10.1080/08927936.2020.1694316

Andrukonis, A., Hall, N. J., & Protopopova, A. (2020). The impact of caring and killing on physiological and psychometric measures of stress in animal shelter employees: A pilot study. *International Journal of Environmental Research and Public Health, 17*(24), 1–18. https://doi.org/10.3390/ijerph17249196

Arluke, A., & Madfis, E. (2014). Animal abuse as a warning sign of school massacres: A critique and refinement. *Homicide Studies, 18*(1), 7–22. https://doi.org/10.1177/1088767913511459

Arluke, A., Levin, J., Luke, C., & Ascione, F. (1999). The relationship of animal abuse to violence and other forms of antisocial behavior. *Journal of Interpersonal Violence, 14*(9), 963–975. https://doi.org/10.1177/088626099014009004

Ascione, F. R. (1998). Battered women's reports of their partners' and their children's cruelty to animals. *Journal of Emotional Abuse, 1*(1), 119–133. https://doi.org/10.1300/J135v01n01

Ascione, F. R., Weber, C. V., Thompson, T. M., Heath, J., Maruyama, M., & Hayashi, K. (2007). Battered pets and domestic violence: Animal abuse reported by women experiencing intimate violence and by nonabused women. *Violence Against Women, 13*(4), 354–373. https://doi.org/10.1177/1077801207299201

Baglivio, M. T., Wolff, K. T., DeLisi, M., Vaughn, M. G., & Piquero, A. R. (2017). Juvenile animal cruelty and firesetting behaviour. *Criminal Behaviour and Mental Health, 27*(5), 484–500. https://doi.org/10.1002/cbm.2018

Baran, B. E., Allen, J. A., Rogelberg, S. G., Spitzmüller, C., DiGiacomo, N. A., Webb, J. B., Carter, N. T., Clark, O. L., Teeter, L. A., & Walker, A. G. (2009). Euthanasia-related strain and coping strategies in animal shelter employees. *Journal of the American Veterinary Medical Association, 235*(1), 83–88.

Barnard-Nguyen, S., Breit, M., Anderson, K. A., & Nielsen, J. (2016). Pet loss and grief: Identifying at-risk pet owners during the euthanasia process. *Anthrozoös, 29*(3), 421–430. https://doi.org/10.1080/08927936.2016.1181362

Barrett, B. J., Fitzgerald, A., Stevenson, R., & Cheung, C. H. (2020). Animal maltreatment as a risk marker of more frequent and severe forms of intimate partner violence. *Journal of Interpersonal Violence, 35*(23–24), 5131–5156. https://doi.org/10.1177/0886260517719542

Behler, A. M. C., Green, J. D., & Joy-Gaba, J. (n.d.). "We lost a member of the family": Predictors of the grief experience surrounding the loss of a pet. *Human-Animal Interaction Bulletin.* Retrieved January 17, 2021, from https://www.apa-hai.org/haib/download-info/we-lost-a-member-of-the-family-predictors-of-the-grief-experience-surrounding-the-loss-of-a-pet/

Boat, B. W. (2014). Connections among adverse childhood experiences, exposure to animal cruelty and toxic stress: What do professionals need to consider? *National Center for Prosecution of Child Abuse, 24*(4), 1–3.

Boss, L., Branson, S., Hagan, H., & Krause-Parello, C. (2019). A systematic review of equine-assisted interventions in military veterans diagnosed with PTSD. *Journal of Veterans Studies, 5*(1), 23. https://doi.org/10.21061/jvs.v5i1.134

Brelsford, V. L., Meints, K., Gee, N. R., & Pfeffer, K. (2017). Animal-assisted interventions in the classroom—A systematic review. *International Journal of Environmental Research and Public Health.* https://doi.org/10.3390/ijerph14070669

Bright, M. A., Huq, M. S., Spencer, T., Applebaum, J. W., & Hardt, N. (2018). Animal cruelty as an indicator of family trauma: Using adverse childhood experiences to look beyond child abuse and domestic violence. *Child Abuse and Neglect.* https://doi.org/10.1016/j.chiabu.2017.11.011

Bui, E. (Ed.). (2018). *Clinical handbook of bereavement and grief reactions.* Springer International Publishing. https://doi.org/10.1007/978-3-319-65241-2

Bussolari, C., Habarth, J. M., Phillips, S., Katz, R., & Packman, W. (2018). Self-compassion, social constraints, and psychosocial outcomes in a pet bereavement sample. *Omega (United States), 82*(3), 389–408. https://doi.org/10.1177/0030222818814050

Bussolari, C., Habarth, J., Kimpara, S., Katz, R., Carlos, F., Chow, A., Osada, H., Osada, Y., Carmack, B. J., Field, N. P., & Packman, W. (2019). Posttraumatic growth following the loss of a pet: A cross-cultural comparison. *Omega (United States), 78*(4), 348–368. https://doi.org/10.1177/0030222817690403

Campbell, A. M., Thompson, S. L., Harris, T. L., & Wiehe, S. E. (2018). Intimate partner violence and pet abuse: Responding law enforcement officers' observations and victim reports from the scene. *Journal of Interpersonal Violence,* 1–20. https://doi.org/10.1177/0886260518759653

Cavallaro, L. (2016). Employee wellbeing and compassion fatigue among animal caregivers: A hermeneutic phenomenological study. *Dissertation abstracts international: Section B: The sciences and engineering.*

Chang, S. J., Lee, J., An, H., Hong, W.-H., & Lee, J. Y. (2020). Animal-assisted therapy as an intervention for older adults: A systematic review and meta-analysis to guide evidence-based practice. *Worldviews on Evidence-Based Nursing, 18*(1), 60–67.

Collins, E. A., Cody, A. M., McDonald, S. E., Nicotera, N., Ascione, F. R., & Williams, J. H. (2018). A template analysis of intimate partner violence survivors' experiences of animal maltreatment: Implications for safety planning and intervention. *Violence Against Women*. https://doi.org/10.1177/1077801217697266

Conversano, C., Ciacchini, R., Orrù, G., Di Giuseppe, M., Gemignani, A., & Poli, A. (2020). Mindfulness, compassion, and self-compassion among health care professionals: What's new? A systematic review. *Frontiers in Psychology*. https://doi.org/10.3389/fpsyg.2020.01683

Cooney, K. A., Kogan, L. R., Brooks, S. L., & Ellis, C. A. (2020). Pet owners' expectations for pet end-of-life support and after-death body care: Exploration and practical applications. *Topics in Companion Animal Medicine, 43*, 100503. https://doi.org/10.1016/j.tcam.2020.100503

Cotoc, C., An, R., & Klonoff-Cohen, H. (2019). Pediatric oncology and animal-assisted interventions: A systematic review. *Holistic Nursing Practice, 33*(2), 101–110. https://doi.org/10.1097/HNP.0000000000000313

Davies, E., & James, S. (2018). The psychological responses of amateur riders to their horses' injuries. *Comparative Exercise Physiology, 14*(2), 135–142. https://doi.org/10.3920/CEP180009

DeViney, E., Dickert, J., & Lockwood, R. (1983). The care of pets within child abusing families. *International Journal for the Study of Animal Problems, 4*(4), 321–329. http://search.proquest.com/docview/616882281?accountid=11233%5Cn; http://sfx.scholarsportal.info/guelph?genre=article & sid=ProQ: & atitle=The careofpetswithinchildabusingfamilies. & title =InternationalJournalfortheStudyofAnimalProblems & issn=0195-755

Dickinson, G. E. (2019). US and UK veterinary medicine schools: Emphasis on end-of-life issues. *Mortality, 24*(1), 61–71. https://doi.org/10.1080/13576275.2017.1396970

Dimolareva, M., & Dunn, T. J. (2020). Animal-assisted interventions for school-aged children with autism spectrum disorder: A meta-analysis. *Journal of Autism and Developmental Disorders*, 0123456789. https://doi.org/10.1007/s10803-020-04715-w

Djelantik, A. A. A. M. J., Smid, G. E., Mroz, A., Kleber, R. J., & Boelen, P. A. (2020). The prevalence of prolonged grief disorder in bereaved individuals following unnatural losses: Systematic review and meta regression analysis. *Journal of Affective Disorders, 265*, 146–156. https://doi.org/10.1016/j.jad.2020.01.034

Doka, K. J. (1999). Disenfranchised grief. *Bereavement Care, 18*(3), 37–39.

Dow, M. Q., Chur-Hansen, A., Hamood, W., & Edwards, S. (2019). Impact of dealing with bereaved clients on the psychological wellbeing of veterinarians. *Australian Veterinary Journal, 97*(10), 382–389. https://doi.org/10.1111/avj.12842

Dunn, J., Best, C., Pearl, D. L., & Jones-Bitton, A. (2019). Mental health of employees at a Canadian animal welfare organization. *Society & Animals*, 1–37. https://doi.org/10.1163/15685306-00001709

Eckerd, L. M., Barnett, J. E., & Jett-Dias, L. (2016). Grief following pet and human loss: Closeness is key. *Death Studies, 40*(5), 275–282. https://doi.org/10.1080/07481187.2016.1139014

Eisma, M. C., & Stroebe, M. S. (2020). Emotion regulatory strategies in complicated grief: A systematic review. *Behavior Therapy, 52*(1), 234–249. https://doi.org/10.1016/j.beth.2020.04.004

Ferguson, C. J. (2009). An effect size primer: A guide for clinicians and researchers. *Professional Psychology: Research and Practice, 40*(5), 532–538. https://doi.org/10.1037/a0015808

Fine, A. H., Beck, A. M., & Ng, Z. (2019). The state of animal-assisted interventions: Addressing the contemporary issues that will shape the future. *International Journal of Environmental Research and Public Health, 16*(20), 3997. https://doi.org/10.3390/ijerph16203997

Fitzgerald, A. J., Barrett, B. J., Stevenson, R., & Cheung, C. H. (2019). Animal maltreatment in the context of intimate partner violence: A manifestation of power and control? *Violence Against Women, 25*(15), 1806–1828. https://doi.org/10.1177/1077801218824993

Gee, N. R., & Mueller, M. K. (2019). A systematic review of research on pet ownership and animal interactions among older adults. *Anthrozoös, 32*(2), 183–207. https://doi.org/10.1080/08927936.2019.1569903

Glenk, L. M. (2017). Current perspectives on therapy dog welfare in animal-assisted interventions. *Animals (Basel), 7*(2), 7. https://doi.org/10.3390/ani7020007

Green, C., Kangas, M., & Fairholm, I. (2018). Investigating the emotion regulation strategies implemented by adults grieving the death of a pet in Australia and the UK. *Journal of Loss and Trauma, 23*(6), 484–501. https://doi.org/10.1080/15325024.2018.1478934

Habarth, J., Bussolari, C., Gomez, R., Carmack, B. J., Ronen, R., Field, N. P., & Packman, W. (2017). Continuing bonds and psychosocial functioning in a recently bereaved pet loss sample. *Anthrozoös, 30*(4), 651–670. https://doi.org/10.1080/08927936.2017.1370242

Hartman, C., Hageman, T., Williams, J. H., Mary, J. S., & Ascione, F. R. (2019). Exploring empathy and callous – Unemotional traits as predictors of animal abuse perpetrated by children exposed to intimate partner violence. *Journal of Interpersonal Violence, 34*(12), 2419–2437. https://doi.org/10.1177/0886260516660971

Harvey, L. C., & Cameron, K. E. (2020). Stress and compassion fatigue in veterinary nurses in New Zealand. *The Veterinary Nurse, 11*(1). https://doi.org/10.12968/vetn.2020.11.1.42

Hawkins, E. L., Hawkins, R. D., Dennis, M., Williams, J. M., & Lawrie, S. M. (2019a). Animal-assisted therapy for schizophrenia and related disorders: A systematic review. *Journal of Psychiatric Research, 115*, 51–60. https://doi.org/10.1016/j.jpsychires.2019.05.013

Hawkins, R. D., McDonald, S. E., O'Connor, K., Matijczak, A., Ascione, F. R., & Williams, J. H. (2019b). Exposure to intimate partner violence and internalizing symptoms: The moderating effects of positive relationships with pets and animal cruelty exposure. *Child Abuse and Neglect, 98*(August), 104166. https://doi.org/10.1016/j.chiabu.2019.104166

Hess-Holden, C. L., Jackson, D. L., Morse, D. T., & Monaghan, C. L. (2019). Understanding non-technical competencies: Compassion and communication among fourth-year veterinarians-in-training. *Journal of Veterinary Medical Education, 46*(12), 506–517. https://doi.org/10.3138/jvme.0917-131r1

Hill, E. M., LaLonde, C. M., & Reese, L. A. (2019). Compassion fatigue in animal care workers. *Traumatology, 26*(1), 96–108. https://doi.org/10.1037/trm0000218

Hoagwood, K. E., Acri, M., Morrissey, M., & Peth-Pierce, R. (2017). Animal-assisted therapies for youth with or at risk for mental health problems: A systematic review. *Applied Developmental Science, 21*(1), 1–13. https://doi.org/10.1080/10888691.2015.1134267

Hoffer, T., Hargreaves-Cormany, H., Muirhead, Y., & Meloy, J. R. (2018). *Violence in animal cruelty offenders*. Springer.

Human-Animal Bond Research Institute. (2021). *No title*. https://habri.org/

Johannsen, M., Damholdt, M. F., Zachariae, R., Lundorff, M., Farver-Vestergaard, I., & O'Connor, M. (2019). Psychological interventions for grief in adults: A systematic review and meta-analysis of randomized controlled trials. *Journal of Affective Disorders, 253*, 69–86. https://doi.org/10.1016/j.jad.2019.04.065

Joinson, C. (1992). Coping with compassion fatigue. *Nursing, 22*(4), 116–118.

Joubert, D., Welsh, K., & Edward, L. J. (2021). Validity of the MacDonald triad as a forensic construct: Links with psychopathology and patterns of aggression in sex offenders. *Legal and Criminological Psychology, 26*(1), 103–116. https://doi.org/10.1111/lcrp.12183

Kazdin, A. E. (2010). Establishing the effectiveness of animal-assisted therapies: Methodological standards, issues, and strategies. In P. McCardle, S. McCune, J. A. Griffin, & V. Maholmes (Eds.), *How animals affect us: Examining the influences of human–animal interaction on child development and human health* (pp. 35–51). American Psychological Association. https://doi.org/10.1037/12301-002

Kemp, H. R., Jacobs, N., & Stewart, S. (2016). The lived experience of companion-animal loss: A systematic review of qualitative studies. *Anthrozoös, 29*(4), 533–557. https://doi.org/10.1080/08927936.2016.1228772

Klass, D., Silverman, P. R., & Nickman, S. (2014). *Continuing bonds: New understandings of grief*. Taylor & Francis.

Klimova, B., Toman, J., & Kuca, K. (2019). Effectiveness of the dog therapy for patients with dementia - A systematic review. *BMC Psychiatry, 19*(1), 276. https://doi.org/10.1186/s12888-019-2245-x

Kogan, L., & Erdman, P. (2020). *Pet loss, grief, and therapeutic interventions: Practitioners navigating the human-animal bond*. Taylor & Francis.

Kogan, L. R., Wallace, J. E., Schoenfeld-Tacher, R., Hellyer, P. W., & Richards, M. (2020). Veterinary technicians and occupational burnout. *Frontiers in Veterinary Science, 7*, 328. https://doi.org/10.3389/fvets.2020.00328

Lai, N. M., Chang, S. M. W., Ng, S. S., Tan, S. L., Chaiyakunapruk, N., & Stanaway, F. (2019). Animal-assisted therapy for dementia. *The Cochrane Database of Systematic Reviews, 2019*(1), CD013243. https://doi.org/10.1002/14651858.CD013243.pub2

Laing, M., & Maylea, C. (2018). "They burn brightly, but only for a short time": The role of social workers in companion animal grief and loss. *Anthrozoös, 31*(2), 221–232. https://doi.org/1 0.1080/08927936.2018.1434062

Lee, S. A. (2020). Does the DSM-5 grief disorder apply to owners of deceased pets? A psychometric study of impairment during pet loss. *Psychiatry Research, 285*, 112800. https://doi.org/10.1016/j.psychres.2020.112800

Levitt, A. L., & Gezinski, L. B. (2020). Compassion fatigue and resiliency factors in animal shelter workers. *Society and Animals, 28*(5–6), 633–650. https://doi.org/10.1163/15685306-12341554

Littlewood, K. E., Beausoleil, N. J., Stafford, K. J., Stephens, C., Collins, T., Fawcett, A., … Zito, S. (2020). How management of grief associated with ending the life of an animal is taught to Australasian veterinary students. *Australian Veterinary Journal, 98*(8), 356–363. https://doi.org/10.1111/avj.12960

Longobardi, C., & Badenes-Ribera, L. (2019). The relationship between animal cruelty in children and adolescent and interpersonal violence: A systematic review. *Aggression and Violent Behavior, 46*, 201–211. https://doi.org/10.1016/j.avb.2018.09.001

Maber-Aleksandrowicz, S., Avent, C., & Hassiotis, A. (2016). A systematic review of animal-assisted therapy on psychosocial outcomes in people with intellectual disability. *Research in Developmental Disabilities, 49–50*, 322–328. https://doi.org/10.1016/j.ridd.2015.12.005

Macdonald, J. M. (1963). The threat to kill. *American Journal of Psychiatry, 120*(2), 125–130. https://doi.org/10.1176/ajp.120.2.125

Matijczak, A., McDonald, S. E., O'Connor, K. E., George, N., Tomlinson, C. A., Murphy, J. L., … Williams, J. H. (2020). Do animal cruelty exposure and positive engagement with pets moderate associations between children's exposure to intimate partner violence and externalizing behavior problems? *Child and Adolescent Social Work Journal, 37*(6), 601–613. https://doi.org/10.1007/s10560-020-00702-3

McArthur, M. L., Andrews, J. R., Brand, C., & Hazel, S. J. (2017). The prevalence of compassion fatigue among veterinary students in Australia and the associated psychological factors. *Journal of Veterinary Medical Education, 44*(1), 9–21. https://doi.org/10.3138/jvme.0116-016R3

McDonald, S. E., Collins, E. A., Nicotera, N., Hageman, T. O., Ascione, F. R., Williams, J. H., & Graham-Bermann, S. A. (2015). Children's experiences of companion animal maltreatment in households characterized by intimate partner violence. *Child Abuse and Neglect, 50*, 116–127. https://doi.org/10.1016/j.chiabu.2015.10.005

McDonald, S. E., Cody, A. M., Booth, L. J., Peers, J. R., O'Connor Luce, C., Williams, J. H., & Ascione, F. R. (2018). Animal cruelty among children in violent households: Children's explanations of their behavior. *Journal of Family Violence, 33*(7), 469–480. https://doi.org/10.1007/s10896-018-9970-7

McKinney, K. (2019). Emotion work of coping with the death of a companion animal. *Society and Animals, 27*(1), 109–125. https://doi.org/10.1163/15685306-12341586

Monaghan, H., Rohlf, V., Scotney, R., & Bennett, P. (2020). Compassion fatigue in people who care for animals: An investigation of risk and protective factors. *Traumatology*. https://doi.org/10.1037/trm0000246

Moses, L., Malowney, M. J., & Wesley Boyd, J. (2018). Ethical conflict and moral distress in veterinary practice: A survey of North American veterinarians. *Journal of Veterinary Internal Medicine, 32*(6), 2115–2122. https://doi.org/10.1111/jvim.15315

Musetti, A., Schianchi, A., Caricati, L., Manari, T., & Schimmenti, A. (2020, August). Exposure to animal suffering, adult attachment styles, and professional quality of life in a sample of Italian veterinarians. *PLoS ONE, 15*(8), 1–18. https://doi.org/10.1371/journal.pone.0237991

National Coalition Against Domestic Violence. (n.d.). *Pets and domestic violence.* https://www.sheriffs.org/publications/NCADV-Pets-DV.pdf

O'Haire, M. E., Guérin, N. A., & Kirkham, A. C. (2015). Animal-assisted intervention assisted intervention for trauma: A systematic literature review. *Frontiers in Psychology, 6*, 1121. https://doi.org/10.3389/fpsyg.2015.01121

Packman, W., Carmack, B. J., Katz, R., Carlos, F., Thérapeute, T., Field, N. P., & Landers, C. (2014). Online survey as empathic bridging for the disenfranchised grief of pet loss. *Omega (United States), 69*(4), 333–356. https://doi.org/10.2190/OM.69.4.a

Packman, W., Bussolari, C., Katz, R., Carmack, B. J., & Field, N. P. (2017). Posttraumatic growth following the loss of a pet. *Omega (United States), 75*(4), 337–359. https://doi.org/10.1177/0030222816663411

Parfitt, C. H., & Alleyne, E. (2020). Not the sum of its parts: A critical review of the MacDonald triad. *Trauma, Violence, and Abuse, 21*(2), 300–310. https://doi.org/10.1177/1524838018764164

Park, R., & Royal, K. (2020). A national survey of companion animal owners' self-reported methods of coping following euthanasia. *Veterinary Sciences, 7*(7). https://doi.org/10.3390/VETSCI7030020

Patterson-Kane, E. G., & Piper, H. (2009). Animal abuse as a sentinel for human violence: A critique. *Journal of Social Issues, 65*(3), 589–614. https://doi.org/10.1111/j.1540-4560.2009.01615.x

Peak, T., Ascione, F., & Doney, J. (2012). Adult protective services and animal welfare: Should animal abuse and neglect be assessed during adult protective services screening? *Journal of Elder Abuse and Neglect, 24*(1), 37–49. https://doi.org/10.1080/08946566.2011.608047

Perret, J. L., Best, C. O., Coe, J. B., Greer, A. L., Khosa, D. K., & Jones-Bitton, A. (2020). Prevalence of mental health outcomes among Canadian veterinarians. *Journal of the American Veterinary Medical Association, 256*(3), 365–375. https://doi.org/10.2460/javma.256.3.365

Polachek, A. J., & Wallace, J. E. (2018). The paradox of compassionate work: A mixed-methods study of satisfying and fatiguing experiences of animal health care providers. *Anxiety, Stress and Coping, 31*(2), 228–243. https://doi.org/10.1080/10615806.2017.1392224

Reisbig, A. M. J., Hafen, M., Siqueira Drake, A. A., Girard, D., & Breunig, Z. B. (2017). Companion animal death: A qualitative analysis of relationship quality, loss, and coping. *Omega (United States), 75*(2), 124–150. https://doi.org/10.1177/0030222815612607

Rohlf, V. I. (2018). Interventions for occupational stress and compassion fatigue in animal care professionals-a systematic review. *Traumatology, 24*(3), 186–192. https://doi.org/10.1037/trm0000144

Roth, A., & Fonagy, P. (2005). *What works for whom: A critical review of psychotherapy research* (2nd ed., pp. vii, 661). Guilford Publications.

Rowan, A., & Kartal, T. (2018). Dog population & dog sheltering trends in the United States of America. *Animals (Basel), 8*(5), 68. https://doi.org/10.3390/ani8050068

Schroeder, K. (2019). Grieving the equine companion: Implications for mental health care practitioners. In L. Kogan & P. Erdman (Eds.), *Pet loss, grief, and therapeutic interventions: Practitioners navigating the human-animal bond* (pp. 175–187). Taylor & Francis.

Scotney, R. L., McLaughlin, D., & Keates, H. L. (2015). A systematic review of the effects of euthanasia and occupational stress in personnel working with animals in animal shelters, veterinary clinics, and biomedical research facilities. *Journal of the American Veterinary Medical Association, 424*(August), 928–929. https://doi.org/10.2460/javma.247.10.1121

Scotney, R. L., McLaughlin, D., & Keates, H. L. (2019). An investigation of the prevalence of compassion fatigue, compassion satisfaction and burnout in those working in animal-related occupations using the Professional Quality of Life (ProQoL) Scale. *The Veterinary Nurse, 10*(5). https://doi.org/10.12968/vetn.2019.10.5.276

Serpell, J., McCune, S., Gee, N., & Griffin, J. A. (2017). Current challenges to research on animal-assisted interventions. *Applied Developmental Science, 21*(3), 223–233. https://doi.org/10.108 0/10888691.2016.1262775

Shear, M. K., Simon, N., Wall, M., Zisook, S., Neimeyer, R., Duan, N., Reynolds, C., … Keshaviah, A. (2011). Complicated grief and related bereavement issues for DSM-5. *Depression and Anxiety, 28*(2), 103–117. https://doi.org/10.1002/da.20780

Smith, N. (2016). A questionnaire based study to assess compassion fatigue in UK practising veterinary nurses. *The Veterinary Nurse, 7*(7). https://doi.org/10.12968/vetn.2016.7.7.418

Spain, B., O'Dwyer, L., & Moston, S. (2019). Pet loss: Understanding disenfranchised grief, memorial use, and posttraumatic growth. *Anthrozoös, 32*(4), 555–568. https://doi.org/10.108 0/08927936.2019.1621545

Srinivasan, S. M., Cavagnino, D. T., & Bhat, A. N. (2018). Effects of equine therapy on individuals with autism spectrum disorder: A systematic review. *Review Journal of Autism and Developmental Disorders, 5*(2), 156–175. https://doi.org/10.1007/s40489-018-0130-z

Stevenson, R., Fitzgerald, A., & Barrett, B. J. (2018). Keeping pets safe in the context of intimate partner violence: Insights from domestic violence shelter staff in Canada. *Affilia - Journal of Women and Social Work, 33*(2), 236–252. https://doi.org/10.1177/0886109917747613

Tomasi, S. E., Fechter-Leggett, E. D., Edwards, N. T., Reddish, A. D., Crosby, A. E., & Nett, R. J. (2019). Suicide among veterinarians in the United States from 1979 through 2015. *Journal of the American Veterinary Medical Association, 254*(1), 104–112. https://doi.org/10.2460/javma.254.1.104

Villafaina-Domínguez, B., Collado-Mateo, D., Merellano-Navarro, E., & Villafaina, S. (2020). Effects of dog-based animal-assisted interventions in prison population: A systematic review. *Animals, 10*(11), 1–19. https://doi.org/10.3390/ani10112129

Walters, G. D. (2019). Animal cruelty and bullying: Behavioral markers of delinquency risk or causal antecedents of delinquent behavior? *International Journal of Law and Psychiatry, 62*(October 2018), 77–84. https://doi.org/10.1016/j.ijlp.2018.11.008

Walton-Moss, B. J., Manganello, J., Frye, V., & Campbell, J. C. (2005). Risk factors for intimate partner violence and associated injury among urban women. *Journal of Community Health, 30*(5), 377–389. https://doi.org/10.1007/s10900-005-5518-x

Wijker, C., Leontjevas, R., Spek, A., & Enders-Slegers, M. J. (2020). Effects of dog assisted therapy for adults with autism spectrum disorder: An exploratory randomized controlled trial. *Journal of Autism and Developmental Disorders, 50*(6), 2153–2163. https://doi.org/10.1007/s10803-019-03971-9

World Health Organization. (2019). *International statistical classification of diseases and related health problems* (11th ed.). Author.

Yakimicki, M. L., Edwards, N. E., Richards, E., Beck, A. M., & Professor, A. (2019). Animal-assisted intervention and dementia: A systematic review. *Clinical Nursing Research, 28*(1), 9–29. https://doi.org/10.1177/1054773818756987

Young, R. L., & Thompson, C. Y. (2020). Exploring empathy, compassion fatigue, and burnout among feral cat caregivers. *Society and Animals, 28*(2), 151–170. https://doi.org/10.1163/15685306-00001704

Zhang, Y., Yan, F., Li, S., Wang, Y., & Ma, Y. (2020). Effectiveness of animal-assisted therapy on pain in children: Systematic review and meta-analysis. *International Journal of Nursing Sciences.* https://doi.org/10.1016/j.ijnss.2020.12.009

Chapter 16
Veterinary Social Work Across Diverse Cultures

Sana Loue

Introduction

Veterinary social work as a distinct branch of social work practice is a relative new-comer to the profession of social work. One of the earliest training programs in veterinary social work was developed only as recently as 1990 (Brackenridge, Hacker, and Pepe, this volume). Veterinary social workers are employed in a wide range of contexts including veterinary hospitals, private psychotherapy practices, academia, child or adult welfare agencies, domestic violence programs, courthouse services, and homeless shelters. In these contexts, they are likely to work with colleagues and clients who self-identify as members of diverse groups.

As a new subspeciality within social work, VSW is in the process of both developing standards and competencies for the profession and becoming recognized as a distinct subspeciality in the United States and other countries. However, like all social workers, regardless of the context in which they practice or train, VSWs are expected to comport with the ethical principles of the profession. Both national and international codes of ethics enunciate ethical principles that govern social work practice across cultures. The ethical standards in the Code of Ethics of the National Association of Social Workers (United States) relating to diversity provide in pertinent part:

1.05 Cultural Awareness and Social Diversity

(a) Social workers should understand culture and its function in human behavior and society, recognizing the strengths that exist in all cultures.

S. Loue (✉)
Department of Bioethics, Case Western Reserve University School of Medicine,
Cleveland, OH, USA
e-mail: Sana.Loue@case.edu

(b)   Social workers should have a knowledge base of their clients' cultures and be able to demonstrate competence in the provision of services that are sensitive to clients' cultures and to differences among people and cultural groups.

(c)   Social workers should obtain education about and seek to understand the nature of social diversity and oppression with respect to race, ethnicity, national origin, color, sex, sexual orientation, gender identity or expression, age, marital status, political belief, religion, immigration status, and mental or physical ability.

(d)   Social workers who provide electronic social work services should be aware of cultural and socioeconomic differences among clients and how they may use electronic technology. Social workers should assess cultural, environmental, economic, mental or physical ability, linguistic, and other issues that may affect the delivery or use of these services (National Association of Social Workers, 2017).

The Global Social Work Statement of Ethical Principles of the International Federation of Social Workers (2018) embodies various principles that speak to the value of and respect for diverse persons and diversity:

1.   Recognition of the Inherent Dignity of Humanity
Social workers recognize and respect the inherent dignity and worth of all human beings in attitude, word, and deed. We respect all persons, but we challenge beliefs and actions of those persons who devalue or stigmatize themselves or other persons.

2.   Promoting Human Rights
Social workers embrace and promote the fundamental and inalienable rights of all human beings. Social work is based on respect for the inherent worth, dignity of all people and the individual, and social/civil rights that follow from this. Social workers often work with people to find an appropriate balance between competing human rights.

3.   Promoting Social Justice
Social workers have a responsibility to engage people in achieving social justice, in relation to society generally, and in relation to the people with whom they work. This means:

3.1.   Challenging Discrimination and Institutional Oppression
Social workers promote social justice in relation to society generally and to the people with whom they work.
Social workers challenge discrimination, which includes but is not limited to age, capacity, civil status, class, culture, ethnicity, gender, gender identity, language, nationality (or lack thereof), opinions, other physical characteristics, physical or mental abilities, political beliefs, poverty, race, relationship status, religion, sex, sexual orientation, socioeconomic status, spiritual beliefs, or family structure.

3.2.   Respect for Diversity
Social workers work toward strengthening inclusive communities that respect the ethnic and cultural diversity of societies, taking account of individual, family, group, and community differences (International Federation of Social Workers, 2018).

We must look, then, at how these principles can be embodied and effectuated in veterinary social work.

Practicing Veterinary Social Work Across Cultures

Reports suggest that more than two-thirds of all households in the United States include at least one animal member (American Pet Products Association, 2021), as do 41 percent of Canadian households (Canadian Animal Health Institute, 2019), 38 percent of all households in the European Union (European Pet Food Industry, 2020), and 44 percent of all UK households (Royal Society for the Prevention of Cruelty to Animals, 2021). Worldwide, dogs are the most commonly kept pets, followed by birds, cats, and other animals (Gray & Young, 2011). Although statistics relating to the high prevalence of animals within households do not provide information about how these or any other animals may be viewed within or across countries, these high proportions suggest that human-animal relationships exist across diverse groups. Animals may be regarded as companions; as cherished family members; as siblings among children; as a means of production, such as a farm animal; as a source of food; or as an instrument to be utilized in pursuit of a goal, such as a hunting animal (Archer, 1997; Gray & Young, 2011; Irvine & Cilia, 2017; Seps, 2010). Depending on both the specific animal and individuals' views about animals, the animal may live inside the home or be relegated to an outdoor shelter, may be maintained within the home regardless of their behaviors or illnesses, or may be relinquished to a shelter or euthanized for unwelcome behavior or incurable illness. Across families and communities, the meaning of harming animals varies, ranging from viewing it as a game to feeling horror, guilt, and grief when witnessed (Arluke, 2002, 2006; Atwood-Harvey, 2007; Pagani et al., 2007). Indeed, in some communities, exposure to animal abuse is so frequent as to be considered normative (Pagani et al., 2007).

Attitudinal Differences and Similarities Across Groups and Societies

Research suggests that attitudes toward animals may vary across societies (Brown, 1985). Researchers conducting a questionnaire study with 297 Romanian respondents and 302 respondents from Mexico City, all of whom were adults, reported significant differences between the two groups, with responses all in the same direction, with respect to attitudes toward farm animals, animal feeling and sentience, and keeping animals as pets (Rusu et al., 2018). The authors explained that they had wanted to translate a questionnaire into Spanish and Romania, but did not provide a reason for their selection of participants from these two countries. The authors noted that many of the Romanian respondents were psychologists, veterinarians, or veterinary students, suggesting that the two samples may not have been comparable.

A study conducted by Prokop et al. (2009) found that Turkish students participating in their study had more positive attitudes toward snakes than did the Slovakian students. However, they did not offer an explanation of how or why this might be the case. Many factors could explain this result including methodological issues, e.g., the nature of the sample from which participants were drawn and the analytic strategy, previous experience with animals, and variations in religious attitudes toward animals. A study conducted by Miura et al. (2002) with young adult participants in Japan and in the United Kingdom found that the British students were more likely to have positive attitudes toward animals and greater concern for animal welfare than did their Japanese counterparts, which the researchers attributed to more positive childhood experiences with pets.

Researchers conducting a study with high school students in Belgium and the Netherlands analyzed 358 questionnaires from participants between the ages of 12 and 21, inclusive (Martens et al., 2019). They noted an increased concern for animals among females, those who did not eat meat, and Belgian students. They did not offer an explanation as to why a difference might exist between the two nationalities apart from hypothesizing that "Belgian respondents may be somewhat more passionate about these issues than Dutch students" (p. 9). They also reported a weak relationship between opposition to the killing of animals or the violation of their integrity and greater importance of religion in the students' lives.

Prokop et al. (2010) compared the attitudes of high school students in Slovakia and South Africa toward spiders. Although they raised the possibility that a cultural factor might explain the lower level of fear among Slovakian students, they concluded that their findings did not allow them to draw any conclusions with respect to underlying cultural factors. However, they noted that South Africa and Slovakia vary greatly in their approach to science education and students' attitudes toward spiders could be associated with the educational approach.

Brown (2002) sought to assess the "ethnic variations in animal companion ('pet') attachment" (p. 250) among 133 white and African American students enrolled in a school of veterinary medicine. She found from her analysis of the completed surveys that white students were more likely to have more pets and more kinds of pets, more likely to allow pets to sleep on their beds, and appeared to be more attached to their pets. Brown acknowledged that because her sample was confined to veterinary students, her findings could not be generalized. Nevertheless, she concluded:

> Different racial or ethnic cultures within the United States have their own unique, anthropomorphic views of animals. Whites may tend to have a sentimental, anthropomorphic view of animals while African Americans may have a more instrumental or utilitarian view of animals ... This view probably is due partially to economics because keeping a pet as a companion requires money above and beyond resources for survival. However, it is possible that these differences are *cultural customs* passed down from one generation to the next. (Brown, 2002, p. 260) (emphasis added)

This conclusion suggests that race/ethnicity constitutes a distinct culture; however, significant diversity exists even among individuals who identify as members of the same racial or ethnic group. Indeed, individuals who self-identify within the same group may differ with respect to many factors that may be relevant to their perspectives about animals, such as age, educational level, economic status, religion, and so forth. Like Brown, Sheade and Chandler (2012) in their discussion of animal-assisted counseling similarly attributed specific attitudes toward animals to individuals' race or ethnicity.

Fehlbaum and colleagues conducted a study to compare the attitudes of 3000 randomly selected French-speaking and German-speaking Swiss adults toward animals. The study was a smaller component of a larger research project that sought to "better understand the magnitude of the effects of culture and religious differences" (Fehlbaum et al., 2010, p. 286). They found from the returned 193 French questionnaires and 319 German questionnaires that the French speakers were more likely to endorse the benefits of maintaining a pet, to find eating pork and beef acceptable, and to oppose the idea that people should refrain from eating meat. The authors did not explain what might differ culturally between French- and German-speaking Swiss persons and why those cultural differences would shape their attitudes toward animals.

In contrast to the previously mentioned studies, Phillips and McCulloch (2005) suggested that religious and other traditions may play a role in individuals' perceptions of animal sentience and their attitudes toward animal suffering. Their cross-cultural study examined the beliefs of 425 students of 17 different nationalities with respect to animal sentience and the use of animals, noting that "[c]ultural differences in students' attitudes towards animals need to be better understood and respected in order to promote tolerance in multicultural biological education" (p. 17). The questionnaire results indicated that students from the United States and European countries were more likely than Asian students to oppose animal cruelty and to disapprove of animal use for the testing of shampoos and cosmetics. US students were less likely than others to indicate a belief that hunting of deer and foxes is both cruel and unnecessary. Unfortunately, the researchers did not report students' religious beliefs and their possible effect on their findings. Phillips et al. (2012) similarly found from their questionnaire study with 3433 students from 103 countries that European students evidenced greater concern for animals' welfare than did their Asian counterparts, a finding that the researchers attributed to the European students' greater affluence.

Attitudes toward the use of animals in research have been found to differ across countries. Pifer et al. (1994) conducted an analysis of questionnaire data collected from 15 different countries: 2000 individuals interviewed by phone in Canada; 1457 individuals interviewed in person in Japan; 13,024 individuals from various European countries, some of whom were interviewed in person; and 2001 individuals from the United States. Women were found to be more likely to oppose animal research than men. The researchers reported that the European participants indicated high levels of opposition to animal research, in contrast to the study participants in the United States, Canada, and Japan. The researchers did not find a consistent relationship between scientific knowledge or lack of scientific knowledge and opposition to animal research. The authors hypothesized that the differences seen across countries with respect to (non)opposition to animal research could be related to the level of industrialization and urbanization within each country.

A relatively small body of research has examined the relationship between religious beliefs and views of animals. Religious fundamentalism and a higher frequency of attendance at church services have been found to be associated with a greater emphasis on animal utility (Bowd & Bowd, 1989; Driscoll, 1992; Kellert & Berry, 1980). The sanctity of cows among religious Hindus and the prohibition against the ingestion of pork among observant Muslims and Jews serve as examples of the potential effect of religious beliefs on individuals' views of animals (Douglas, 1966; Harris, 1978). Other religious precepts may also impact individuals' acceptance of and attitudes toward animals.

Judaism posits that God is concerned for the welfare of animals. The idea of *imitatio dei*, of having been made in God's image, is a governing principle, one that urges the individual toward the highest moral behavior. Individuals are expected to perform acts of justice, mercy, and wisdom (Kalechofsky, 1992), and human beings' relations with animals are governed by the principle of *tsa'ar ba'alei chayim*, referring to the pain of living creatures (Bleich, 1986; Kalechofsky, 1992), whether due to concerns that the performance of cruel acts toward animals would cause humans to habitually act in a cruel manner (Maimonides, 1956 [1204]) or out of concern for the animal itself (Kalechofsky, 1992). Despite the concern for animals' well-being and the principle of *tsa'ar ba'alei chayim*, Judaism gives priority to the needs of humans, as in the case of animal experimentation.

There is no uniform view across Christian denominations with respect to animals and the relationship between animals and humans. Indeed, it has been suggested both that the "Christian tradition is curiously ambivalent about animals and their place in theology and ethics" (Gilmour, 2015, p. 254) and that it is "relentlessly anthropocentric" in its outlook (Gaffney, 1986, p. 151). Aquinas, for example, asserted that animals are not worthy of ethical attention specifically because of their irrationality, their inability to exercise freedom of choice, and the fact that they are not social persons (Gaffney, 1986). Charity shown to animals, according to Aquinas, was not to be for the sake of the animal, but rather for the sake of the humans who care for that animal (Francione, 2000; Gaffney, 1986).

It was thought in the past that Genesis 1:28 conferred on humans the right of dominion over other creatures, such that power could be effectuated without limit or responsibility (Linzey, 1986), essentially an interpretation of "dominion" as "domination." More recently, it has been suggested dominion means that humans are to serve as agents for the care and cultivation of creation, including animals; that all creations in nature have value, although that precise value may not be known to humans; and that animals are considered by God to be good simply because God brought them into existence (Yarri, 2005). Rather than relying on the creation stories and the concept of dominion to justify ruthlessness toward animals, these passages are instead to be interpreted as mandating benign stewardship (Gaffney, 1986; Montefiore, 1970; Yarri, 2005). Yarri (2005), noting that the covenant of God following the flood applied not only to Noah, but to all creatures in the ark, has argued that a covenant exists between God and all of God's creatures.

The Qur'an, which is the central source of law in Islam, indicates that animals have value; indeed, the Qur'an considers man to be a beast as others. Additionally, passages of the Qur'an indicate that nonhuman beings have a spiritual dimension and an awareness of Allah, who created them (Abdoul-Rouf, 2010). Islam not only prohibits cruelty to animals but also places upon humans responsibility for the welfare of all living beings (Masri, 1986). Although the Qur'an makes clear that animals have "divinely given lives" (Tappan, 2017) and are not to be treated cruelly or killed randomly, it also advises that animals may be used for food, clothing, and transport.

Implications for Veterinary Social Work and Veterinary Social Workers

Many of the studies noted above hint at possible differences between groups with respect to attitudes and behaviors toward animals. Unfortunately, much of this research lacks the methodological rigor that would allow VSWs to rely on the research findings for definitive guidance when working with specific groups. For example, the research has frequently failed to adequately define culture, to identify specific components of culture relevant to the research question at hand, or to present a coherent hypothesis regarding the relationship between specific aspects of a culture and attitudes toward animals. Additionally, a number of researchers have equated race and ethnicity with culture, which ignores the differences across these concepts and suggests that each such group is homogenous, although there is great diversity even within groups, e.g., by educational level, religion, socioeconomic status, previous experience with animals, and so forth.

These methodological deficiencies indicate the need for additional, methodologically rigorous research to assess the acceptability and effectiveness of VSW in various contexts in diverse societies. As an example, it is possible that individuals or communities that believe that animals do not belong in the home may reject animal-assisted psychotherapy in an office setting, but may be more amenable to the idea of equine therapy. It may be inadvisable in some settings to rely on specific animals that are generally viewed within a community as a source of nutrition or are regarded with disgust. The absence of such research diminishes the possibilities for the successful expansion and adoption of VSW within diverse societies.

The absence of an adequate research foundation underscores the need for social workers to exercise cultural humility in their efforts to introduce VSW into settings unfamiliar with the practice. Unlike cultural competence, which suggests that one is "competent" to engage across cultures and groups following the acquisition of a specified body of knowledge, cultural humility posits that there is something that is unknown in every interaction (Tervalon & Murray-Garcia, 1998). Indeed, there is now broad understanding that someone cannot truly be competent in someone else's culture (Chavez, 2018; Isaacson, 2014; Minkler et al., 2012; Murray-Garcia & Tervalon, 2014). In contrast, cultural humility requires that an individual both develop an accurate view of him- or herself, including the limits to one's own knowledge and awareness, and adopt an other-oriented perspective (Davis et al., 2020). It is only by putting aside one's preconceptions and biases that an individual is able to connect and engage with others authentically. In doing so, the balance of power shifts (Tervalon & Murray-Garcia, 1998); the VSW recognizes that it is the client—whether a veterinarian, a pet owner, or a psychotherapy client—who holds the knowledge that is needed to help move the relationship forward productively. The VSW must create the space for this to occur.

Various techniques are available to VSWs to nurture cultural humility. First and foremost, it is important to recognize one's own biases and triggers, which may interfere with one's ability to understand a situation or a client. It is critical to distinguish between what is being seen and the interpretation and judgment that often precedes an accurate appraisal of what is being seen. In an effort to process information quickly, it is common to jump immediately to interpretation and judgment of a scenario or person, without actually seeing them. Finally, cultural humility is a lifelong process (Tervalon & Murray-Garcia, 1998) that requires openness, curiosity, respect, and accountability (Grauf-Grounds & Rivera, 2020; Fahlberg et al., 2016).

Diversity Within the VSW Profession

A 2017 demographic profile of social workers in the United States indicates that there are approximately 850,000 individuals in the country who define themselves as social workers (George Washington University Health Workforce Institute and School of Nursing, 2017). However, only a proportion of these hold at least a bachelor's degree (650,000), and even fewer hold an active social work license (approximately 350,000). The report noted that the majority of social workers (88.3%) are female and slightly more than two-thirds (68.8%) are white, suggesting that the social work profession itself lacks significant diversity. Data from a recent report of the US Bureau of Labor Statistics (2019) that counted social workers in three categories—child, family, and school social workers, healthcare social workers, and other social workers—indicated that in each of these categories, the majority of social workers are white women. Slightly more than one-quarter of healthcare workers are African American or Black and slightly more than one-fifth identified as Hispanic or Latino. Asian individuals account for a small proportion of social workers in each of these categories.

A similar lack of diversity exists in the European social work workforce. A report of the European Social Network that focused on the social services workforce in Europe noted a lack of men in the workforce and difficulties recruiting and retaining a culturally diverse workforce (Baltruks et al., 2017). Identified impediments include low wages, nonrecognition of workers' credentials issued by another country, and complex registration processes for social service workers credentialed in other countries. Additionally, the establishment of social work education programs in some countries has occurred relatively recently (Rutgers University Center for International Social Work, 2008), which may also contribute to a lack of diversity in the workforce.

One cannot assume that because a provider is of the same nationality, race, or ethnicity as a client, who may be a veterinarian, a shelter worker, a pet owner, or a person seeking psychotherapy, among others, that the provider will necessarily share the values or understand the client's particular situation. However, although research results have not been consistent, some US-based research suggests that some clients may prefer therapists of their own race, perceive therapists of their own race somewhat more positively than other therapists (Cabral & Smith, 2011), and experience a stronger therapeutic alliance and greater levels of participation in treatment when it is provided by a therapist of the same race or ethnicity (Sue, 1977; Sue et al., 1991). It is not known whether similar preferences exist among individual in other societies with diverse ethical/racial populations.

Implications for Veterinary Social Work and Veterinary Social Workers

Enhancing diversity and supporting inclusion within VSW calls first for greater diversity and inclusion within the social work profession itself, both in the United States and elsewhere. Diversity and inclusion may be defined differently in different locales and across different societies; foundational work is needed to better understand existing perspectives. Research is needed, as well, to elucidate at the community and societal levels perspectives about animals and the human-animal relationship so that VSWs can better understand the role that they may be able to fill in specific contexts.

Conclusion

The practice of VSW across cultures is challenging but offers significant opportunities for growth as well. VSWs must consider not only the affinities and preferences of individual clients, whether they are veterinarians, persons seeking counseling, shelter workers, or others, but also the norms and preferences of organizations, communities, and larger societies. In doing so, however, the VSW must be careful to avoid superimposing preconceived judgments and ideas on the clients and their communities and must, additionally, work toward greater self-awareness, openness, and attunement to others.

The lack of diversity within VSW, and, indeed, within the social work profession itself, presents additional concerns. Because of the limited number of social workers who are familiar with specified cultures and/or are fluent in the languages of potential clients, individuals in need of services may be unable to access appropriate services, suggesting that additional approaches are needed to recruit individuals into the profession of social work and, specifically, into VSW. (For a discussion of the development of VSW programs and internships, see Chaps. 1 and 14 in this volume.)

References

Abdoul-Rouf, H. (2010). *Schools of Qur'anic exegesis: Genesis and development*. Routledge.

American Pet Products Association. (2021). *Pet industry market size, trends and ownership statistics*. https://www.americanpetproducts.org/press_industrytrends.asp. Accessed 28 March 2021.

Archer, J. (1997). Why do people love their pets? *Evolution and Human Behavior, 18*, 237–259.

Arluke, A. (2002). Animal abuse as dirty play. *Symbolic Interaction, 25*, 405–430.

Arluke, A. (2006). *Just a dog: Understanding animal cruelty and ourselves*. Temple University Press.

Atwood-Harvey, D. (2007). From touchstone to tombstone: Children's experiences with the abuse of their beloved pets. *Humanity and Society, 31*, 379–400.

Baltruks, D., Hussein, S., & Lara Montero, A. (2017). *Investing in the social service workforce*. European Social Network. https://www.esn-eu.org/sites/default/files/publications/Investing_in_the_social_service_workforce_WEB.pdf. Accessed 02 April 2021.

Bleich, D. J. (1986). Judaism and animal experimentation. In T. Regan (Ed.), *Animal sacrifices* (pp. 61–114). Temple University Press.

Bowd, A. D., & Bowd, A. C. (1989). Attitudes towards the treatment of animals: A study of Christian groups in Australia. *Anthrozoös, 3*, 20–24.

Brown, D. (1985). Cultural attitudes towards pets. *Veterinary Clinics of North America: Small Animal Practice, 15*(2), 311–317.

Brown, S. E. (2002). Ethnic variations in pet attachment among students at an American school of veterinary medicine. Society & Animals: Journal of Human-Animal Studies, 10(3), 249–266.

Cabral, R., & Smith, T. B. (2011). Racial/ethnic matching of clients and therapists in mental health services: A meta-analytic review of preferences, perceptions, and outcomes. *Journal of Counseling Psychology, 58*, 537–554.

Canadian Animal Health Institute. (2019). *Latest Canadian pet population figures released*. https://www.cahi-icsa.ca/press-releases/latest-canadian-pet-population-figures-released. Accessed 28 March 2021.

Chavez, V. (2018). Cultural humility: Reflections and relevance for CBPR. In N. Wallerstein, B. Duran, J. Oetzel, & M. Minkler (Eds.), *Community-based participatory research for health: Advancing social and health equity* (3rd ed., pp. 357–362). Jossey-Bass.

Davis, D., DeBlaere, C., Hook, J. N., & Owen, J. (2020). *Mindfulness-based practices in therapy: A cultural humility approach*. American Psychological Association.

Douglas, M. (1966). *Purity and danger*. Penguin Books.

Driscoll, J. S. (1992). Attitudes towards animal use. *Anthrozoös, 5*, 32–39.

European Pet Food Industry. (2020). *European facts & figures 2019*. https://fediaf.org/images/FEDIAF_facts_and_figs_2019_cor-35-48.pdf. Accessed 28 March 2021.

Fahlberg, B., Foronda, C., & Baptiste, D. (2016). Cultural humility: The key to patient/family partnerships for making difficult decisions. *Nursing, 46*(9), 14–16.

Fehlbaum, B., Waiblinger, E., & Turner, D. C. (2010). A comparison of attitudes towards animals between the German- and French-speaking part of Switzerland. *Schweizer Archiv für Tierheilkunde, 152*(6), 285–293.

Francione, G. L. (2000). *Introduction to animal rights: Your child or the dog?* Temple University Press.

Gaffney, J. (1986). The relevance of human experimentation to Roman Catholic ethical methodology. In T. Regan (Ed.), *Animal sacrifices* (pp. 149–170). Temple University Press.

George Washington University Health Workforce Institute and School of Nursing. (2017). *Profile of the social work workforce: A report to the Council on Social Work Education and National Workforce Initiative Steering Committee*. https://www.cswe.org/Centers-Initiatives/Initiatives/National-Workforce-Initiative/SW-Workforce-Book-FINAL-11-08-2017.aspx. Accessed 01 April 2021.

Gilmour, M. J. (2015). C.S. Lewis and animal experimentation. *Perspectives on Science and Christian Faith, 67*(4), 254–262.

Grauf-Grounds, C., & Rivera, P. M. (2020). The ORCA-stance as a practice beyond cultural humility. In C. Grauf-Grounds, T. Schermer Sellers, S. Edwards, et al. (Eds.), *A practice beyond cultural humility: How clinicians can work more effectively in a diverse world* (pp. 8–25). Routledge.

Gray, P. B., & Young, S. M. (2011). Human-pet dynamics in cross-cultural perspective. *Anthrozoös, 24*(1), 17–30.

Harris, M. (1978). *Cannibals and kings*. Collins.

International Federation of Social Workers. (2018). *Global social work statement of ethical principles*. https://www.ifsw.org/global-social-work-statement-of-ethical-principles/. Accessed 28 March 2021.

Irvine, L., & Cilia, L. (2017). More-than-human families: Pets, people, and practices in multispecies households. *Sociology Compass, 11*, e12455. https://doi.org/10.1111/soc4.12455

Isaacson, M. (2014). Clarifying concepts: Cultural humility or cultural competency. *Journal of Professional Nursing, 30*, 251–258.

Kalechofsky, R. (1992). Jewish law and tradition on animal rights: A usable paradigm for the animal rights movement. In R. Kalechofsky (Ed.), *Judaism and animal rights: Classical and contemporary responses* (pp. 46–55). Micah Publications.

Kellert, S. R., & Berry, J. K. (1980). *Phase III: Knowledge, affection and basic attitudes towards animals in American Society*. United States Department of the Interior, Fish and Wildlife Service.

Linzey, A. (1986). The place of animals in creation: A Christian view. In T. Regan (Ed.), *Animal sacrifices* (pp. 115–148). Temple University Press.

Maimonides, M. (1956 [1204]). *Guide of the perplexed, Book III* (trans. M. Friedländer). Dover Publications.

Martens, P., Hansart, C., & Su, B. (2019). Attitudes of young adults toward animals—The case of high school students in Belgium and the Netherlands. *Animals, 9*, 88. https://doi.org/10.3390/ani9030088

Masri, A.-H. B. A. (1986). Animal experimentation: The Muslim viewpoint. In T. Regan (Ed.), *Animal sacrifices* (pp. 171–197). Temple University Press.

Minkler, M., Pies, C., & Hyde, C. A. (2012). Ethical issues in community organizing and capacity building. In M. Minkler (Ed.), *Community organizing and building for health and welfare* (3rd ed., pp. 110–129). Rutgers University Press.

Miura, A., Bradshaw, J. W. S., & Tanida, H. (2002). Childhood experiences and attitudes towards animal issues: A comparison of young adults in Japan and the UK. *Animal Welfare, 11*, 437–448.

Montefiore, H. (1970). *Can man survive? (The question mark and other essays)*. Fontana.

Murray-Garcia, J., & Tervalon, M. (2014). The concept of cultural humility. *Health Affairs, 33*(7), 1303.

National Association of Social Workers. (2017). *Code of ethics*. https://www.socialworkers.org/About/Ethics/Code-of-Ethics/Code-of-Ethics-English. Accessed 28 March 2021.

Pagani, C., Robustelli, F., & Ascione, F. R. (2007). Italian youths' attitudes toward, and concern for, animals. *Anthrozoös, 20*(3), 275–293.

Phillips, C. J. C., Izmirli, S., Aldavood, S. J., Alonso, M., Choe, B. I., Hanlon, A., … Rehn, T. (2012). Students' attitudes to animal welfare and rights in Europe and Asia. *Animal Welfare, 21*, 87–100.

Phillips, C. J. C., & McCulloch, S. (2005). Student attitudes on animal sentience and use of animals in society. *Journal of Biological Education, 40*(1), 17–24.

Pifer, R., Shimuzu, K., & Pifer, L. (1994). Public attitudes toward animal research: Sme international comparisons. *Society & Animals, 2*(2), 95–113.

Prokop, P., Özel, M., & Uşak, M. (2009). Cross-cultural comparison of student attitudes towards snakes. *Society and Animals, 17*, 224–240.

Prokop, P., Tolarovičová, A., Camerik, A. M., & Peterková, V. (2010). High school students' attitudes towards spiders: A cross-cultural comparison. *International Journal of Science Education, 32*(12), 1665–1688.

Royal Society for the Prevention of Cruelty to Animals. (2021). *Facts and figures*. https://www. rspca.org.uk/whatwedo/latest/facts. Accessed 28 March 2021.

Rusu, A. S., Pop, D., & Turner, D. C. (2018). Geographically apart, attitudinally very close: A comparison of attitudes toward animals between Romania and Mexico City. *People and Animals: The International Journal of Research and Practice, 1*(1), 2. https://docs.lib.purdue. eu/paij/vol1/iss1/2.

Rutgers University Center for International Social Work. (2008). *Social work education and the practice environment in Europe and Eurasia. United States Agency for International Development.* http://www.socialserviceworkforce.org/system/files/resource/files/Social_ Work_Education_and_the_Practice_Environment_in_Europe_and_Eurasia_1.pdf. Accessed 02 April 2021.

Seps, C. D. (2010). Animal law evolution Treating pets as persons in tort and custody disputes. *University of Illinois Law Review, 2010*(4), 1339–1374.

Sheade, H. E., & Chandler, C. K. (2012). Cultural diversity considerations in animal assisted counseling. *VISTAS Online, 76*. https://www.counseling.org/docs/ default-source/vistas/article_76. pdf?sfvrsn=3. Accessed 28 March 2021.

Sue, S. (1977). Community mental health services to minority groups: Some optimism and pessimism. *American Psychologist, 32*, 616–624.

Sue, S., Fujino, D. C., Hu, L., Takeuchi, D. T., & Zane, N. W. S. (1991). Community mental health services for ethnic minority groups: A test of the cultural responsiveness hypothesis. *Journal of Consulting and Clinical Psychology, 59*(4), 533–540.

Tappan, R. (2017). Islamic bioethics and animal research: The case of Iran. *Journal of Religious Ethics, 45*(3), 562–578.

Tervalon, M., & Murray-García, J. (1998). Cultural humility versus cultural competence: A critical distinction in defining physician training outcomes in multicultural education. Journal of Health Care for the Poor and Underserved, 9(2), 117–125.

United States Bureau of Labor Statistics. (2019). *Labor force statistics from the Current Population Survey*. https://www.bls.gov/cps/cpsaat11.htm. Accessed 01 April 2021.

Yarri, D. (2005). *The ethics of animal experimentation: A critical analysis and constructive Christian proposal*. Oxford University Press.

Index

Printed in Great Britain
by Amazon

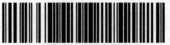

56767091R00216